A Primer on Prostate Cancer

The Empowered Patient's Guide

Stephen B. Strum, MD, FACP

and

Donna L. Pogliano

Second Edition

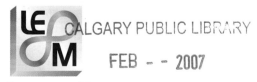

LIFE EXTENSION MEDIA

Book and Cover Design
Diana J. Garnand, Visual Purple Graphics

Illustration (except where indicated)
Diana J. Garnand, David B. Hargreaves, and Stephen B. Strum, MD, FACP

A Primer on Prostate Cancer may be purchased for personal, educational, business, or sales promotional use. For ordering information, please contact:

The Life Extension Foundation
P.O. Box 229120, Hollywood, Florida 33022-9120
1-866-820-7457
www.lefprostate.org

Second Edition

ISBN: 0-9658777-7-9

About the Cover

The cover photograph was taken by Dr. Stephen Strum, whose passion for sailing is his respite from the world of prostate cancer. The sun rising over Pitcairn Island in the Pacific is an appropriate image to express the vision of the authors in writing this book. *A Primer on Prostate Cancer* has been a labor of love for each of them for over two years. The authors hope that their efforts in introducing this book into the world of prostate cancer will bring a new day of enlightenment to the struggles of individual patients and to the practice of many medical professionals who work in the field of prostate cancer.

The power and momentum of the sailboat slicing through the water serves as a metaphor for the empowerment of the patient whose education will result in the power to choose his own destiny. This empowerment through education will serve him well in creating the momentum that will enable the man and his family to overcome his disease. The man on the deck, although appearing isolated, is not really alone, since the supporting crew needed to reach the destination is close at hand, just out of view, but ready to take action if needed.

Finally, the image includes the power of God's sunrise and the hope it connotes as an ongoing symbol of the hope and faith of the prostate cancer patient that a cure for prostate cancer is just over the horizon.

About The Publisher

Most books are published for the purpose of generating a profit for the company that invested in researching, writing, editing, and printing the book.

The motivations for this book are quite different.

Through direct contact with its members, the Life Extension Foundation (LEF) recognized that many of those afflicted with prostate cancer had developed advanced disease because their oncologist had failed to employ therapies that were substantiated in the peer-reviewed published literature. The consequence was that men were needlessly suffering and dying, even though effective approaches for treating their illness were available, but had not been used.

The LEF is a non-profit organization established in 1980 for the purpose of funding scientific research and educating the public about better ways of preventing and treating disease.

The LEF provided critical support for this book because of their realization that a vital need existed to communicate information to prostate cancer patients that was too often overlooked by their treating physicians.

The LEF has over 78,000 members who are committed to following strict scientific principles as it relates to their healthcare. You can access all of Life Extension's information at no charge by logging on to their Web site, www.lefprostate.org. If you don't have a computer, call 1-866-820-7457 and they will mail you information at no charge.

THIS BOOK IS DEDICATED:

*To the people of the prostate cancer community
whom we are privileged to serve and educate, and*

*To the men and women touched by prostate cancer
who are constantly educating, amazing and inspiring us.*

—*Stephen and Donna*

*To Robert Vaughn Young, Webmaster of Phoenix5, my mentor, my
beloved friend and my inspiration. Robert taught me how to post
messages to the discussion lists and how to stick out my tongue on
email. He was my editor-in-secret, my confidant, my financial
advisor, my most ardent fan and my most steadfast benefactor.
Because of Robert's life and the legacy he left, we have cause to
celebrate. Let us celebrate life, love, laughter, hope, courage and the
spirit of those who refuse to be beaten into submission by the
vagaries of circumstance.*

—*Donna Pogliano*

*To Wil de Jongh. I never met Wil. Yet, through many communications
with him, I witnessed his ceaseless dedication to his brothers with
PC from around the world. I marveled at his humanity, and his
passionate devotion towards improving the welfare of countless lives.
I never met the man, face-to-face, yet I knew him, heart-to-heart.
Wil, you are dearly missed.*

*Let us honor Wil's memory, and our other brothers and sisters who
have shown extraordinary self-sacrifice. Let our actions become the
story of how PC was conquered in our time.*

—*Stephen Strum*

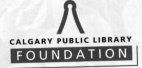
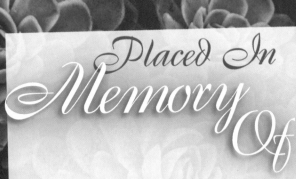

A Primer on Prostate Cancer

Table of Contents

---

* *Page citations locate description and illustration of forms.*

Appendix F: Useful Forms *(cont.)*

Appendix G: Clinical Stages of PC Illustrated

Appendix H: Figures, Tables, Physician's Notes, and Forms Listed

Index

How to Use This Book

If you are a patient newly diagnosed with prostate cancer, you will learn more from *A Primer on Prostate Cancer* if you don't try to read it like a novel, cover to cover in one sitting. If you are unfamiliar with the terminology and concepts involved in books about prostate cancer, reading *The Primer* may tend to discourage and overwhelm you with more information than you can absorb all at once. The authors suggest that you read enough at one time to discover and absorb a few new concepts and then perhaps take the time to discuss them with your significant other, fellow patients, or others close to you.

We have provided you with an area for notes at the bottom of most pages so you can write down any thoughts or questions that may come to you as you are reading. Throughout *The Primer*, you will find bold face print emphasizing sentences of special importance. The **bold green** sentences relate to proactive issues, the **bold blue** ones denote areas of concern, and the **bold red** ones serve as cautionary notes.

Interspersed throughout the text are Physician's Notes written by Dr. Stephen Strum. These include case studies used as examples to reinforce the concepts in the text. The authors hope this book will provide educational opportunities for physicians and patients alike.

Don't be dismayed if you are not a medical professional and are unable to completely understand every single topic and concept presented within *The Primer*. Some knowledge of the principles of biochemistry and other complex areas of learning may be needed to accomplish this. If such expertise is not within your realm of experience, don't despair. This book is written with many levels of understanding in mind.

To direct you to as many wonderful resources as possible, we have created a resource section in **Appendix A**.

For the serious student of prostate cancer, we have included an "If You Want to Know More" section in **Appendix B**. This appendix provides detailed back-up data for some of the subjects presented in the basic chapters. This appendix contains its own reference section, independent of the rest of *The Primer*.

Appendix C contains the 2001 version of the Partin Tables.

To help you comprehend medical terms used in *The Primer*, we have added a "Glossary of Definitions" (**Appendix D**). To facilitate an understanding of the clinical stages of prostate cancer, a description of the TNM staging system as it relates to prostate cancer is also presented in the Glossary.

The references for *The Primer* are found in **Appendix E**.

Appendix F contains forms that you will find useful such as the American Urological Association (AUA) Urinary Symptom Score, etc.

Appendix G contains illustrations that are pertinent to the clinical stage designations most commonly used in PC medicine. There will be overlap with the T stage portion of the TNM staging system described in the Glossary in Appendix D.

We hope that you will find this book helpful in charting a successful course and in safely navigating your way through your experience with prostate cancer.

A Primer on Prostate Cancer

An Overview

A Primer on Prostate Cancer is a basic resource for a man, his family and his loved ones. It is a valuable resource in any of the following circumstances:

- Abnormal levels of prostate specific antigen (PSA) in the blood
- Accelerated increase in PSA
- Abnormal digital rectal exam (DRE)
- A recent diagnosis of prostate cancer (PC)

The Primer is not intended to replace consultation with members of the medical profession, but rather to be a starting point to increase your knowledge of prostate cancer (PC). This *Primer* is not all-inclusive, and new information is constantly being published. Your reading of the literature on PC, your interaction with others, and your ongoing research will produce new insights.

If you are leaning toward a specific treatment, you should strive to find specific information regarding the response rates as well as side-effects, both physical and emotional, for the treatment(s) you are considering. **You will need to consult with your physician to determine if the proposed treatment(s) are appropriate for your particular situation as expressed by the biologic manifestations of the PC.** These biologic expressions include, but are not limited to such findings as the:

- Clinical stage (via physical examination, laboratory testing, radiology studies)
- Baseline PSA (via laboratory testing)
- Gleason score (via pathology evaluation)
- Percentage of biopsy cores involved with PC (via pathology evaluation) and the
- Pathologic stage (via pathology evaluation).

These findings represent the detective work needed to understand your particular situation. Careful analyses of these findings tell us about the *nature* of and the *aggressiveness* of the PC and increase our understanding of the *extent of disease* in your particular situation.

You can become a superb medical detective and actually, although it may be hard to believe, understand this disease almost as well as any physician. But, you have to do your homework. This is optimally done in concert with your significant other and/or family and friends. (See Physician's Note 1.) In the best of all worlds, this too involves working together with your fellow PC survivors in the context of support groups and other forums and having a collegial relationship with your physician(s) and other involved members of the healthcare profession.

> **Physician's Note 1:**
>
> **"Profile the Disease and Obtain a Superior Outcome."**
>
> Virtually every complicated-sounding test or study that a doctor orders is intended to increase an understanding about the nature of the cancer by means of "Profiling." A "Profile" of the tumor cell population enables a good detective to understand the aggressiveness and extent of the prostate cancer better. **Proper testing profiles prostate cancer.**

There is logic and reason to understanding the biology of PC. Once you understand the basics, you will find yourself much more at ease in your communication with your medical co-partners (physicians). In addition, you will be able to discuss your diagnosis and your treatment plans with your loved ones

_____

_____

_____

and develop a strategy that will optimize the probability of a successful outcome for you (Fig. 1).

After treatment, you will need to be vigilant about monitoring your PSA, probably for the rest of your life. Fortunately, we have this simple test—the PSA—to monitor the disease, to monitor the response to treatment and to give early warning if the PC returns, allowing for earlier and more diverse

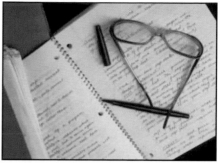

Figure 1: An Empowered Patient is Involved in His Own Outcomes. *An empowered patient feels this way because he has attained a knowledge base that allows him to feel secure enough to communicate freely and with less anxiety with physicians and other healthcare personnel. A less anxious patient is a happier patient who can expend his energy to more appropriate goals directed at achieving successful outcomes.*

treatment opportunities. The PSA is a wonderful tool. Prostate cancer is a disease that is very well understood when we learn to use this tool and others that will be discussed in *The Primer*.

There is no quick-fix solution to a diagnosis of PC. Moreover, at times there may be difficulties encountered in distinguishing between which cancers are "in remission" and those which may be "cured."

This document incorporates the input of a great many people; all have been touched in some way by PC. Some are battling the disease, others are spouses or partners of men who are fighting PC, and others are physicians or health-care providers insistent on seeing an end to prostate cancer. The contributors to *The Primer* are both subscribers and contributors to various Internet e-mail PC discussion groups. They share their knowledge and support with others who are feeling bewildered, alone and frightened—much the same as you may be feeling right now. Know that you are not alone and that there are many out there in the same boat, struggling to stay afloat, battling similar storms, learning new ways to guide them through these challenging passages in an effort to find safe harbors.

PC is a disease of epidemic proportions. The annual incidence for new prostate cancer patients in the USA has ranged from 170,000 to more than 230,000, with over 230,000 Americans diagnosed with PC in 2004. In the USA alone, the total number of men with PC is estimated at between three and five million. As a result of the incidence and mortality rates for PC throughout the world, this disease has

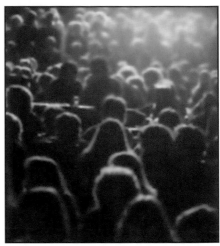

Figure 2: PC Impacts the Lives of Tens of Millions of People. *PC is not a disease of "old" men. It affects men as young as their thirties. With the better understanding of this disease achieved by routine PSA testing, we would estimate that PC probably starts when a man is in his 30s to 40s but only becomes clinically manifest fifteen to twenty years later. The impact of this disease on the family unit and on the productivity of our society is staggering. Although men are stricken with the disease, their women also suffer the fallout, both emotionally and economically.*

had a staggering impact on men and their circle of family and friends. **PC is thus a global disease involving millions of men that has been blatantly ignored relative to other major health issues.** A working co-partnership of patients and physicians is mandatory if we wish to change this. We are only as strong as we are united, as weak as we are divided (Fig. 2). ■

Chapter

How To Proceed

Move Beyond Panic

A ny diagnosis of cancer is likely to cause panic, primarily because of lack of knowledge and fear of the unknown. However, great strides have been made in the treatment of prostate cancer. As never before, you have options, and those who have "been there, done that" universally recommend that you move beyond the panic and gain knowledge. Knowledge is power. We recommend that you take your time, do your research and arrive at the best treatment decision for YOU and your family, based on the characteristics of your total health situation.

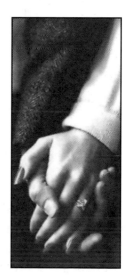

Figure 3: "Friendship is one mind in two bodies." —Mencius

Synergize Your Efforts

PC is a "couple's disease." It affects not only the man, but also his partner and his other loved ones as well. **Stress and depression are common consequences of dealing with the diagnosis, the treatment decision, the treatment itself, and the side-effects of the treatment.** If depression becomes severe and overwhelming, it is appropriate to seek professional help. People deal with life crises in their own ways. It is especially important for you to remember during your ups and downs with PC to be good to yourself, to the people whom you care about, and to those who care about you. In doing this, you are united in the effort to overcome the disease. This focused, reasoned, and calm attitude will be an asset in dealing with the day-to-day pressures all of you will face. Remember, *our humanity lies in our human unity* (Fig. 3).

After you have studied all your options, trust your instincts along with the knowledge you have gained. If any treatment really doesn't feel right, it isn't. If any treatment feels right, it probably is. Ask questions until you understand your options. (See Physician's Note 2.)

Understand Your Options

Be realistic. If a man is not generally in good health, surgery is probably not the best option.

12

Surgery of any kind is hard, and recovery is easiest when a person is in good shape. If a man has existing bowel or bladder problems, radiation of any kind may make them worse. Fortunately for most patients there are a number of options, including various forms of surgery, radiation therapy, cryo-surgery, hormone therapy, and a combination of treatments. In addition, during these exciting times in medicine, new and novel treatment approaches are being developed in our attempts to cure or control PC.

Question your doctors thoroughly regarding the treatment(s) you are considering and what side-effects they may produce. Some treatment side-effects are temporary and some are, or may become, permanent. These vary from individual to individual, depending on the physical condition, age and sensitivity of the patient to various treatment modalities. There are medications to help patients cope with bowel or bladder problems resulting from treatment and a vast array of measures to cope with partial or even total impotence. **An active role on the part of the PC patient in understanding these supportive aspects of PC medical care is crucial. This often translates into significant advances in regard to quality of life issues.** Your physicians must be focused on such issues for you to benefit from these important advances in medicine. (See Physician's Note 3.)

13

Understand the Inherent Biases

Be aware that some medical specialists will steer you in the direction of their specialty and often will understate the risks involved with their treatment of choice. Urologists tend to favor a surgical option, radiation therapists favor radiation, and medical oncologists may be focused on androgen deprivation therapy (ADT) and/or chemotherapy. Sitting in the doctor's consultation room with his spouse or other supportive person(s), **a patient will be able to detect whether the physician is presenting biased information about his treatment specialty only if the patient and his family have become empowered with knowledge.** The physician involved in your care should be outstanding in his or her knowledge of PC and have a caring personality plus a willingness to enter a co-partnership with you, the patient, in your journey through prostate cancer. "One of the essential qualities of the clinician is interest in humanity, for the secret of the care of the patient is in caring for the patient."*

Know the Tempo of the Disease

The goal of PC treatment, it is often said, is to be sure that the patient lives long enough to die of something else. Many prostate cancers are slow growing. (See Physician's Note 4.) **In most situations, you don't need to make a decision regarding how to deal with your disease in days or even weeks.** Many patients take as long as a few months to look at their options. You need to have time to talk with your family about the results of your research, to discuss the implications of the side-effects, to be prepared to deal with them, and to be sure you have the support you need.

14

Physician's Note 4:

"Intelligent Watchful Waiting Mandates Objectified Observation."

BK was diagnosed in August of 1994. His baseline PSA (bPSA) was 4.2. His Gleason score (GS) read by Jonathan Epstein, M,D., was (3,3). His clinical stage was T1c. His gland volume by transrectal ultrasound was 45 cubic centimeters. He had 2 of 10 cores positive for prostate cancer.

He could not decide what to do so he elected close monitoring of the PC. Over the ensuing two years, his PSA doubling time was calculated at 95 months (almost 8 years). His DRE has remained unchanged. His last PSA was 4.61, six years after his diagnosis of PC. Watchful waiting via objective observation was a good strategy for him.

---

* *Sir Francis Weld Peabody, Lecture to Harvard medical students, 1917.*

Choosing a Doctor and a Treatment

Choosing a doctor is a critical step toward making a treatment decision. Your choice of treatment and who will carry it out is crucial in giving you the best outcome based on the foundation of information provided by your test results. Your choice of treatment should be complementary to your age, life expectancy, lifestyle and general health, and to your expectations for future quality of life.

Patient references given by a doctor may direct you to their successes and not to their failures. Make every effort to verify any information you are given. Ask other patients who have been there and done that. For example, if you are involved in support group meetings, ask those attending about their experiences with a particular physician. "Have any of you had surgery with Dr. X? If so, tell me about your experience." "Was anyone treated with radiation by Dr. Y? How did it go for you?" Also, realize that the doctor who diagnosed your PC may not be the best choice of doctors to perform your treatment. **15** Once you decide on a treatment modality, it is time to search out the experts in that modality.

Consider your priorities. **It is not wise to *overtreat* your disease based on fear of recurrence, nor to *undertreat* your disease based on fear of impotence or other side-effects.** Most people would agree that when numbering your priorities, staying alive is at the top of the list, keeping firmly in mind that dead men don't have erections.

If you are uncomfortable with your doctor, change doctors until you find one you trust, one who will take the time to examine you properly, answer your questions, and address all of your concerns, both physical and emotional. Be sure to write down your questions in advance of your medical appointments, so you can be assured of getting the most out of your patient-physician interactions.

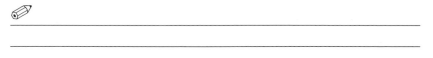

Most importantly, take your partner, wife or a good friend with you to your appointments and consultations (Fig. 4). Doctors expect to see someone present in a supporting role, and most are disappointed if a patient arrives at his appointment alone. Many times, especially in the early phase of adjusting to the harsh reality of a diagnosis of PC, it is that supportive person who has the wherewithal to research the options and question the doctor. This is perfectly appropriate. Two heads are better than one and having someone who is your friend during these trying times is essential.

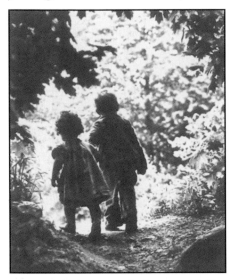

Figure 4: "Friends are God's way of taking care of us."

"We all take different paths in life, but no matter where we go, we take a little of each other everywhere."
—**Tim McGraw**

16

The results of primary treatment are closely linked to the expertise of the doctor performing the treatment, so selecting the very best doctor (an artist) for a given procedure will significantly increase the chance of success. An artist, in contrast to an "average" doctor, is going to have a superior outcome in eliminating the cancer and in minimizing the side-effects of treatment regardless of the treatment modality you choose. Therefore, it is of utmost importance that you decide not only on a treatment choice, but that you seek out the best doctor to perform the procedure. It is not unusual for patients to travel across the country to find the very best medical professionals, some of whom have performed thousands of successful procedures. You have but one life. You deserve the best treatment—the best chance of success. **It is therefore important for you to realize that successful medicine requires special paths that lead to excellent outcomes** (Fig. 5).

The three most important aspects in the successful treatment of a patient are:

- Selection of a treatment(s) appropriate to the patient.
- Preparation of the patient for the intended treatment.
- Choice of an artist or artists throughout the course of the illness.

Remember that the three components necessary to achieve a successful outcome shown above are not listed in chronological order. For example, the choice of an artist early in your course will usually lead to a better match between treatment and patient as well as the proper preparation of the patient.

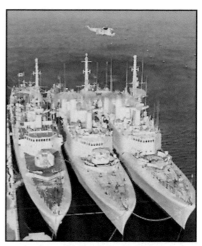

17

Figure 5: Three Components of a Successful Passage.
The selection of a treatment appropriate to the patient, the preparation of the patient for that treatment and the choice of an artist to carry out the treatment are the factors essential to an optimal outcome.

Keep Meticulous Records

Some people tape-record every office visit so they can review what was said later and not be preoccupied with taking notes. To get the most value from this approach, it is necessary to listen to the tapes and take notes about what seems really important. Of course, you should ask the physician if he would object to your taping of such interactions with you. Most physi-

cians who are competent
and confident in their ability will not be offended by
this request and will in fact
view it positively as a sign
of a patient committed to
understanding his illness
and restoring his health.

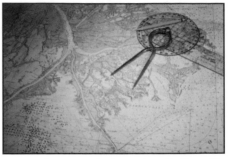

An empowered patient
maintains meticulous med-

Figure 6: Each Patient Should Use His
Medical Chart to Compose a PC Digest.

ical records and obtains copies of the results of all medical, surgical, diagnostic and therapeutic procedures. (See Physician's
Note 5 and Fig. 6.) Ask for these reports as they are done or
after the results are back in the medical chart. This is less labor-
intensive than asking the physician's staff to copy your entire
chart. Remember, either you or your insurance company has
paid for these tests or treatments and you are entitled to have
copies of the results. These results should be sorted in chronological order and should be put into categories such as "Lab",
"Radiology", "Pathology", "Consultations", "Office Visits" and

18

Physician's Note 5:

**"An Empowered Patient Uses Empowerment
Combined with Rationale to Co-Partner With His Physicians."**

At age 69, GB was diagnosed with PC in 8/99. His baseline PSA was 4.2,
his Gleason score (read by David Bostwick, M.D.) was (3,4), and his digital
rectal exam (DRE) revealed his entire right lobe to be rock hard and consistent with clinical stage T3a disease (see Appendix G). He was offered
radiation therapy (RT) but decided to seek additional consultation after
doing much investigation on his own. He began androgen deprivation therapy (ADT) in 11/99 to reduce the PC volume and gland size prior to RT.
After eight months, the DRE had reverted to normal. He then elected to receive intensity modulated RT (IMRT) with BAT guidance (see Chapter 4,
page 115) at the Cleveland Clinic with Pat Kupelian, M.D., starting in 8/00.
ADT was stopped in 12/00. GB has done well and is at 20 months of follow-
up with the recent PSA in 6/2002 at 0.3 and stable. GB chose artists, was
properly prepared, and selected therapy appropriate to his clinical situation.

"Notes." Such notes may relate to conversations with your doctors, medication and diet changes, and other issues pertinent to your medical situation.

A PC Digest depicts the critical events in the diagnosis, evaluation of extent of disease (staging) and treatment of the PC. You can share your PC Digest with your physicians via hard copy or by e-mail if the physician and/or his staff are open to this channel of communication. (See Appendix A, Section V, Item B.) The PC Digest was created by Dr. Stephen Strum in 1994 and is described in detail in the October 1998 and August 2000 issues of the PCRI newsletter *Insights* (articles start on page 4 and 6, respectively). You can access past issues of *Insights* from the PCRI Web site at www.pcri.org (Fig. 7).

Listen to the biology of the prostate cancer, keep organized records that allow you and your co-partners to develop a logical strategy and arrive safe and sound at your desired destination. This is the essence of empowerment.

Note too, that doctors who are experts in the field of PC sometimes volunteer their time to help patients with specific, complex problems on Internet e-mail lists. (See Appendix A, Section V, Item A.) If you ever wish to use such a service, the specifics of your case are most conveniently communicated by the use of the PC Digest. Keep your medical information in a safe place.

Since October 1996, the PCRI (Prostate Cancer Research Institute) in Los Angeles has worked with PC patients and given them individual assistance via its Helpline Staff. You can relate your PC history to the PCRI Helpline staff person via

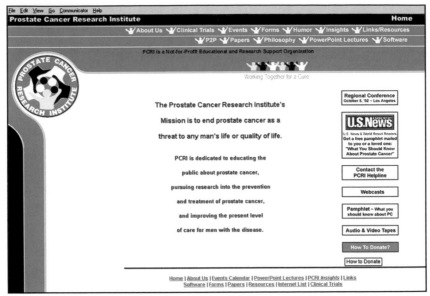

Figure 7: The PCRI Homepage *(www.pcri.org)*. This PC-dedicated Web site has valuable tools to help organize your medical database and analyze your situation. Papers on various aspects of PC, software to evaluate your specific situation, Web casts and PowerPoint lectures on key topics in PC as well as all past issues of the PCRI newsletter Insights are available free of charge.

your PC Digest. They can offer you advice on how to create your PC Digest and can give you general information to facilitate your understanding of what is occurring in your particular situation.

Be Aware of the Financial Side of Your Illness

Many healthcare providers will accept your insurance company's "reasonable and customary reimbursement" as payment in full or may ask you to be responsible for the co-insurance — the difference between what the insurance company allows and actually pays for. **Medicare and Medicare supplemental insurances routinely cover medically necessary testing and treatment for PC, but be sure you know in advance if the treatment you are considering is one of those approved by Medicare.** Ask questions regarding the financial aspect of your treatment. Some procedures and medications are very expensive. You need to put your mind at ease regarding these financial issues so that you can focus your energy on fighting the disease.

Gathering Information

E-mail and Internet access are of great benefit in researching your treatment options and seeking out support. For your convenience, we have provided some of the available Web sites and support group Web sites in the Resource List in Appendix A. The PCRI Web site (Fig. 7) also provides a wealth of information about PC, software to analyze various patient scenarios, PowerPoint slide presentations, Web casts, and links to important Internet sites.

If you do not have computer access, you might want to visit your local library and see what computer resources they can offer. Most libraries now have computers for patron use. Librarians can help you find and print the information you are seeking. You can read these documents at your convenience and have them available for reference. Do not be afraid to ask for help. In addition, do not be afraid to tell the librarian why you need the information. You may find that cancer has also touched that person, and that he or she is willing to give compassion and help. Keeping your diagnosis a secret consumes valuable energy that is better conserved for constructive uses.

You have now inadvertently joined the fraternity of prostate cancer. You have a responsibility to yourself and your loved ones to get the best care and the most information you can. At a time appropriate to you, part of your evolution as a human being afflicted with a potentially life-threatening disease is to become an advocate for more support for PC research, early detection, early cure, appropriate treatment, and supportive care of the PC patient. You will learn that if you mentor those

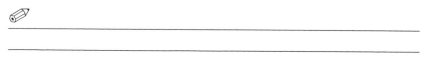

who come after you, as so many others have done, your life will be further enriched and made more meaningful. Know then that you have fulfilled Emerson's definition of success:

"To leave the world a bit better,
whether by a healthy child, a garden patch
or a redeemed social condition;
To know even one life has breathed easier because you lived.
That is to have succeeded."

Nuts And Bolts

It is estimated that 50% of men over 50 and 70% of men over 70 have some form of prostate cancer. Some of these cancers are life threatening, but the majority will grow so slowly as to never be a threat to life, so more men will die "with" prostate cancer than "of" it. (See Physician's Note 6.) Some men have such overwhelming health issues before being diagnosed with PC that treatment is not indicated, or that treatment to diminish symptoms (palliative treatment) is all that is necessary. The intention of palliative treatment is to help the patient deal with the pain and discomfort of the disease and is not intended to cure the disease.

Despite its reputation as an "old man's disease", PC can strike men in their 40s and 50s, and even as young as their 30s. If your life expectancy is more than ten years, more aggressive treatment is usu-

22

> **Physician's Note 6:**
>
> **"Good comprehensive PC management often leads to marked overall health of the patient."**
>
> JB was diagnosed with PC in 7/98. He underwent a radical prostatectomy in 10/98. Two months later, his PSA began to rapidly rise consistent with metastatic PC. Six months later, a bone scan revealed bone metastases. Androgen deprivation therapy (ADT) was begun and a PSA of <0.05 was obtained within two months of starting therapy. During his ongoing care, JB was found to have severe osteoporosis. Additionally, concerns about his cardiac status soon led to a diagnosis of serious cardiac disease requiring coronary artery bypass grafts. JB had an excellent response to ADT with resolution of all bone metastases, improvement in his osteoporosis, a marked improvement in his overall performance ability with a wonderful sense of health that was not felt by him previously.

ally indicated. A family history of PC or breast cancer would suggest that regular PSA blood tests be started at age 35. For other men, annual PSA testing should begin at age 40. ■

What You Should Have Learned From This Chapter

✔ You are the person who has most to gain or lose from this encounter with PC.

✔ There is logic, reason and understanding throughout the entirety of PC.

✔ The results of your physical exam, pathology, lab and radiology tests are all biological manifestations of the interaction between the host (you) and the tumor (the PC).

✔ These biological inputs are used to create a profile that helps to more clearly define the nature of the PC and helps you create a strategy based on biologic reality.

✔ Your empowerment as a patient enables you to help steer the course of your illness and ensure a safe passage.

✔ Despite this threat to your life, those who care for you and about you are here to remind you that there is a synergy of brotherhood; by working in co-partnership with others you will emerge stronger and healthier.

Chapter

The Basics of Prostate Cancer

The prostate gland is part of the endocrine system. It is a walnut-sized gland that sits below the bladder and in front of the rectum at the bottom of the pelvis. The prostate surrounds part of the urethra (Figs. 8 and 9). The urethra is the urinary channel that exits the bladder, then traverses the prostate and enters the penis. The prostate adds vital nutrients and fluid to the sperm, and therefore local treatment of PC impacts upon a man's ability to father children. Because local PC therapies affect prostatic secretion, they also impact upon a man's sexuality, specifically affecting the quantity and quality of ejaculation and orgasm. Only men have prostate glands.

Cancer of the prostate is not contagious or sexually transmitted. It is generally accepted that there is a genetic link that increases the risk of PC, and that a diet high in saturated fat over many years can contribute to the development of PC.[1,2] In many respects, PC and breast cancer (BC) are brother-sister diseases. This appears to be true regarding the hormonal aspects of these diseases, the sites of disease spread, and the striking similarities regarding effective treatments for both. In addition, there is now evidence of a hereditary link between PC and breast cancer in women and vice versa in men. This genetic link makes it wise for a man diagnosed with prostate cancer or a woman with a history of breast cancer to advise their sons and daughters to undertake early and adequate screening for prostate cancer and breast cancer, respectively, as well as to embark upon life style changes known to reduce their risks for PC and BC.

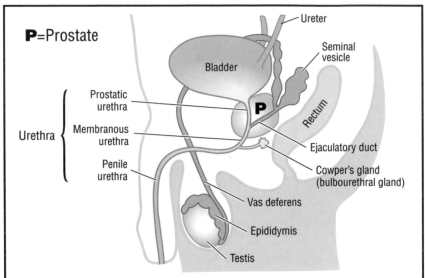

Figure 8: The Prostate Anatomy I. *Note the urethra empties the bladder, then enters the prostate where it is joined by the ejaculatory duct, which delivers sperm and seminal vesicle fluid to nourish the sperm and help liquefy the ejaculate. The urethra then exits the prostate, enters the bulb of the penis and continues through the penis to the glans penis where it ends.*

In a study by Sellers et al, 41,827 women with breast cancer (BC) were evaluated. Of these women, 4,769 (11.4%) had a father or brother with a history of PC. In 6,359 (15.2%), a mother or a sister had a history of BC. In 836, or 2% of the total population, there was a history of both PC and BC in the family. **In this study, the risk of subsequent BC during follow-up was 42% if there was a family history of BC. The risk rose to 71% if there was a family history of both PC and BC.**[3]

Furthermore, the younger a man is at the time of diagnosis of PC and the greater number of paternal relatives with PC (e.g. grandfather, father and uncles), the greater the risk of PC developing in brothers of this PC patient.[4] Black men seem to have the highest prostate cancer incidence, followed by Hispanic men. The causal factors involved in this discrepancy could be genetic, environmental, or a combination of factors and are being investigated. Meanwhile, it would make sense for men in these groups to be vigilant about PSA testing and digital rectal exams (DRE). *If you want to know more about Hereditary Aspects of PC, consult Appendix B, section 2.1.*

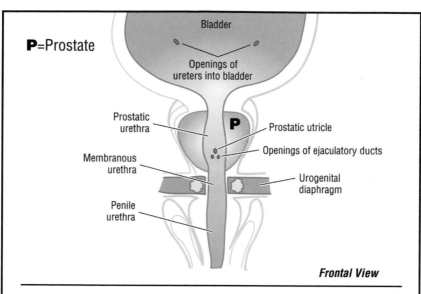

P=Prostate

Bladder

Openings of
ureters into bladder

Prostatic
urethra

P

Prostatic utricle

Openings of ejaculatory ducts

Membranous
urethra

Urogenital
diaphragm

Penile
urethra

Frontal View

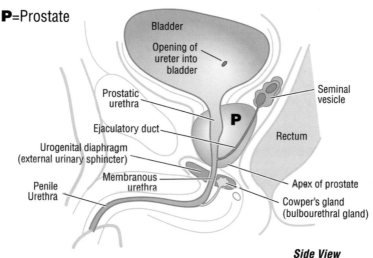

P=Prostate

Bladder

Opening of
ureter into
bladder

27

Prostatic
urethra

Seminal
vesicle

P

Ejaculatory duct

Rectum

Urogenital diaphragm
(external urinary sphincter)

Membranous
urethra

Penile
Urethra

Apex of prostate

Cowper's gland
(bulbourethral gland)

Side View

Figure 9: The Prostate Anatomy II: *The upper frame of this figure is a frontal view; it depicts the prostate and regional anatomy as if the patient were standing in front of you. The three components of the urethra are again shown (also see Fig. 8) in this view. The yellow structures lying within the urogenital diaphragm on either side of the membranous urethra are the Cowper's glands.*

The lower frame is a lateral or side view and depicts the same anatomy as if the patient were standing with his left side facing you. The position of the seminal vesicles above and behind the prostate is shown, along with the ejaculatory duct entering the prostatic urethra. The urethra leaves the prostate at its apex and passes through the urogenital diaphragm (external urinary sphincter) where it is called the membranous urethra. The proximity of the rectum to the prostate, as shown in this side view, allows the physician to feel the posterior and lateral aspects of the prostate gland.

How Does Prostate Cancer Work?

Every cancer, including prostate cancer, is a disordered and abnormal cell growth. Cancer cells have lost the ability to network and communicate in the way that normal cells do, and they no longer function as normal cells are intended to function in the overall framework of body chemistry (Fig. 10). They also do not die as they should, through normal cell death and replacement, and they grow beyond their normal borders. Eventually, they can overwhelm the system.

Some cancers are slow-growing and not typically life-threatening. Some are aggressive, fast-growing cancers. There is a lot

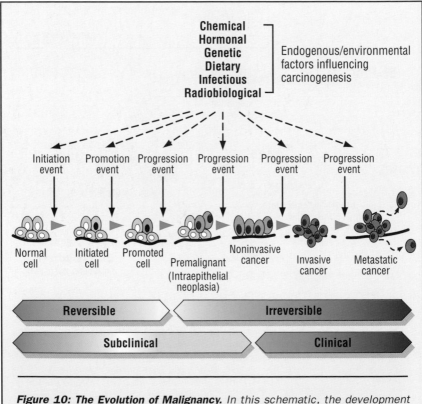

Figure 10: The Evolution of Malignancy. *In this schematic, the development of malignancy is seen resulting from a combination of "hits" on the cell. Initial factors that lead to cancer production (carcinogenesis) are shown at the top. Ongoing promotional and progression events eventually lead to premalignant changes (in this case PIN or prostatic intraepithelial neoplasia) to noninvasive cancer and finally to invasive cancer. If not diagnosed early and eradicated, metastatic cancer may eventually occur.*

of variation. Either you or your doctor can calculate how fast your prostate cancer is growing. The PSA blood test allows us to approximate such factors by determining PSA doubling time (PSADT) and PSA velocity (PSAV).

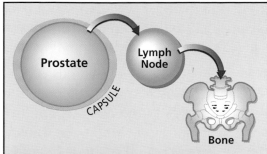

Figure 11: The Orderly Spread of PC.
Most malignancies spread by contiguity—from tissue to nearby tissue. This is true for PC as well. However, mutated PC, often associated with a high Gleason score and aneuploidy, will often invade vascular structures and will metastasize to distant sites. As with other malignancies, an earlier diagnosis improves the probability of eradicating the cancer before it has had a chance for such spread to take place.

Prostate cancer that is confined within the gland itself is called "organ-confined" prostate cancer or "organ-confined disease." When PC has not penetrated the perimeter of the gland (referred to as the prostate capsule), it is very treatable with intent to cure. In such a setting, options such as surgery or various forms of radiation therapy typically result in ten or more years of being disease-free. In this context, disease-free refers to an absence of a progressive rise in PSA in the years following treatment. Some people consider this long-term remission while others equate this with "cure."

If the cancer spreads before local treatment can be undertaken, it usually has penetrated the capsule. If continued growth goes unchecked, it may spread to the seminal vesicles, lymph nodes, and to bones (Fig. 11). When bone involvement occurs, it most often involves the pelvis, spine and ribs. PC can directly invade the bladder wall and rectum and can also involve vital organs such as the liver and the lungs. When it reaches this advanced stage, it usually, but not invariably, has a fatal outcome.

The spread of PC is usually an orderly process. The disease starts in the prostate gland–the primary site–and with increased growth spreads to the capsule, and from there to the seminal vesicles, lymph nodes and bone. **Biologic factors expressed in the Gleason score, PSA, digital rectal examination and core percentage involvement, among others, relate to such probabilities of spread.** (See Physician's Note 7.) ■

Physician's Note 7:

"An early diagnosis is important to prevent an advanced presentation of PC. If diagnosed 'late', PC will often show evidence of spread to nearby structures such as the seminal vesicles, lymph nodes, and bone."

EH was diagnosed in November 1997 at 54 years of age with a baseline PSA of 67. At the time of diagnostic biopsy, six of six tissue cores showed evidence of PC. The Gleason score, read by Jonathan Epstein, M.D., was (5,4). The DRE (digital rectal examination) revealed findings consistent with T3c disease (seminal vesicle involvement). A CT scan showed a mass in front of the sacrum that was consistent with enlarged internal iliac lymph nodes. There was also a 2 cm external iliac node with tumor extension to the left sidewall of the pelvis. This presentation of extensive PC at diagnosis would be eliminated or its chances markedly diminished using routine PSA testing starting at age 40 and at 35 in high-risk men. Despite the findings above, EH was treated with ADT (androgen deprivation therapy) and reached an undetectable PSA of < 0.05 with normalization of his CT scan findings. As of March 2002, he remains on ADT and continues to have an undetectable PSA.

✔ Understanding the anatomy of PC is helpful to reinforce the need for early diagnosis. The prostate gland is in a strategic location with strategic functions affected by its removal or treatment.

✔ PC and breast cancer are so alike that we can learn much about both diseases by sharing our understanding of either. The genetic link between the two also relates to an increased risk of either disease when one disease is present in the family history.

✔ Carcinogenesis or cancer development is believed to require multiple cell "insults" to drive the cell from its normal state through a premalignant condition to full-fledged malignancy. This provides an opportunity for prevention if we understand the factors involved in predisposing a man to PC.

31

✔ PC spreads in an orderly fashion, from gland to surrounding tissues (regional spread) and from there to lymph nodes and then to bone. An early diagnosis, prompted by routine PSA testing and DRE, can prevent a situation where the initial diagnosis reveals advanced disease. We have already seen such benefits of PSA testing, but even more progress can be made if annual or biannual PSA testing is done.

Chapter

Diagnosis and Testing

To achieve the desired goal of eradicating prostate cancer and curing the patient, a rational strategy must be employed by the patient-physician co-partnership. An accurate assessment of (1) the nature of the PC, and (2) the extent or stage of the PC is essential for this strategy to be victorious. **Various testing procedures are available to correctly assess the character and spread of PC, and these should be individualized to the specific patient's situation.** Most patients will not need all the tests that are available. Most physicians will honor an informed patient's requests for testing that seems reasonable. However, some insurance companies or HMOs may not agree to pay for certain tests.

Scientifically and psychologically, it is vital that everything appropriate that can be known about your cancer be discovered *before* you make a treatment decision. This establishes a baseline that indicates what your status was prior to the time that treatment was initiated. Follow-up studies after treatment has begun can then be compared with the baseline studies to document evidence that the therapeutic modality(ies) has been appropriate for your individual situation, and that the treatment you have chosen has shown evidence of efficacy.

Many doctors will stress that with the current available treatment options you have the best chance at a cure if you have organ-confined disease (OCD). **Your physician co-partners should provide explicit guidance to determine the presence or absence of OCD, and then discuss with you the pros and cons of the treatment options available.** Your doctor should not be responsible for making the ultimate choice of treatment for you since this is your decision, and you need to live with the consequences of this decision for the rest of your life.

A *risk assessment* unfolds for a particular patient as more and more information becomes available through various levels of investigation. The first level relates to information discerned at the time of diagnosis of prostate cancer. Table 1 presents an overview of the entire scope of *possible* investigations, although not in a specific order of testing. The investigations that most likely would be considered "non-standard" by the majority of physicians are shown in bold italics. In some circumstances, we find these studies to be helpful in clarifying a strategy for the individual patient. Because they are non-standard, most insurance companies will not agree to pay for these. The decision to obtain such tests needs to be made by you, with input from your physician. However, please realize that many physicians will discount medical examinations that they do not employ in a standard fashion rather than seek information about them.

A detailed discussion of these layers or levels of investigation follows. Additional information on "Biomarkers and Tests for Prostate Cancer" is available on the Internet. After the results of testing have been obtained, and prior to a treatment decision, you and your doctor should utilize the "Partin Tables" and other algorithms that assess the probability of organ-confined disease, probability of extra-capsular extension, spread to the seminal vesicles, and probability of lymph node involvement using your individual test results. See further discussion of the Partin Tables in the Radiation Therapy (brachytherapy section) of Chapter 4. These tables and others that are used to assess your risk at diagnosis or after RP are presented as user-friendly software programs on the Prostate Cancer Research Institute (PCRI) Web site at www.pcri.org. The new Partin Tables for

Table 1: Overview of All Possible Investigations for PC Risk Assessment.	
Type of Investigation	Details of Investigation
Laboratory Testing	Biomarkers like **PSA** and its subunits: **free PSA** and complexed PSA
	PAP and other biomarkers of more aggressive disease activity such as **CGA, NSE** and **CEA**
	Routine complete blood count (**CBC**)
	Chemistry panel that evaluates kidney, liver, bone and electrolyte status
	Markers of bone breakdown like **Pyrilinks-D™ (Dpd)** or **Metra™ DPD**
Physical Examination	Digital Rectal Examination (**DRE**)
	Examination for any enlarged lymph nodes
Pathology Evaluation	**Second opinion of diagnostic biopsy slides** (validation of Gleason score by an expert)
	Evaluation of tumor DNA with **ploidy** analysis
	Assessment of cell growth and repair regulators like **bcl-2** and **p53**
	Assessment of angiogenesis, e.g., **microvessel density** or **VEGF** * levels
Radiology Exams	**Bone scan**
	ProstaScint scan or **ProstaScint-CT-PET fusion** studies
	Endorectal MRI of the prostate **with spectroscopy**
	CT scan
	PET scan
	Bone mineral density with **quantitative CT scanning (QCT)**
*Vascular endothelial growth factor	

2001 are also presented in Appendix C. An overview of PC evaluation and treatment strategy is shown in Physician's Note 8.

The PSA and the Free PSA Percentage

The first major breakthrough in laboratory testing for the diagnosis and evaluation of PC has been the *prostate specific antigen* blood test, simply abbreviated as PSA. Blood is drawn and the amount of PSA is quantified. PSA is actually an enzyme made by prostate tissue. PSA has many biological effects but its main purpose is to liquefy the gelatinous semen so that sperm can be sufficiently mobile to accomplish fertilization.

In some medical practices, an investigation to determine if cancer is present is usually recommended if the PSA exceeds a value of 4.0. However, we know that baseline-testing starting at least at the age of 40 (35 if there is a family history of prostate or breast cancer) will reveal changes in the PSA consistent with PC at values far less than 4.1. It is reasonable to consider first-time PSA values of 2.0 or higher as reasons for further evalua-

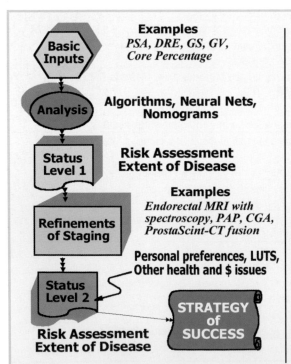

Physician's Note 8:

This strategy is a methodology or process. It must be enacted within a context that involves the supportive care of the patient, a real co-partnership with the healthcare team, and a healthy sense of empowerment and belief. An in-depth discussion of this Strategy of Success is presented in the July 2002 issue of the PCRI newsletter *Insights* (www.pcri.org).

tion and closer scrutiny to rule out PC.[5,6]

The dynamics of PSA or the changes in PSA over time are clues to the presence of malignancy. This makes sense if we understand that the tumor cell population involved in PC is making PSA in amounts consistent with the tumor cell volume. As the tumor cell population or clone grows, so does its quantitative expression of PSA. The PSA doubling time or PSADT and the PSA velocity or PSAV (alluded to in Chapter 2) are clues to significant biologic changes that indicate malignancy. The PSADT also provides a clue as to the extent of PC. This will be discussed in more detail later in this chapter.

PSA is made up of several sub-types of PSA. The two major ones are complexed PSA and free PSA (Fig. 12). Complexed PSA is associated with PC and is in contrast to free PSA, which is associated with benign prostatic cell proliferation. (The free PSA divided by the total PSA, when expressed as a percent, is the free PSA percentage.) The free PSA percentage is a useful

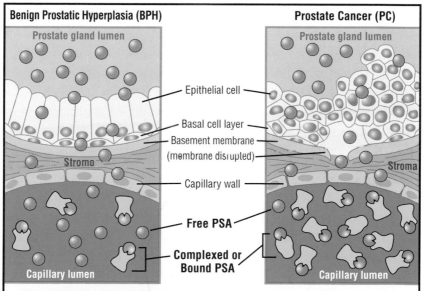

Benign Prostatic Hyperplasia (BPH)   **Prostate Cancer (PC)**

Prostate gland lumen

Prostate gland lumen

Epithelial cell

Basal cell layer

Basement membrane

(membrane disrupted)

Stroma

Stroma

Capillary wall

Free PSA

Complexed or
Bound PSA

Capillary lumen

Capillary lumen

Figure 12: The Free PSA. *In benign processes (such as benign prostatic hyperplasia shown on the left side of the figure), free PSA leaves the prostate gland lumen and gains access to the blood stream (capillary). In PC (shown on the right side of the figure), free PSA enters the capillary via disruption of the basement membrane; this disruption does not occur in benign processes such as BPH. In PC, most of the free PSA (blue spheres) is bound to alpha chymotrypsin (ACT) (shown in gold), and is called complexed PSA or bound PSA. In PC, the free PSA percentage is therefore low. Free PSA percentage = (Free PSA ÷ [Free PSA + Complexed PSA]) x 100.*

tool to evaluate patients with pretreatment PSAs in the 4 to 10 range and even at lower total PSA levels ranging from 2.51 to 4.0 ng/ml.[7]

Before undergoing a biopsy, you should have your PSA tested several times. There can be considerable variation in test results depending on the lab and assay used, so you need several readings using the same laboratory to arrive at an average.[8] Since ejaculation will elevate the PSA, refrain from sexual activity for 48 hours before the PSA testing, and do not do anything else that massages the gland (such as riding a bicycle or a motorcycle) for one week prior to the blood draw. These activities may temporarily raise your PSA and could result in unnecessary concern and/or inappropriate testing based on falsely elevated PSA results.[9-11]

In addition, after the first elevated PSA and before a biopsy, some experts recommend that you exclude prostatitis, or inflammation of the prostate, as a possible explanation for the elevated PSA. Prostatitis can be a non-cancerous cause of an elevated PSA. However, prostatitis can result in low free PSA percentages that make laboratory distinction from PC treacherous. If prostatitis is confirmed, it sometimes responds to treatment with an antibiotic such as Cipro®, usually given for 4-8 weeks. Be sure to allow at least six weeks of antibiotic treatment before rechecking the PSA.[12]

Benign Prostate Hyperplasia (BPH) results in a non-malignant enlargement of the prostate. This can also increase PSA levels. Symptoms of slowness in urinary flow, difficulty in starting the urine stream, and getting up at night to urinate are common to both BPH and PC. The DRE in men with BPH reveals an enlarged but smooth prostate gland. The free PSA percentage is usually 25% or higher in patients with BPH who do not have PC.

In the setting of PC, low levels of free PSA are found. (See

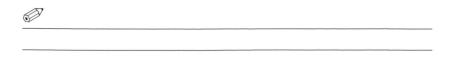

Physician's Note 9.) The PSA is complexed to a protein called alpha-1 chymotrypsin or ACT. The free PSA percentage is therefore *low* in men having PC, usually less than 15%. Lower free PSA percentages, in multiple studies, have been shown to correlate with greater risk for non-organ-confined PC.[13-17]

Another approach to PSA evaluation considers the biologic process inherent to cancer growth. Cancer cells grow and divide from one to two, two to four and so on. There is cancer cell loss or attrition along the way but for the most part, the growth is exponential. In addition, malignant processes not only relate to persistent cell growth but to the production of specific proteins by the malignant cell population. With PC, PSA production is the biomarker most commonly monitored. If the rate of doubling of the PSA (PSA doubling time or PSADT) or the rate of increase in PSA (PSA velocity or PSAV) is abnormal, then PC is *more likely* present than not (Fig. 13). **A PSADT**

shorter than twelve years and a PSA velocity greater than 0.75 ng/ml/year (nanograms per milliliter per year) relates to a greater probability of a malignant condition. These are adjunctive tests, and although they are not absolute criteria for or against malignancy, they are valuable tools. These basic principles apply to all malignancies.

In the context of a patient with a confirmed diagnosis of PC, PSA is a biologic marker (biomarker) that generally reflects the amount and extent of prostate cancer activity.

Patient CE had multiple PSADT results ranging from 7.02 to 21.32 months; such findings were clearly consistent with PC. Software tools that simplify PSADT calculations are accessible

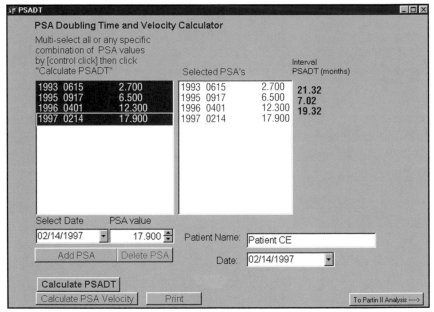

Figure 13: PSA Doubling Time (PSADT) Quantifies the Biologic Process. These are the inputs for patient CE discussed in Physician's Note 9.The PSA values and their dates are highlighted in blue in the far left panel. The three PSADT determinations for these sets of data are shown in bolded black on the right side of the figure under the column "Interval PSADT (months)". The interval between doubling time calculations should be at least six months for accuracy. A persistent progressive rise in PSA should be regarded as prostate cancer until proven otherwise.

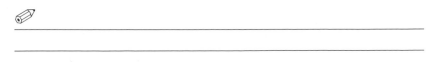

via the PCRI Web site at www.pcri.org and also via Dr. Israel Barken's Prostate Cancer Research and Education Foundation at http://members.cox.net/jfistere/MultiGraphIntro.htm.

Digital Rectal Exam (DRE)

The DRE is used to:

- Estimate the prostate gland volume.
- Detect abnormalities in the quality of the gland (hard areas or significant asymmetry) that suggest the presence of PC.
- Discern any extension of PC outside of the gland if the interface between the gland and adjacent tissues is obliterated.
- Evaluate the possibility of prostatitis if the gland is highly tender and/or mushy.

The doctor will insert a gloved finger inside the rectum to feel the gland (Fig. 14). This is not as bad as it sounds if the DRE

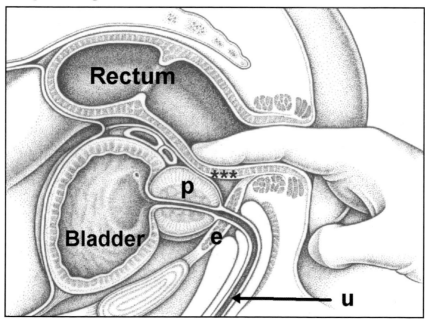

Figure 14: The DRE. In this schematic of a patient bent over for a DRE, the physician's gloved finger is seen palpating the **prostate** (**p**) through the **anterior rectal wall** (***). The prostate sits between the **bladder** above and the **external urinary sphincter** (**e**) below. The **urethra** (**u**) is shown as it exits the bladder, transits the external urinary sphincter (also called the urogenital diaphragm) and enters the penis. The portion of the urethra inside the prostate is aptly called the "prostatic urethra", while the part that goes through the urogenital diaphragm is called the "membranous urethra." Figs. 8 and 9 show additional anatomical details.

is done properly. The physician should use ample lubricant, allow the rectal sphincter to adjust to the pressure of the gloved finger, and gently insert the finger into the rectum to palpate or feel the prostate.

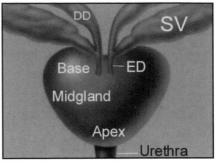

Figure 15: Prostate Regions and Associated Structures. *View this schematic and refer to Figures 8, 9, and 14. The ductus deferens (DD) carries sperm from the testicles and joins the seminal vesicles (SV) to become the ejaculatory duct (ED). The orientation of the prostate on DRE and during the sextant biopsy is often viewed as an upside down triangle with a base, midgland and apex. The prostatic portion of the urethra ends in the apical portion of the gland.*

The patient should be aware of the physician's finger feeling the left and then the right sides (lobes) of the prostate and systematically evaluating the upper portion or *base*, the *midgland* and the lower portion or *apex* of the gland (Fig. 15). The gland is given these designations because anatomically it resembles an upside-down triangle (without the acute angles), with a base and an apex.

The DRE therefore allows the physician to act as a "digital realtor" and assess the "landscape" of the prostate gland to feel for lumps, bumps and/or hardness consistent with malignancy (Fig. 16). Although this is a crude means of evaluating tumor

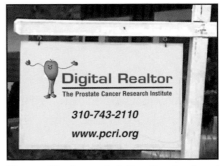

Figure 16: Assessing the Geography of the Prostate. *The DRE enables the examining physician to assess the "landscape" of the gland. This is a reflection of tumor volume, extent of disease, response to androgen deprivation therapy (ADT) and often an indicator of disease recurrence. The DRE is as critical a part of the evaluation of the prostate cancer patient as a breast exam is to a breast cancer patient.*

42

volume, it is an indicator to the physician when the DRE is consistent with PC, that a significant tumor volume is present and that a lower probability of organ-confined PC is likely.

The DRE is the major input in determining the *Clinical Stage* of the cancer, which will help to assess your situation and enable you to describe your condition in a way that others familiar with staging will understand. The *TNM* system is used internationally at this time to describe the cancer and its stage. *"T" describes the tumor*, whether or not it can be felt (is it palpable?), how much it involves one lobe of the prostate, and whether it occupies one or both lobes of the prostate or extends beyond the capsule or invades the seminal vesicles. *"N" stands for nodes* and describes whether or not the cancer has spread to the lymph nodes. Do not confuse nodes with lobes. Nodes or lymph nodes are tissues that belong to the immune system. This filtering system is normally scattered around the entire body. PC can spread to the nodes near the prostate and to more distant nodes far from the prostate (Fig. 17). *"M"* 43

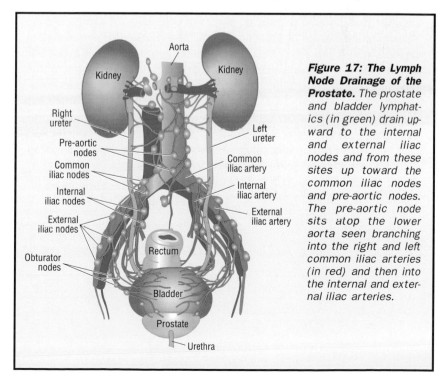

Figure 17: The Lymph Node Drainage of the Prostate. *The prostate and bladder lymphatics (in green) drain upward to the internal and external iliac nodes and from these sites up toward the common iliac nodes and pre-aortic nodes. The pre-aortic node sits atop the lower aorta seen branching into the right and left common iliac arteries (in red) and then into the internal and external iliac arteries.*

stands for metastasis, and indicates whether or not the cancer has spread to other organs or tissues, usually bone, but on more rare occasions, to the liver or lungs. A full description of TNM staging designations is available in Appendix D (see "Staging"). Additional resources that discuss and/or illustrate Staging are given in Appendix A, Section IV.

The clinical stage of PC is essentially the T stage within the TMN classification. Due to the earlier diagnosis of PC now made possible by annual PSA testing,[18,19] the vast majority of

---

Physician's Note 10:

"Listen to the Biology of PC." If you pay attention to all the clues provided to the student of PC, you can predict with a far greater degree of certainty the natural history of this disease. In most patients with PC, the spread of disease, when it occurs, is orderly from prostate gland into the capsule and from there to the seminal vesicles and then to lymph nodes and bones. Fortunately, with PSA testing at regular intervals in conjunction with the DRE, advanced presentations of PC are no longer common in the United States. However, in countries where such practices are not taken seriously, lymph node and bone involvement is often found at diagnosis.

Patient RR was found to have an abnormal DRE with a 1 cm nodule involving the left lobe of the prostate (clinical stage T2a). His PSA had almost doubled from 4.0 to 7.6 in a six-month period. A transrectal ultrasound of the prostate with biopsies in 5/99 indicated PC in four of eight cores with a Gleason score of 10 (read by UroCor). A bone scan was reported as negative for metastases but a CT scan of the pelvis showed an enlarged left common iliac lymph node. Exploratory laparotomy with lymph node sampling indicated involvement of the right internal iliac node and the left common iliac node upon pathologic examination. RR's short PSA doubling time, his high Gleason score, and the high core percentage involvement by PC (50%) all were high-risk factors for advanced PC with lymph node involvement in a pattern typical for PC. His TNM stage was T2aN2M0.

44

men now diagnosed with PC in the USA do not have evidence of metastasis to bone or lymph nodes, nor does a DRE detect palpable disease. (See Physician's Note 10.)

Biopsy of the Prostate and the Gleason Score

In the past, prostate biopsy involved obtaining at least six cores of tissue. This was called the *sextant* biopsy and related to the prostate anatomy as shown in Figure 18A. The typical sextant biopsy involves sampling the base, midgland and apex from each side for a total of six core biopsies. Any additional suspicious lesions seen on TRUSP (Transrectal Ultrasound of the Prostate) or felt on DRE are also biopsied. **To maximize our understanding of a specific patient's situation, the biopsy specimens should be placed in separate, clearly labeled vials so the pathologist can draw conclusions based on the locations from which the samples were taken.**

Recent studies indicate that biopsing additional regions increases PC detection by as much as 35%. One such approach, **45** the *5-region biopsy technique*, involves taking additional samples from the midline tissue of the prostate and the far lateral zones on either side of the prostate. Figure 18 compares the

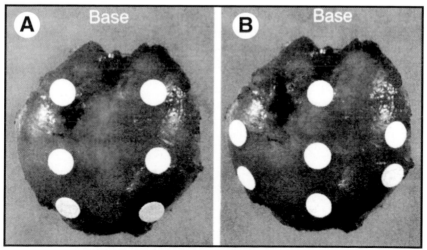

Figures 18A and 18B: The 5-Region Biopsy Technique. The old "standard" sextant biopsy with the six sites shown on the left with the additional seven sites involving the lateral portions and midline of the prostate comprise the 5-region biopsy approach. Reprinted with permission from Lippincott Williams and Wilkins from Eskew LA, Bare, RL, McCullough DL: Systematic 5 region prostate biopsy superior to sextant method for diagnosing carcinoma of the prostate. J Urol 157:199-202, 1997, figure 1, page 200.

prostate areas sampled with the "standard" sextant biopsy approach (A) and shows the seven additional sites biopsied with the 5-region technique (B). Many experts believe the 5-region biopsy approach should be the standard biopsy technique used today. Use of the 5-region biopsy would reduce the physical and emotional trauma to the patient by minimizing the need for repeat biopsy procedures and would reduce healthcare costs while expediting an earlier diagnosis of PC.[20]

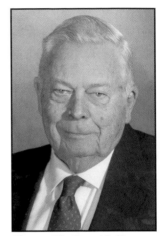

The biopsy results yield much information about the biology of the patient's PC that is unique to that specific patient. **The Gleason score is one of the most important pathologic determinants.** Our understanding of the pathology of PC and how the biologic manifestations of PC under the microscope relate to the aggressiveness of the disease is founded in the pioneering work of Donald Gleason, M.D. (Fig. 19). The Gleason score is an analysis by a pathologist of how the PC appears in the diagnostic biopsies (or in the RP specimen) as compared to the normal cellular architecture.

Figure 19: Donald Gleason, M.D. In 1974, this pioneer observed features of biologic aggressiveness during microscopic examination of countless biopsies of human PC and developed a rating system. The Gleason score is another facet of cancer "profiling" based on the degree of loss of the normal glandular tissue architecture (i.e. the shape, size and distribution of the glands). The classic Gleason scoring system shows five basic tissue patterns that are technically defined as "grades."

The following are characteristics of the Gleason system.

- The Gleason score consists of two numbers: a primary Gleason grade and a secondary grade.

46

- Each Gleason grade is assigned a value between 1 and 5, the higher numbers indicating a more aggressive cancer (Fig. 20).
- The first number indicates the predominant grade; the second number is the second most predominant grade.
- The predominant (primary) grade, by definition, has to be at least 51% of the total picture seen under the microscope. The secondary grade has to be at least 5% of this same picture but less than 50% of the total pattern seen under the microscope, i.e. 5% to 49%.

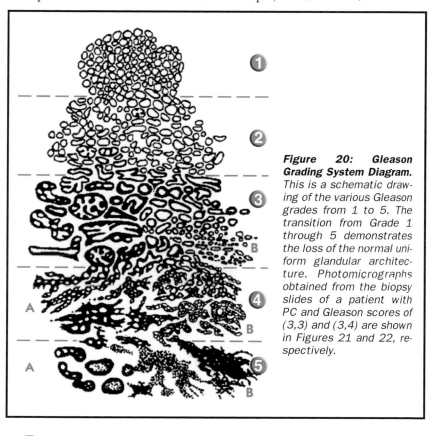

Figure 20: Gleason Grading System Diagram. *This is a schematic drawing of the various Gleason grades from 1 to 5. The transition from Grade 1 through 5 demonstrates the loss of the normal uniform glandular architecture. Photomicrographs obtained from the biopsy slides of a patient with PC and Gleason scores of (3,3) and (3,4) are shown in Figures 21 and 22, respectively.*

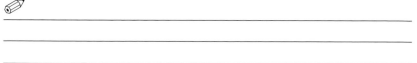

- The Gleason "score" indicates these two grades in the format of (primary grade, secondary grade) as for example: (3,4).
- The most common Gleason score is (3,3). This is illustrated in Figure 21.
- A Gleason score [e.g. (3,4)] indicates that anywhere from 51% to 95% of the specimen is Gleason grade 3 disease and that anywhere from 5% to 49% of the specimen has a secondary pattern of Gleason grade 4 disease (Fig. 22).

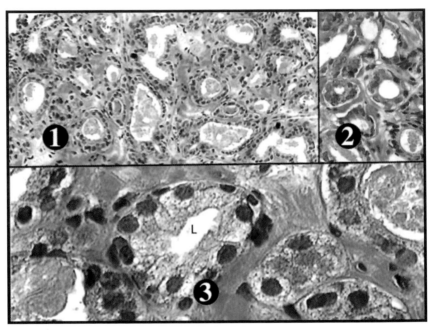

Figure 21: Gleason score (3,3) Photomicrographs. *These are composite photos from three different patients, each with a GS of (3,3). Areas 1 and 2 show the prominent infiltrative glandular pattern with variation of size and shape of the glands. Area 3 is a higher power view to point out the cell structure with the individual dark nuclei of the cells that comprise each gland. Just to the left of center of Area 3 is a clearer defined gland with a central opening or lumen (L).*

- The amount of Gleason grade 4 and/or 5 disease is an important NEGATIVE prognostic finding that usually relates to more extensive disease and to a more aggressive course.

Tissue samples taken during biopsies or at radical prostatectomy (RP) are preserved and retained, making it possible to send the samples to an expert PC pathologist for review and confirmation. Experts in assessing prostate cancer biopsies are available at specific labs (*UroCor and Dianon*) and at certain major

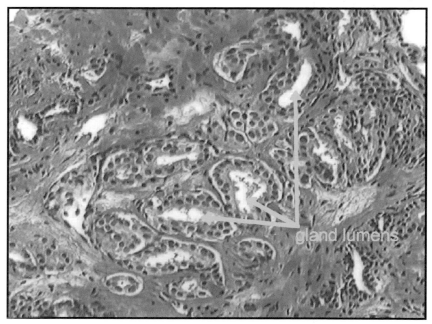

49

Figure 22: Sample Photomicrograph of Gleason score (3,4). *The predominant Gleason grade in this patient's prostate biopsy was grade 3. This is characterized by an infiltrative glandular pattern with individual glands showing significant variation in shape with elongated and angulated glands present. The glandular structure defines what we call adeno (gland) carcinoma. The central opening in the gland is the lumen. The epithelial cells that make PSA and other cell products surround the lumen. The dark blue dots are the cell nuclei. Three glands with obvious lumens are shown (yellow arrows).*

medical centers under the guidance of specific artists in the area of PC pathology. Samples from anywhere in the world can be sent to these artists for "second opinions." Do not be afraid to ask for this additional assurance that your Gleason score is accurate, because this is a *major* factor in your decision-making process. **If your Gleason score has been given an interpretation that is lower or higher than that rendered by an expert, you may undertreat or overtreat your cancer based on erroneous information!** Some of the *expert PC pathologists* and two of the expert laboratories in the United States who can be consulted to confirm your Gleason score are:

David Bostwick (Virginia):	(800) 214-6628
Francisco Civantos (Florida):	(305) 325-5587
Jon Epstein (Maryland):	(410) 955-5043
David Grignon (Michigan):	(313)-745-2520
John McNeal (California):	(650) 725-5534
Jon Oppenheimer (Tennessee):	(888) 868-7522
Dianon Laboratories:	(800) 328-2666
UroCor:	(800) 411-1839

(UroCor and Dianon have recently merged into one company)

Some of the experts in PC pathology in Europe are:

Prof. Dr. B. Helpap at the Chefarzt Institut fur Pathologie, Hegau Klinikum
Virchowstrasse 10, 78224 Singen/Htwl.
Tel: 07731/892100; Fax: 07731/892105

Prof. Dr. med Helmut Bonkhoff
Prof. of Pathology
Tietzenweg 129
12203 Berlin, Germany, or:
P.O.B. 450211, 12172 Berlin, Germany
Tel: +49-30-84317882
E-mail: info@prostapath.de

Prof. Dr. Wernert at the Uniklinik Bonn, Pathologie
Sigmund-Freud-Strasse 25, 53127 Bonn
Tel: 0228/2875030
E-mail: wernert@meb.uni-bonn.de

We suggest that you call one of these pathologists or national laboratories. Speak to them about the procedure for obtaining a second opinion. Your physician should be willing to work with you on this matter—if not, do not be afraid to initiate a call yourself. Such initiative reflects your active role in the co-partnership with your physician(s) and affirms that you expect to play a major part in this liaison. Obtaining a *validated* Gleason score is a highly important step in analyzing the biologic manifestation of PC.

Prostatic Acid Phosphatase (PAP)

The *PAP* should be a part of your baseline PC evaluation. However, as with PSA, the PAP may also be elevated due to the trauma caused by the prostate biopsies. Therefore, you need to wait at least five weeks after the biopsy procedure before testing for PAP unless this test was ordered prior to the diagnostic biopsies. Ideally, both PSA and PAP testing should not be done for at least 48 hours after any sexual activity involving ejaculation or 48 hours after DRE.[21]

Most physicians and patients consider the PSA and PAP to be simply "blood tests." However, the biologic reality is that PC cells elaborate numerous chemical substances that are vital to their growth and well-being and are often related to their function. Many of these cell products are enzymes important to the growth and spread of the cancer. PAP and PSA are just two of many enzymes that should be regarded beyond that of merely representing commercial laboratory tests. The results of PAP and PSA testing add to the biologic "profile" that an astute patient-physician team uses to accurately decipher the real status of the patient's disease. (See Physician's Note 11.) Answering the question: "Is the PC confined to the prostate gland or not?" should be the first order of business for men newly diagnosed with PC.

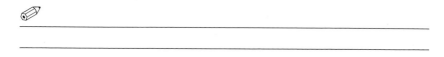

PP had never had routine PSA testing and when he was diagnosed with PC his baseline (bPSA) was 108. His PAP at that time was 13.5. He had a Gleason score of (3,3), but this was not reviewed by an expert in PC pathology. He was advised to have a radical prostatectomy. His RP specimen, when reviewed by an expert in PC pathology (David Bostwick, M.D.), indicated a GS of (4,3) with the Gleason grade 4 component approximated at 70% of the specimen. Extensive perineural invasion (PNI), a high risk factor for capsular penetration, was present at RP. The left lobe of the gland contained a PC nodule that was 3.5 cm in diameter. One of 10 lymph nodes showed PC. Capsular penetration and surgical margins (apex of gland) were positive for PC, and seminal vesicle involvement was present on the left. PSA recurrence post-RP was noted within six months of surgery. The bPAP, bPSA, and validated Gleason score were all risk factors for his suboptimal clinical course.

The PAP is useful for predicting a higher risk of PSA recurrence. In a study by Moul et al, men who were monitored after a radical prostatectomy (RP) had a **PSA recurrence (PSAR) rate at four years of 61.2% if the baseline PAP was 3 ng/ml or higher. The PSAR rate of those with a PAP of less than 3.0 ng/ml was 21.2% (Fig. 23).** These findings held when the pretreatment PSA was less than 10 ng/ml (p = 0.047) as well as when the baseline PSA was 10 ng/ml or greater (p = 0.012). A baseline PAP (bPAP), therefore, adds valuable prognostic information to pretreatment PSA (bPSA) values and is an independent predictor of recurrence.[22]

PAP elevation is also a high-risk factor for patients likely to have PSA relapse (biochemical failure) after seed implantation. In a series of 124 consecutive patients treated with palladium and supplemental external beam irradiation for clinically localized, high-risk prostate carcinoma, (i.e. clinical stages T2a–T3), **the strongest predictor of biochemical failure was an elevated baseline PAP (p = 0.02)**, followed by the Gleason score (p = 0.1), and PSA (p = 0.14).[23] In this study, PAP was a more accurate indicator of micrometastatic disease than bPSA.

These reports by Moul and Dattoli et al mandate the addition of baseline testing with PAP. Both reports indicate that PAP elevation at diagnosis signifies a higher risk that the PC is outside the prostate and is likely to be outside either the surgical field or RT treatment port. Such patients are most likely to fail local therapies and probably require adjuvant or supplemental systemic therapy to eradicate metastatic disease. The finding of a PAP elevation is a biological clue that the PC is more aggressive and less likely to be organ-confined. Such findings should also lead the patient-physician co-partnership to use other evaluative procedures such as the ProstaScint scan or the endorectal MRI, as well as obtaining blood samples for other biologic markers (biomarkers) such as NSE, CEA, CGA, and TGF-ß$_1$. *If you want to know more about PAP see Appendix B, Section 3.1.*

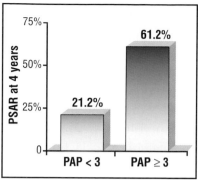

Figure 23: The Importance of Baseline PAP (bPAP) Testing. A simple blood test, the PAP, is a major guide to the patient-physician team in assessing the patient's probability of having a successful radical prostatectomy. In the study by Moul et al, if the baseline PAP (bPAP) was ≥ 3.0, the probability of PSA recurrence post radical prostatectomy was almost triple that of men with bPAP values less than 3.0.

53

ProstaScint Scan

ProstaScint is a staging tool in which a radioactive isotope is attached to an antibody. What makes this approach unique is the use of a monoclonal antibody (mAb), which by definition is *targeted against a specific cancer protein* (antigen). In other words, the isotope-monoclonal antibody cocktail is injected into the bloodstream and seeks that specific cancer protein and then attaches to it. Four days later, the patient is scanned with a special camera that detects gamma radiation emitted from the isotope-mAb-protein "sandwich", which serves to localize the specific cancer protein. The ProstaScint scan uses a mAb called 7E11 anti-prostate specific membrane antibody (anti-PSMA mAb), which seeks to find *prostate specific membrane antigen* (PSMA) associated with PC.

PSMA is a distinctly different protein from PSA. While PSA is found within the prostate cell and is secreted into the blood stream in easily detectable quantities, PSMA is essentially a

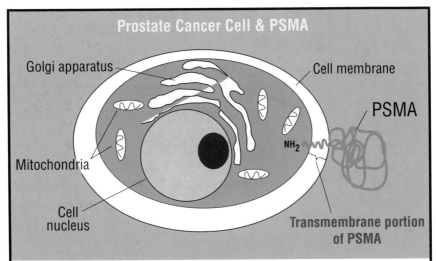

Figure 24: PSMA and the ProstaScint Scan. *A prostate cancer cell and its relationship with prostate specific membrane antigen (PSMA) is shown. PSMA is a **transmembrane** antigen and a portion of this protein is shown oriented across the cell membrane (brackets), while the tail end dangles outside the cell in the extracellular fluid. During ProstaScint scanning, a specific antibody to PSMA tagged with the radioactive isotope Indium[111] attaches to the intracellular amino terminal (NH_2) portion of PSMA. Prostate tissue expressing PSMA (not PSA) is therefore targeted by the ProstaScint monoclonal antibody scan.*

transmembrane protein: part of it is inside the prostate cell but it extends through the cell membrane with a large amount of the antigen dangling outside the cell (Fig. 24). Relatively tiny amounts of PSMA are detectable in the blood stream of PC patients.

If a patient is ascertained at diagnosis to be at a high risk for extra-prostatic disease by PC that involves *soft tissue* (such as the seminal vesicles or lymph nodes), the ProstaScint scan may be a valuable tool to refine treatment strategy. If the ProstaScint shows seminal vesicle or lymph node involvement, local treatment options (e.g. RP, RT or cryosurgery) would proba-

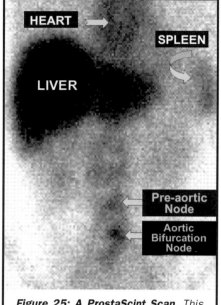

Figure 25: A ProstaScint Scan. *This is an actual ProstaScint scan showing uptake of the mAb-isotope complex in at least two nodal areas: (1) a pre-aortic node and (2) the common iliac node at the bifurcation of the right and left common iliac arteries (aortic bifurcation node). Figure 17 illustrates these lymph node sites and shows their relationship to the prostate.*

55

bly not be curative options, although they could still be used as treatments to eradicate local disease. The ProstaScint is also used in the context of PSA recurrence (PSAR) after local therapy to determine if cancer activity is limited to the prostate area or whether there is metastatic disease involving lymph nodes (Fig. 25).[24]

Just as the interpretation of a Gleason score requires especially talented pathologists, so does the ProstaScint scan require expertise in its technique and interpretation. The ProstaScint scan demands meticulous preparation of the patient. The intestinal tract must be thoroughly cleansed with the use of NuLytely®, GoLytely® or a similar cathartic since fecal material interferes with the reading of this monoclonal antibody scan. The preparation of the patient is identical to that used for colonoscopy. Moreover, the nuclear medicine equipment must involve the use of at least a dual-headed gamma camera, and the nuclear medicine personnel must be able to subtract the effect of the blood pool from the images obtained.

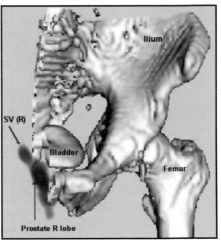

PC patients need to network through their support groups or speak with people of special talent in this field to find out who are the "artists" doing ProstaScint scanning. In the last few years, ProstaScint scan findings have been co-registered or fused with other radiologic imaging techniques such as the CT scan of the pelvis, PET (positron emission tomography) scans, and bone scans. This graphic presentation technique has been labeled "Fusion Technology." An example of co-registration of the CT

Figure 26: Co-registration or "Fusion" of ProstaScint and CT Imaging. In this approach, computer software integrates the images generated by both the ProstaScint scan and the CT scan, which are fused into one output. The image shown has been obtained from a patient going to surgery for a radical prostatectomy. Unfortunately for this patient, the pathology findings confirmed those of the ProstaScint fusion study, i.e. PC was present in the right lobe of the prostate with extension to the right seminal vesicle. (Image shown with permission from Drs. Bruce Sodee and Zhenghong Lee, Department of Nuclear Medicine, University Hospitals of Cleveland. Dr. Lee rendered this 3D image from the fusion study.)

scan and the Prosta-Scint is shown in Figure 26.[25]

Endorectal MRI

Endorectal MRI is also a relatively new radiologic advance that is used to image the prostate, the prostatic capsule and the lymph nodes in the region of the prostate. This technique provides input about the degree of involvement (volume of PC) and the extent of involvement (stage of PC). Two centers (University of California at San Francisco and Memorial Sloan Kettering in New York City) are employing this tool in combination with spectroscopy of the prostate gland. The spectroscopy or spectrographic analysis involved utilizes the

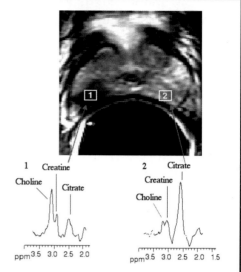

Figure 27: Endorectal MRI with Spectroscopy. *This is an endorectal MRI from a 58-year-old man with pathologic stage pT3a prostate cancer. It is a corrected T2-weighted image (T2WI) through the mid-portion of the gland using an endorectal coil placed in the rectum (the black area below locations 1 and 2). MR spectroscopy of area 1 shows an elevated choline:citrate ratio consistent with PC, whereas area 2 shows a normal spectroscopy pattern with the citrate peak dominant and no abnormal elevation in choline. In this T2WI, prostate cancer has a low signal intensity; therefore, we see a darker area in area 1 consistent with malignancy. The findings of MR imaging and MR spectroscopy were concordant. In other words, we have two biologic inputs indicating malignancy: MR imaging and MR spectroscopy. Concordance is associated with greater accuracy.*

57

finding that prostate tissue *involved by prostate cancer* is high in the amino acid "choline" while low in the amino acid citrate as contrasted to *benign prostate tissue*, which is low in choline and high in citrate (Fig. 27). Thus, spectroscopy determines relative amounts of choline and citrate and is used as a differential test to confirm the findings of magnetic resonance imaging or MRI.

This technique is far superior to a routine pelvic MRI and is associated with a 75% to 90% accuracy rate when there is agreement (*concordance*) between both spectroscopy and MRI modalities of imaging.[26] This fifty minute procedure, therefore, is used to help determine the probability of organ-confined disease. It is also useful in determining if PC has spread to seminal vesicles and regional lymph nodes.[27] It can also be extremely useful in detecting the site(s) of PC in men who are suspected of having PC but who have not yet been positively diagnosed despite previous transrectal ultrasound guided biopsies.[28] Such patients undergo "targeted" needle biopsies of the prostate using the findings of endorectal MRI with spectroscopy to direct the needle to sites most likely to contain PC.

58 DNA Ploidy

DNA analysis or DNA ploidy is a pathological examination performed on PC tissue obtained from the diagnostic biopsy or radical prostatectomy specimen. **Ploidy provides additional information on the aggressiveness of PC and its probable responsiveness to androgen deprivation therapy (ADT) described in Chapter 4.**

Ploidy is a term used to describe the chromosome content of the cell population of a tumor. A ploidy analysis of cancer cells determines whether they are either diploid or aneuploid. Diploid PC cells have the normal number of chromosome pairs, are more often associated with Gleason scores of 6 or less, tend to grow more slowly, and respond well to ADT. Aneuploid tumors have abnormal numbers of chromosomes, are more often associated with high Gleason scores of 8 to 10, are more aggressive in their growth, and do not respond as well to hormonal therapies.[29] In light of these unfavorable characteristics, aneuploid PC has a greater risk of being non-organ-confined. Hence, ploidy is of special interest to patients considering ADT since it relates to the likelihood that such treatment will be effective. Ploidy is yet another facet of tumor profiling that provides additional information that enhances risk assessment and affects treatment strategy.

Positron Emission Tomography (PET) Scan

A PET scan is a relatively new tool in the evaluation and management of PC. Current PET scanning most commonly uses ^{18}F-deoxyglucose: a glucose molecule (fluorodeoxyglucose) that contains a radioactive isotope, in this case fluorine 18 (^{18}F). ^{18}F-deoxyglucose is localized within biologically active PC because tumor cells utilize glucose as an energy source. The ^{18}F isotope then begins to decay, emitting a nuclear particle called a positron—essentially a positive electron. The emitted positron collides with a free electron, and the interaction of these two subatomic particles results in a conversion of matter to energy in the form of two gamma rays. These high-energy gamma rays emerge from the collision point in opposite directions and are detected by an array of detectors that surround the patient. **PET scans, therefore, not only can locate tumors in the above manner but also can provide information on the metabolic activity of the cancer.** This allows for a "live look" at how tumors are responding to treatment, rather than providing a static image, as do most other imaging techniques.

59

In Figure 28, a whole body PET scan shows areas of abnormal isotope uptake in the right axilla, the right and left femora, the left pelvic bone and the ribs. Four months after chemotherapy, the femora, right axilla and pelvic abnormalities are devoid of activity. Normal or physiologic uptake is seen in the brain, heart, liver, kidneys and bladder.

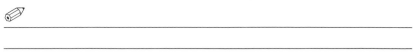

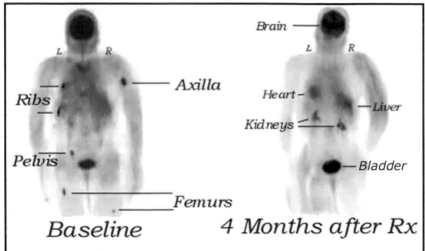

Baseline   4 Months after Rx

Figure 28: The PET Scan. *The PET scan is a functional scan in that it shows areas of metabolic uptake of the specific isotope-tagged molecule by the tumor. The isotope utilized here was fluorine 18 that "tags" the fluorodeoxyglucose molecule. In this figure, the patient is positioned with his back to us. As you can see, the brain, heart and liver show major glucose utilization. Increased isotopic activity in the urinary bladder is due to excretion of the isotope.*

Bone Scan

The bone scan involves the use of a radioactive isotope (technetium-99) that is picked up at sites within the bone in the presence of significant bone metastases. **Bone scanning should routinely be done as part of your baseline evaluation if the PSA is over 10.** Since uptake of the technetium isotope also occurs at sites of arthritis or trauma to the bone, routine x-rays, CT scans or MRI scans may be used to evaluate areas of uptake seen on the bone scan. If these studies explain the uptake of the isotope based on past trauma or arthritis, the bone scan is considered to be "negative"—showing no evidence for metastatic disease. **If, on the other hand, there is no explanation for the isotopic uptake on any of these studies, the bone scan must be presumed abnormal and consistent with PC until proven otherwise.**

In patients newly diagnosed with PC, a PSA of less than or

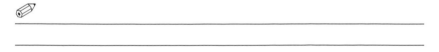

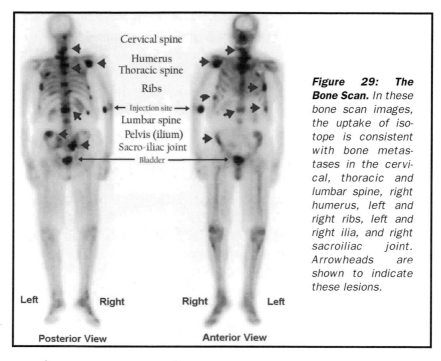

Cervical spine
Humerus
Thoracic spine
Ribs
← Injection site →
Lumbar spine
Pelvis (ilium)
Sacro-iliac joint
Bladder

Figure 29: The Bone Scan. In these bone scan images, the uptake of isotope is consistent with bone metastases in the cervical, thoracic and lumbar spine, right humerus, left and right ribs, left and right ilia, and right sacroiliac joint. Arrowheads are shown to indicate these lesions.

Left   Right   Right   Left

Posterior View   **Anterior View**

equal to 10 is associated with an abnormal bone scan in only one of 200 (0.5%) patients.[30] In the United States alone, at least $60 million per year is spent performing unnecessary bone scans.[31] These healthcare dollars could be used for more appropriate testing or for research. Therefore, your physician may decide to forego a bone scan if your PSA is 10 or less and your Gleason score, validated by an expert, is 6 or less. **Patients with Gleason scores of 7, 8, 9 and 10 may have prostate cancers that make relatively less PSA because such PC cell populations are associated with a smaller leak of PSA into the blood.**[32] In such settings, the PSA is a less reliable indicator of disease volume and the risk of extra-prostatic spread is still significant despite a baseline PSA of 10 or less. Therefore, if your Gleason score is in this range, your physician should consider a bone scan as part of your initial evaluation.

CT (Computerized Tomography) Scan or CAT Scan

Unfortunately, a CT scan of the *pelvis* and of the *abdomen* is routinely ordered in virtually all newly diagnosed men with PC. However, it is our contention, based on published literature, that this is a serious waste of healthcare dollars while exposing the patient to unnecessary radiation and inconvenience.[33-35] The biological profile at the time of the patient's initial presentation dictates whether or not such studies are necessary. This is true for virtually every imaging study that is being done in men with PC. For at least 90% of men undergoing baseline staging procedures, a CT scan of the pelvis is not indicated. **In 99.9% of all newly diagnosed patients with PC, a CT of the abdomen is definitely not needed. The CT scan of the pelvis requires high volume PC to enable detection of disease in the lymph nodes. In the context of a newly diagnosed patient, a pelvic CT is valueless in detecting extra-prostatic extension such as capsular penetration or seminal vesicle involvement, unless a late diagnosis has been made and bulky disease has become established.**

62 However, high Gleason scores may warrant a CT scan. A study by Lee et al of 544 newly diagnosed patients with PC who had routine CT scans of the pelvis and abdomen revealed that 36 (6.6%) had abnormal CT pelvic findings, as shown in Table 2. **Not surprisingly, none of the 244 men presenting with a PSA less than or equal to 15 with a validated Gleason score of 7 or less and a clinical stage of T2b or less had an abnormal CT scan.** Moreover, in the 174 men with a PSA at diagnosis greater than 15 and/or a clinical stage of T2c or higher, only eight of 174 (5%) had an abnormal CT scan if the Gleason score was less than or equal to 7. **However, of those 126 men with**

Table 2: Incidence of Abnormal Pelvic CT Scan Based on Biologic Findings at Diagnosis.			
Gleason Score	**PSA**	**Clinical Stage**	**CT Scan Findings**
2-7	≤ 15	≤ T2b	0/244 (0%)
2-7	>15 and/or clinical stage > T2b		8/174 (5%)
8-10	Any value	Any value	28/126 (22%)
Totals			36/544 (6.6%)
At diagnosis, the CT scan can be omitted in men presenting with a validated Gleason score of 2-7, a baseline PSA of less than or equal to 15 and a clinical stage of less than or equal to T2b. Modified after Lee et al.[36]			

Gleason scores of 8-10, a total of 28 (22%) had positive pelvic CT scan findings.[36]

USPIO Particle Scanning and Assessment of Lymph Node Metastasis

Of particular interest in the assessment of patients at significant risk for lymph node metastasis due to prostate cancer is USPIO (ultrasmall superparamagnetic iron oxide) particle scanning. This radiologic imaging technique was the subject of a lead article in the New England Journal of Medicine.* USPIO particle scanning is a non-invasive staging procedure employing high-resolution MRI imaging after the intravenous injection of the patient with magnetic nanoparticles. Currently, the most accurate approach to determining if PC has spread to lymph nodes is surgical sampling of lymph nodes either by laparoscopy or at the time of radical prostatectomy. Both of these latter procedures are invasive, costly and not without a significant risk of morbidity. In the assessment of lymph nodes measuring 5-10 millimeters (mm), USPIO has an accuracy rate of 98.9% with a sensitivity of 96.4%, and specificity of 99.3%. Even for lymph nodes < 5 mm, USPIO was found to have a specificity of 98.1%. This staging technique should be applicable to all tumors where lymph node metastasis is a common pathway for the spread of cancer. Hopefully, with the input of empowered patients and partners, USPIO will receive FDA approval shortly.

63

Chromogranin A (CGA)

The plasma CGA level is used to help identify patients with an aggressive form of PC. In such patients, the CGA elevations should be documented as *progressively* increasing and not just a sporadic or stable elevation. This is not as complicated as it may sound. Prostate tissue, both benign and malignant, is comprised of at least four different cell types: basal cells, epithelial cells, neuroendocrine cells and stromal cells. CGA testing involves the measurement of blood levels of chromogranin A, a protein synthesized by the neuroendocrine cell type (i.e. of neurogenic origin with endocrine functions) found in prostate cancer. Neuroendocrine cells in PC are not dependent on androgens as are the epithelial cells (also called luminal cells), which are the cells most commonly involved in PC growth.

Harisinghani MG, Barentsz J, Hahn PF, et al: Noninvasive Detection of Clinically Occult Lymph-Node Metastases in Prostate Cancer. N Engl J Med 348:2491-2499, 2003.

Serial CGA testing can help track the patient's response to treatment, especially if serum PSA and/or PAP expression is low. **Low PSA levels may be seen despite significantly high tumor volumes in situations where the PC has mutated to an aggressive cell type; this is characterized by a high Gleason score of 8-10.**[32] In fact, obtaining a full baseline set of bio-markers in situations associated with such an aggressive picture often reveals elevation(s) in plasma CGA, neuron specific enolase (NSE), carcinoembryonic antigen (CEA) and/or prostatic acid phosphatase (PAP) (Fig. 30). When a progressive increase in any of these biomarkers is documented, there is invariably evidence of mutated aggressive PC.[37] These findings should always be placed in context with the rest of the clinical and pathological picture. (See Physician's Note 12.)

In a study by Kadmon et al, almost 50% of clinical stage D2 patients (advanced PC patients in which cancer has spread to

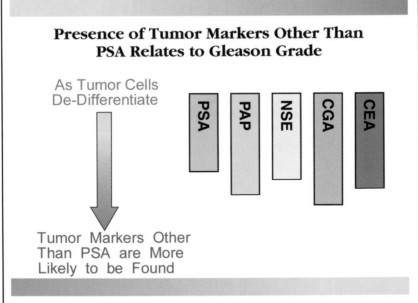

Figure 30: High Gleason Grade PC Means De-Differentiated PC. *As tumor cells become more de-differentiated (less mature) in appearance, they may show biologic expression of other enzymes and peptides in the blood that can be used as parameters or markers of disease activity. Therefore, in the presence of any Gleason* **grade** *4 or 5 disease (Gleason score of 7-10) we should obtain a baseline set of such biomarkers and periodically recheck such values pending the patient's clinical course.*

Physician's Note 12:

"The Importance of Comprehensive Tumor Marker Analysis in the Setting of Gleason Scores of 8 to 10." It is important to realize that the biology of PC is highly varied and that the context of the biologic milieu often mandates an altered approach to the evaluation and management of PC. The clinical findings presented here emphasize the need for more comprehensive biologic marker studies in high Gleason score situations. Other tumor markers like CGA, NSE, CEA and PAP may provide clues to disease activity when the PSA is very low or even undetectable in settings characteristic of a tumor cell population that is becoming or has become de-differentiated.

Patient OG presented with advanced PC indicating bone metastases at age 68 despite a baseline PSA of 8.4. He had seven out of eight core biopsies showing PC with a Gleason score of (5,4). Treatment with ADT using Casodex and Lupron resulted in a transient drop in PSA to < 0.05 for one month followed by a rise in PSA. A diagnosis of androgen-independent PC was made and different chemotherapeutic agents were given with no significant response. Enlarged pelvic nodes were seen on CT compressing the left ureter, and the base of the bladder was felt to be involved by PC. Meanwhile, on ADT, a repeat bone scan showed resolution of the previously documented abnormalities. After much deliberation, neutron beam RT was elected at the FermiLab in Batavia, Illinois to treat the prostate, bladder base and pelvic nodes. This was started in January of 2000. One year later, a repeat CT pelvis and abdomen showed no lymph node enlargement. A PSA was < 0.1, PAP was 1.0 and CEA was 2.7. However, a plasma CGA which was normal at 7.6 in 11/22/98 had risen to 67 in 10/01. The CEA on that date had increased to 4.2. The patient has been advised to repeat these markers and also obtain an NSE level along with repeat staging studies to include a ProstaScint-PET-CT fusion study.

the bones) were found to have significant elevations of plasma chromogranin A.[38] Although the normal range of plasma CGA used in this study was 43 ± 17 ng/ml, the authors elected to use a more conservative cut-off point of 100 ng/ml. If the authors had selected an upper limit of normal of 60 ng/nl, then almost 70% of the population studied would have shown CGA elevation. This study also showed that 50% of those patients with elevated CGA had PSA levels that ranged from 0.2 to 5.6 (mean of 2.08 ng/ml) and all had normal PAP levels.[38] *If you want to know more about CGA, go to Appendix B, Section 3.2.*

Transforming Growth Factor Beta 1 (TGF-ß₁)

The processes of health maintenance and cancer development are associated with the balance and communication between cells. "Cell signaling" and "signal transduction" are some of the terms used to describe these internal control mechanisms. **TGF-ß₁ is believed to be one of the most important regulators of prostate growth, acting under normal circumstances to inhibit proliferation of cells by inducing programmed cell death (apoptosis) of the prostatic epithelial cell.** TGF-ß₁ maintains this profile as an *inhibitory* growth factor through the action of its docking sites or receptors: transforming beta receptor type I and type II (TßR-1 and TßR-II). In this particular setting, TGF-ß₁ is the "ligand," the substance that interacts with the receptor to form a key and lock mechanism that activates cell functions.

In the genesis of a malignancy such as PC, there is loss of expression or function of this receptor: TßR I and II. In response to the decrease in function or expression of the TGF beta 1 receptor, the thermostatic mechanisms of the body try to compensate by overexpressing TGF-ß₁. In other words, cell-cell communication and balance has been disrupted. This is a common occurrence in PC as well as other malignancies. Published studies have correlated loss of expression of the TßR-1 receptor with clinical tumor stage, PSA recurrence post RP, and four-year survival rates.[39,40]

An example of this phenomenon can be seen in the setting of blockade of the androgen receptor with drug therapy involving an anti-androgen. The body tries to compensate by increasing androgen production (the ligand) in an attempt to restore balance. Conversely, in the presence of decreased levels of the ligand (androgen), the cellular mechanisms of balance (homeostasis) try to compensate by increasing the number of androgen receptors. These attempts to restore balance or homeostasis of either ligand or its receptor are commonplace in thousands of bodily functions.

As a result of the loss or function of its receptors, the overexpression of TGF-ß$_1$ has significant biological consequences. **Increased TGF-ß$_1$ levels have been shown to induce angiogenesis, inhibit the immune function of the host, promote cell motility and thus metastasis as well as affect cellular differentiation.**[41] Increased TGF-ß$_1$ expression has been associated with tumor grade, pathologic stage, and lymph node metastases in PC patients.[42] In a highly significant paper by Lee ct al, TGF-ß$_1$ overexpression was shown to have a significant immunosuppressive effect, altering the host-tumor interaction, and thus facilitating tumor growth.[43]

A landmark study by Shariat et al involving 120 men undergoing radical prostatectomy (RP) for clinically localized PC (T1-2 clinical stage), demonstrated that plasma levels of TGF-ß$_1$, obtained preoperatively, were highly correlated with PC progression after RP.[44] *If you want to know more about TGF, see Appendix B, section 3.3.*

uPM3 Urine Test

The uPM3™ test, patented by DiagnoCure, Inc. (http://www.diagnocure.com/anglais/section3/sec33-2.htm) is the first urine-based genetic test for PC detection. uPM3 is based on the PCA3 gene that is profusely expressed in prostate cancer tissue. On average, the incidence is 34 times greater in malignant prostate tissue as opposed to benign prostate tissue. No other human tissues have ever been shown to produce PCA3. ∎

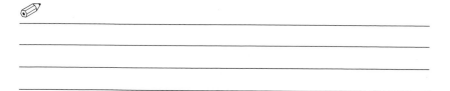

✔ Every test that you are subjected to, be it a physical examination, blood or urine testing, radiology imaging, and/or pathological evaluation, is done, or should be done, for a reason or purpose. At the time of diagnosis of PC, as well as afterwards, much of that purpose equates with "tumor profiling".

✔ This profiling characterizes the cancer by providing information about the nature (degree of aggressiveness) and the extent (stage) of the PC. These are essential first steps for the patient-physician team to win the war against PC. If you don't know the strength and location of your enemy, your chances of winning the battle are diminished greatly.

✔ Of the laboratory tests currently commercially available, the serum PSA level stands out as the major tool in the optimal management of the man with PC. The PSA serves as a marker or indicator of PC activity all throughout the course of PC. The PSA informs us of the quality of response to all major therapies directed against PC. These characteristics make the PSA the single most important product produced by the prostate cancer cell.

✔ However, despite the incredible value of PSA and the importance of PSA dynamics, there are pitfalls in solely relying on PSA measurements. This relates to an understanding of the degree of aggressiveness and the stage of PC. When a Gleason score of 8-10 has been initially interpreted and/or validated by an expert in PC pathology, the PSA loses much of its value as a tumor marker. In such settings, other indicators of disease activity must be checked such as PAP, CGA, CEA, and NSE. These laboratory tests are biomarkers that reflect cellular activity of a more aggressive, and less differentiated (or de-differentiated) tumor cell population.

✔ The dynamics of PSA such as PSA velocity (PSAV) and PSA doubling time (PSADT) are reflections of cell growth (kinetics). A high PSAV and a short PSADT are more consistent with systemic disease. This is true in situations at the time of diagnosis of PC and also in situations of PSA recurrence after any form of treatment.

Chapter

Treatment Options

Today, there a number of different treatment options available. Among them are: surgery, cryosurgery, radiation, androgen deprivation, observation, and several new approaches coming on the scene. Each of these treatment options has its proponents. As a general rule, urologists will lean toward surgery, radiation therapists will favor one or more of the radiation options, cryosurgeons will prefer cryosurgery, and so on.

Unfortunately, it is difficult if not impossible to generalize which is the "best" treatment for all men. It depends upon each individual patient's medical situation and personal preferences. However, we believe that in the attempt to cure prostate cancer there is a correct approach to individualize evaluation and treatment for each man diagnosed with this disease. The selection of the treatment most likely to achieve cure should be based upon an understanding of key concepts in the evaluation and treatment of prostate cancer.

A key concept of prime importance relates to the extent or stage of PC. If our attempts to cure PC are to be successful then the selected local treatment must be a ***biologically appropriate match*** to the true extent of the disease. If the cancer is not confined within the prostate gland, then the likelihood of RP curing the patient is dramatically diminished. If PC has spread to nearby tissues outside the scope of the urologist's scalpel, PSA recurrence after RP is virtually a certainty. If PC is not confined to local and nearby regional tissues, then eradication of PC with radiation therapy or cryosurgery is also unlikely. Too often, we see patients being treated with local therapies such as radical prostatectomy, radiation therapy or cryosurgery with intent to cure when there is no significant probability that the prostate cancer is still confined to the prostate gland or to tissue in close proximity to the gland. Additional concepts such as the importance of tumor volume, the relevance of urinary symptomatology and the biological aggressiveness of the prostate cancer (or lack thereof) are described in detail within this chapter.

As described in Chapter 3, there are various testing procedures available today to enhance our assessment of the extent of PC, and these can and should be individualized to the specific patient's situation. In this way, we can optimize our understanding about a newly diagnosed patient's cancer *before* a treatment decision is made. **This foreknowledge can make the difference in achieving a favorable outcome with the selected treatment because—rather than the patient naively selecting a treatment—he is instead directed towards the selection of a treatment that is biologically appropriate to the specific nature of his disease.**

Patients understandably want to know which treatment has been shown to produce the most favorable outcome. Comparative studies have been made for different treatments to predict *statistically* what the survival or freedom from relapse rate will be at some point in the future. (Usually, the standard is five years.) However, such statistical reports are based upon historical cases that often ignore the wide variation in individual patient conditions and also may or may not have used what we would consider today to be an appropriate treatment.

Adding to the doubts raised about the validity of statistical extrapolation of treatment outcomes are the rapidly evolving technological advances that have been made in recent years. Not only has the widespread use of PSA screening changed PC

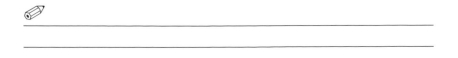

diagnosis dramatically, but also the tools available to practitioners have changed significantly. For example, individual radiation oncologists and institutions have been using different equipment, different doses, different selection criteria for treatment and different criteria for definition of success or failure of treatment. Many of these same factors complicate discussions of any aspect of the primary treatment of PC. Additionally, patients assume the results reported by a small percentage of highly skilled physicians coming from academic institutions will be matched by those of their local practitioners. Too often, this is wishful thinking.

Yet, this is the reality that PC patients have encountered and continue to face. All patients need to realize that medicine is a dynamic field, undergoing changes too rapid for data analyses to keep pace with. Patients must therefore try to choose the form of therapy most appropriate to their particular medical, psychological and financial situations and delivered by the most dedicated staff of artistic practitioners within their specialty. This indeed is a challenge.

Hence, we question the reliability of these statistical prognoses and urge each patient and his physician to seek the "best" treatment for him by developing a rational strategy guided by the diagnostic and staging tools described in Chapter 3 for his particular situation. Furthermore, he should weigh the side-effects of each treatment option carefully, as their effect on his quality of life may well be a determining consideration.

The balance of this chapter describes each of the leading PC treatments with the advantages and disadvantages of each. Thus, depending upon the diagnosis and testing results, it is hoped that each patient and his doctor can select the optimum treatment—and follow-up care—for his individual case.

The authors of this *Primer* have no identifiable bias favoring

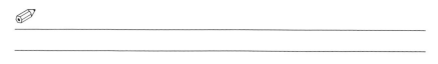

any particular treatment for the man with PC. Rather, this is our credo:

The best outcome for any individual patient is achieved by:

- **Obtaining the best understanding of the biological "truths" of each patient's disease.**
- **Matching those "truths" with the appropriate treatment strategy.**
- **Selecting an "artist" to deliver the chosen therapy(ies).**

Radical Prostatectomy (RP)

Radical prostatectomy (RP) is a surgical procedure involving the removal of the prostate gland and seminal vesicles. It has a long track record with peer-reviewed medical publications reporting follow-up outcomes out to 15 years. Obviously, RP has diminished effectiveness as *curative therapy* if there is microscopically documented evidence of cancer beyond the borders of the surgically removed specimen. When such involvement is present, the surgical specimen is said to exhibit "positive surgical margins."

Lymph node sampling, when appropriate, is done early in the RP procedure. If evidence that the cancer has spread to the lymph nodes is detected, then the surgical removal of the prostate is often aborted in favor of other treatment options because the procedure is not considered curative. However, convincing studies from the Mayo Clinic have shown that despite lymph node involvement by PC, patients undergoing radical prostatectomy who have diploid (normal DNA) prostate cancer do exceptionally well with androgen deprivation therapy (ADT). In such patients, removing the prostate despite the presence of lymph node involvement by PC affords significant survival benefit.[45] Another report from Duke University also showed that RP resulted in a significant survival advantage when no more than two lymph nodes removed at RP showed

72

PC involvement.[46] *If you want to know more about the Duke Study, refer to Appendix B, Section 4.1.*

Pathological Examination

RP permits the most comprehensive understanding of the biology of the PC process since the surgical specimen is subjected to a full pathological examination that includes the removed prostate, seminal vesicles and sampled lymph nodes. Obviously, RP does not give a full representation of the extent of the disease, i.e. the absence or presence of *distant* metastases. In contrast to the RP specimen, biopsies obtained at the time of diagnosis represent only tiny core samples of the prostate (Fig. 31).

Pathology material obtained at the time of RP is also subject to more accurate analysis of the Gleason score. Prostate

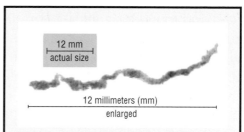

Figure 31: Core Biopsy From Patient with PC. This is the appearance of a single prostate core biopsy specimen, 12 millimeters in length, after staining of the tissue with hematoxylin and eosin (H&E). Traditionally, six such specimens have been obtained for diagnostic and prognostic purposes. Currently, newer biopsy techniques utilize an 11-13 core specimen approach. Slide courtesy of Junqi Qian.

cancer tissue from the RP specimen can also be used to assess ploidy, microvessel density, and the presence of tumor-promoting oncogenes such as mutated p53, bcl-2, and HER-2/*neu* and of tumor suppressor genes such as p21 and p27. **In a study by Bauer et al, over-expression of bcl-2 in the RP specimen was associated with a more than two-fold increase in the 5-year failure rate (67.0% versus 30.7%).** The same was also true for mutated p53 expression in the RP specimen with a failure rate at 5 years of 51.1% if p53 was expressed versus 22% in p53

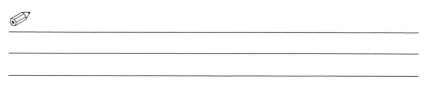

negative patients. If both bcl-2 and p53 were expressed in the RP specimen, the 5-year failure rate rose to 75.3% compared to 20.4% when neither oncogene was expressed.[47]

Some laboratories (Bostwick and Dianon Laboratories) are also performing such studies using the diagnostic biopsy material. Special immunologic studies (immunostaining) are done on the tumor samples from the retained tissue blocks (not the glass slides) assuming there is a sufficient quantity of tumor to permit this. One study evaluated the diagnostic biopsy slides for bcl-2 and found a significant correlation between bcl-2 expression and a more advanced clinical stage (T stage). This would suggest that bcl-2 expression in the diagnostic biopsy might be of help in discriminating locally advanced PC from organ-confined PC.[48] These special pathologic investigations are presently not considered routine studies, and most insurance companies do not now cover the costs for these tests. However, the findings of such studies could preclude unnecessary surgery, an important factor particularly for older men. *If you want to know more about Special Pathology Studies, refer to Appendix B, Section 4.2.*

Debulking the Tumor

From a cancer standpoint, RP quickly debulks a significant amount of tumor. This conceivably may restore immunologic balance between the patient and any residual tumor. Moreover, the prostate cancer within the gland itself represents the oldest portion of the tumor cell population and thus the portion of the tumor at high risk for mutation to a more resistant cell type. Therefore, surgical removal of potentially androgen-independent prostate cancer (AIPC) may have important long-term benefits. Lastly, the removal of the prostate by RP significantly diminishes or eliminates the concern for local spread of the disease to the bladder and/or rectum. Local extension of PC to these sites, if it should occur, would seriously degrade the quality and quantity of life of the patient.

Addressing Lower Urinary Tract Symptoms

These very important benefits of RP mentioned above should not be ignored. Furthermore, it is also important to emphasize that RP is an excellent local therapy option for PC patients presenting with lower urinary tract symptoms (LUTS) such as difficulty in starting urination, slowness of the urinary stream, incomplete emptying of the bladder, frequency of urination, and getting up at night to urinate. If LUTS are present at a moderate to severe degree, radiation therapy (RT) will cause a further increase in these symptoms adversely affecting the patient's quality of life. In contrast, RP removes the prostatic urethra—the portion of the urethra going through the prostate (see Figs. 9 and 14)—and establishes a connection or anastomosis between the bladder neck and penile urethra, providing the patient with a new urinary channel and dramatically improving urinary flow. An objective measurement of LUTS involves the use of the American Urological Association (AUA) Symptom Score. This is an important baseline input that should be part of any treatment strategy involving the decision on whether to choose RT or RP. (See Appendix F, pages F14–15, for an AUA Symptom Score form for you to complete.)

Risk of Impotence

On the downside, a major drawback to RP is that it may result in impotence. The need to eliminate all of the cancer means that it may also be necessary to sacrifice the nerves that control erection, thereby resulting in impotence (Fig. 32). The neurovascular bundles, composed of nerves and vessels that control erection, travel closely around the prostate gland on their way to the penis.[49,50]

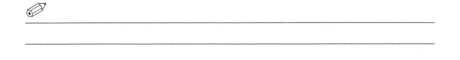

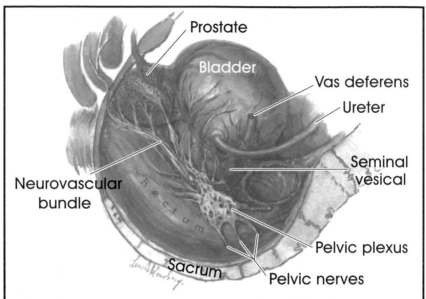

Figure 32: Neurovascular Bundle (NVB) and its Anatomic Relations. *In this view of a hypothetical patient lying on his back with his left side facing you, the pelvic contents (rectum, bladder and prostate) are seen lying within the curve of the sacrum. The NVB is formed by the capsular veins and arteries of the prostate along with the cavernous nerves that are derived from branches of the pelvic plexus. The cavernous nerves supply the penis and are essential for unassisted erectile ability. Art work reproduced with kind permission from Lippincott Williams and Wilkins from Schlegel PN and Walsh PC: Neuro-anatomical approach to radical cystoprostatectomy with preservation of sexual function. J Urol 138:1402-1406, 1987. This graphical presentation (Fig. 1, page 1403) has been modified from its orginal rendering by Leon Schlossberg.*

A surgical procedure called "nerve-sparing radical prostatectomy" can, in selected cases, permit removal of the cancer without the need to sacrifice either one or both of the neurovascular bundles. Moreover, a few hospitals are now using a new nerve grafting procedure performed at the time of the RP. Using a small section of the sural nerve taken from near the patient's ankle, a bridge is created to replace the section of the cavernous nerve removed during the RP.[51] This procedure of nerve grafting is only considered when nerve sparing is not possible and usually when both neurovascular bundles are sacrificed at the time of RP. It is important to emphasize, however, that Pat Walsh, M.D., the pioneer of the nerve-sparing RP, has raised significant issues about the necessity of nerve grafting. ***If you want to know more about Nerve Grafting, refer to Appendix B, Section 4.3.***

Unfortunately, the appropriateness of performing a nerve-sparing RP cannot be determined with certainty prior to the RP. In addition, sural nerve grafting is in its infancy and requires exceptional surgical skills. Moreover, many physicians and many patients believe that the focus of the radical prostatectomy is to remove all the cancer and not be preoccupied with erectile ability. This entire issue is made more complicated because of the wide variation in skill levels among urologists attempting to perform a radical prostatectomy, nerve-sparing or not.

Those physicians who have published their results with a nerve-sparing RP indicate that more men are able to achieve erections unassisted, or with the use of Viagra® or other similar drugs if bilateral nerve-sparing or unilateral nerve-sparing operations are performed. As shown in Table 3, 71% of men having a bilateral nerve-sparing RP were able to have vaginal intercourse with the use of Viagra versus 50% of men having a unilateral nerve-sparing RP. Of the men who had no nerve-sparing performed at RP, 15.4% were reported to achieve erections with Viagra.[52] In other reports, the overall probability of regaining erectile ability with Viagra after radical prostatectomy was 80% if the patient was 55 years of age or younger and had undergone bilateral nerve-sparing,[53] if he had no erectile diffi-

Table 3: Restoration of Potency with Viagra (50-100 mg dose) in Men Post-RP in Relation to Extent of Nerve-Sparing. Modified after Zippe et al. [52]	
Type of RP	**Erectile potency with Viagra**
Bilateral nerve-sparing RP	71%
Unilateral nerve-sparing RP	50%
No nerve-sparing	15%

culties prior to surgery and if he was sexually active before surgery. The response to Viagra also appears to be dependent upon the time interval between RP and when Viagra is first used. In the study by Zagaja et al, no patient who eventually responded to Viagra did so before 9 months after RP.[53] In a report by Hong et al, treatment satisfaction rate with Viagra was 26% at 6 months after RP but improved to 60% between 18 to 24 months post-RP.[54] Early nonresponders to Viagra should not be discouraged and should continue attempts at its use—perhaps also trying combinations of therapies to restore erectile ability.**

If Viagra or other pharmacologically similar oral medications do not work and/or if both nerves responsible for conducting the impulses resulting in erections have been removed, additional options include:

- Use of a vacuum erection device (VED), which manually draws blood into the penis resulting in an erection. Other terms for this equipment are: vacuum constriction device (VCD), external negative pressure device, and vacuum tumescence device.
- Application to the surface of the penis of medication (usually prostaglandin E_1) that stimulates erection.
- Insertion of a urethral pellet that contains prostaglandin E_1, e.g. Muse®.
- Combination therapy with Muse® and oral erectile agents.
- Injection of a single drug or combinations of drugs into the penis (again, not as bad as it sounds and favored by many over other options); such agents include Papaverine, Phentolamine and prostaglandin E_1.
- A penile implant that is surgically inserted into the shaft of the penis.

***

** *Viagra® and similar medications such as Levitra® or Cialis® can result in significant hypotension if taken within 24 hours of the administration of nitroglycerine (NTG) or other organic nitrate compounds. Moreover, the safe co-administration of any of these compounds with alpha-receptor blocker medications such as Cardura® (doxazosin) or Hytrin® (terazosin) remains controversial in the medical literature. Discussion with your physician regarding such use is strongly advised. Medications such as Nizoral® (ketoconazole) will raise the blood levels of any of these agents significantly. It is highly recommended that patients read the respective package inserts before using any of these agents.*

Two excellent resources authored by prostate cancer survivors that discuss sexual issues involved in PC are the books by Ralph and Barbara Alterowitz and by Aubrey Pilgrim. The full references are in Appendix A, sections IIB and VIIIB.

Penile Shrinkage

A side-effect of RP that occurs commonly but is frequently not discussed with patients preoperatively is that of penile shrinkage. This may be a form of atrophy due to scar tissue formation, or it may be caused by the shortening of the urethra since the prostatic urethra is removed as part of the RP procedure. In a study by Munding et al, 22 of 31 (71%) of the patients had a decrease in penile length that ranged from 0.5 cm to 4.0 cm at three months after RP. The shortening of penile length of 15 of these patients (48%) was greater than 1.0 cm.[55]

Whatever the cause, this becomes permanent at approximately six to eight months after the RP is performed. Exercising the penis daily or every other day to stimulate erections as soon as **79** your doctor will allow and using oral agents such as Viagra®, Levitra® or Cialis®, prostagandin E_1 (PGE_1) injections e.g. Edex® and Caverject®, or a VED can help keep the scar tissue elastic.[56,57] If one or both nerves were spared at the time of surgery and there is hope that natural erections will return, it is wise to continue this exercise at least several times a week to stimulate the blood flow to the penis and reduce the effects of penile atrophy. This approach is in keeping with our knowledge about the body and brain: "use it or lose it."

Dry Orgasms

RP, RT and Cryosurgery, as performed in the overwhelming majority of patients, effectively destroys the glandular tissue of the prostate. After RP, there is no ejaculate because the prostate and seminal vesicles removed at the time of RP no longer make the significant contribution to the liquid component of the

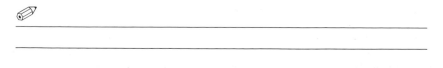

ejaculate. In addition, the ducts (ductus deferens) that carry the sperm to join the seminal vesicles are ligated (tied off with sutures) and thus this contribution to the ejaculate is also lost. Therefore, orgasms that are experienced, either with or without erections, are essentially without ejaculate—they are dry orgasms. It is important to note, that although a man who has undergone prostate cancer treatment may never before in his life have experienced the phenomenon of having an orgasm without an erection, this is entirely possible if stimulation is continued despite the loss or partial loss of the erection. Although this is not ideal, it can provide a level of intimacy that non-orgasmic sexual encounters may lack. Couples need to be aware of this often overlooked aspect of human sexuality as they strive to regain the ability to have unassisted intercourse or intercourse involving erection and penetration using one of the many means available to help stimulate erections, including the simplest: oral sex. Some men do report a small amount of ejaculate after RP that apparently is related to production of fluid from the small sex accessory tissues called the Cowper's glands (see Figs. 8 and 9). The change in ejaculate volume is immediate with RP. With RT, there is a decreasing amount of ejaculate over time because the effects of RT develop over many months, even though the formal treatments have ended. Frequently, these issues are not candidly discussed with the patient prior to or after either RP or RT.

Incontinence

Incontinence is caused by surgical damage to the muscles that control urination. Urinary incontinence may be temporary or permanent. In general, younger patients recover full continence faster, while older patients need to be just that—patient. Stress incontinence, which is characterized by releasing urine involuntarily while lifting, coughing or sneezing, can be a lingering side-effect. In general, incontinence as a result of RP is

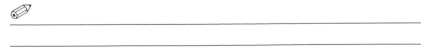

related to the skill of the urologist doing the surgery. In the hands of a talented urologist, permanent incontinence of significant degree resulting from a RP is uncommon (typically less than 2%). During RP, if the primary valve or sphincter situated above the prostate at the bladder neck is injured and incontinence occurs post RP, the use of Kegel exercises (Kegels) can be used to train the secondary valve (sphincter) below the prostate. Other options to regain continence reported to have a durable response include: drug therapies, physical therapy, and biofeedback. If these measures are unsuccessful, surgical implantation of an artificial urinary sphincter or AUS may be performed.[58-62] Another relatively new surgical approach to incontinence involves the urethral sling procedure.[63-65]

Despite maintaining or regaining full continence at all other times, some post-RP patients inevitably leak urine during sexual arousal. Anecdotal evidence seems to indicate that this phenomenon is commonly experienced after RP. This is caused by damage during RP to the primary valve. During erection, normally the primary valve is closed and the secondary value opens to allow flow of the ejaculate via the ejaculatory ducts into the prostatic urethra and out the penis. Kegel exercises, while helping the secondary valve to prevent urine loss during NON-erect states, has no efficacy during erectile states, since the relaxation of the secondary sphincter occurs and overwhelms any constrictive effect of a Kegel maneuver. This is an aspect of RP that doctors seldom discuss with their patients prior to surgery. Once this damage has been done, this is a side-effect that appears to be permanent and irreversible.

81

An excellent resource for those needing information on these topics is the National Association for Continence; their Web site address is www.nafc.org. (See Appendix A, section VIIIA.)

Anastomotic Stricture

After the prostate has been removed, the continuity of the urinary tract must be re-established. The connection or anastomosis between the urine outflow tract—where the bladder empties—with the remaining urethra represents a challenging part of the radical prostatectomy operation. If scar tissue forms at this site of connection, narrowing or stricture of the urethral channel occurs; this is called an anastomotic stricture. As a consequence, hindrance to urine flow occurs requiring medical intervention. This may involve the insertion of catheters of successively larger caliber to expand the urinary channel (dilation) or the need to surgically incise the scar tissue (transurethral incision) or more involved operations. In 868 patients undergoing a radical prostatectomy after 1990, 178 patients (20.5%) reported the need for dilation of the urethra after surgery.[66] Dilation of the urethral channel is the treatment of choice for anastomotic stricture but may be associated with a significant amount of urinary incontinence requiring the use of protective incontinence pads, special undergarments, or the use of urine collection systems. For example, in the study by Park et al, the need to wear protective incontinence pads at one year after RP was reported in 46.2% of the patients who developed an anastomotic stricture compared to 12.5% of patients undergoing RP who did not develop a stricture.[67] In the circumstances of high-volume urinary incontinence, some patients elect a corrective surgical approach such as the urethral sling procedure or the implantation of an artificial urinary sphincter.[68] *If you want to know more about Anastomotic Stricture, refer to Appendix B, Section 4.4.*

Salvage Therapies

In general, if an unfavorable outcome regarding cancer is encountered with local therapy such as RP or RT, there is usually some restorative treatment option or salvage therapy available. For example, following an RP, radiation treatment to the prostate bed can be used *if local recurrence is documented to be restricted to this area only.* Similarly, following local RT failure, salvage RP or salvage cryosurgery may be employed if the recurrence is confirmed to be local rather than systemic. Androgen deprivation therapy is another option for either local or systemic disease activity detected after any local therapy.

The success of a second treatment to control the cancer is significantly dependent upon findings that relate to the initial risk assessment insofar as the probability of organ-confined disease (OCD) at the time of initial local therapy and the meticulous re-evaluation of the patient if PSA recurrence is documented. It must be said, however, that the fewer the intrusions into the human body the better. Therefore, it is important on the first round of treatment to **properly select a treatment for the patient that is most appropriate to him, to prepare the patient for this therapy, and to always choose an artist to perform the procedure.**

83

Cryosurgery (Cryotherapy, Cryoablation)

Cryosurgery uses extremely cold temperatures to destroy PC tissue. This procedure is usually done under ultrasound guidance. Hollow needles (cryoprobes) are inserted through the perineum (the space between the scrotum and the anus) and liquid nitrogen or Argon gas is circulated within these probes to freeze the prostate (Figs. 33–35). Temperature probes (thermocouples) placed within and around the prostate are used to guide the ensuing cryoablation.

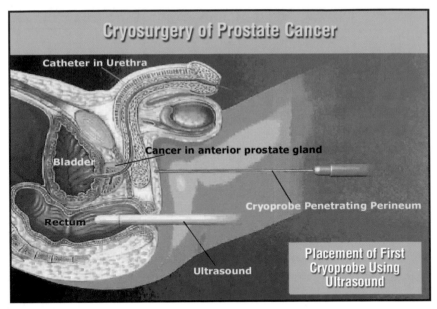

Figure 33: Cryosurgery Procedure. *Under either transrectal ultrasound, MRI or CT guidance, hollow tubes (cryoprobes) are placed in the prostate. Regional anesthesia is used. In these views, the patient is lying supine (on his back) with his legs*

84 *slightly elevated. This is done in the operating room of either a hospital or short-stay outpatient surgery center. Figures 33-35 modified from the January 1999 issue of PCRI* Insights. *Reproduced with permission from Douglas Chinn, M.D.*

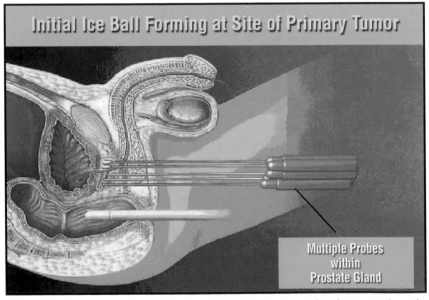

Figure 34: Cryosurgery: Creation of an Ice Ball. *Five cryoprobes have now been introduced. An ice ball is growing around two of the probes involving the anterior portion of the prostate gland.*

The extremely cold temperatures that are achieved create multiple ice balls centered around the probe tips. An ice ball destroys areas of the prostate involved with cancer as well as any normal prostatic tissue within the ice ball (Fig. 35). A "double freeze" is done; i.e. the gland is frozen and then thawed and the process is repeated to ensure adequate destruction or ablation of the gland.

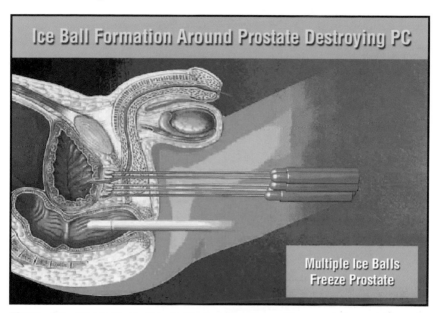

Ice Ball Formation Around Prostate Destroying PC

Multiple Ice Balls Freeze Prostate

Figure 35: Cryosurgery. *Ice balls involve the entire prostate and capsule. Thermocouples are implanted in the prostate to monitor the temperature.*

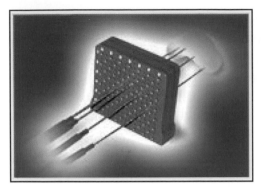

Figure 36: Template Used in Cryosurgery. *Cryoprobes are seen going through specific holes in the template. This approach has been adopted recently by a few cryosurgical companies. The concept makes sense in that the template is specifically created for the individual patient based on anatomical imaging of the prostate.*

Reproduced with permission of Galil Medical (http://www.galilmedical.com/).

Cryosurgery is being used as a salvage procedure after external beam RT (EBRT) and/or brachytherapy in circumstances of recurrent cancer. However, it also is a reasonable primary therapy for organ-confined PC or for prostate cancer with only minimal disease extension outside the prostate.

Recent technical modifications in cryosurgery have involved: (a) the use of MRI of the prostate gland and adjoining tissues to monitor the procedure, (b) the use of Argon gas as a coolant, and (c) the use of a template (Fig. 36), similar to that used in brachytherapy, to guide the cryoprobes. Whether such alterations in procedure will prove beneficial await further clinical experience involving significant numbers of patients.

Some cryosurgeons are performing limited cryosurgery, thereby preserving part of the prostate and neurovascular bundle(s) if extensive biopsies of the gland reveal minimal tumor volume confined to one area of the prostate. This approach is new, and follow-up studies are needed to determine its efficacy. These variations in cryosurgical technique demonstrate that treatments evolve through various stages that often render them potentially more useful to the uniqueness of each patient's situation.

Cryosurgery Centers

There are several centers in the U.S. where cryosurgery is performed. State of the art cryosurgery, as it is presently being performed, usually damages or destroys the neurovascular bundles involved in erection. Men undergoing definitive cryosurgery should be made aware that impotence is a routine occurrence with this therapy but that the use of oral agents like Viagra®, Levitra® or Cialis® and/or injections of prostaglandin (PGE₁) into the penis helps to restore potency in such patients. The July 1999 issue of the PCRI newsletter *Insights* has a review article on cryosurgery written by Douglas Chinn, M.D. Cryosurgery mandates the choice of an artist, as do all treatments for PC.

The premier cryosurgeons that we have identified so far include: Fred Lee in Rochester, Michigan; Duke Bahn in Ventura, California; Gary Onik in Celebration, Florida; Jeffrey Cohen in Pittsburgh, Pennsylvania; Doug Chinn in Arcadia, California; Aaron Katz, Carl Olsson, and Chris Johnson in New York City, New York; and John Long in Boston, Massachusetts.

Although early papers on cryosurgery of the prostate date back to 1970, this field has evolved through many changes with advances such as the transrectal ultrasound to guide the cryoprobes and protection of the urethra from cold (thermal) injury. The latter is accomplished with the use of an indwelling catheter through which warm saline is circulated to act as a urethral warmer. Moreover, monitoring of the temperatures achieved with thermocouples and achieving temperatures of -40°C or less, along with the use of six to eight cryoprobes per procedure and the use of multiple freeze-thaw cycles (two to three) has increased the ability to optimally cryoablate prostatic tissue. These variations on the technique of cryosurgery, which vary from cryosurgeon to cryosurgeon, have made evaluation of the cryosurgical literature problematical. This same reality, however, is inherent throughout much of medicine, including most aspects of prostate cancer evaluation and management.

87

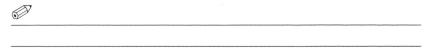

Cryosurgery Results

A multi-institutional retrospective study of 975 patients who were treated with cryosurgery as their initial therapy between 1993 and 1998 was reported by Long et al.[69] The authors pointed out that only a small number of patients were treated with all of the enhancements cited in the previous paragraph. This paper was submitted for publication in May of 2000 and the median follow-up on all patients at the time of publication was only 24 months. Patients were stratified into low-risk, medium and high-risk categories. In the 238 patients defined as low-risk by virtue of a baseline PSA 10 ng/ml or less, a Gleason score of less than 7 and a clinical stage of T2a or less, the actuarial five-year disease-free rate was 76%, using the criterion of a PSA of less than 1.0 as an endpoint.

The medium-risk patient group was defined as patients with any one of the following features: PSA greater than 10 ng/ml, Gleason score 7 or greater, or a clinical stage T2b or greater.

Patients in the high-risk group were defined as those having two or all three of the above features at the time of the procedure. These results, which are shown in Table 4, are compared with results published from well-respected radiation oncologists using external beam RT or permanent seed implants. The choice of the cited literature for comparison was made by Long et al.[69]

Table 4: Pooled Analysis of Cancer-Related Outcomes After Cryosurgery versus Comparable Groups Treated by 3D Conformal RT (3DCRT) and Seed Implantation (SI). Modified after Long et al.[69]			
Treatment Group	**5-Year Biochemical Disease-Free Rate (%)***		
	3D CRT [70]	**SI [71,72]**	**Cryo [69]**
Low-risk T1-2, PSA ≤ 10, GS < 7	85%	87%	76%
Medium-risk > T2, PSA > 10, GS > 6 (1 feature)	65%	32%	71%
High-risk > T2, PSA > 10, GS > 6 (2–3 of above features)	35%	No comparable data given	45%

* PSA criteria = less than1.0 ng/ml

The findings of Table 4 emphasize the importance of comparing patient groups with similar risk factors as indicated by the "Treatment Group" definitions. However, it is important to state that an actuarial analysis is not a substitute for actual follow-up over many years duration. It is hoped that Long et al will submit a four-year follow-up study to see if there has been any deterioration in the early results obtained with cryosurgery.

Of seven patients referred by Dr. Strum for cryosurgery in the early 90s, six have had evidence of stable PSA levels with 10 years of follow-up. Some of these patients presented with PSA levels greater than 10 and also with other adverse risk factors. All of these patients were treated with androgen deprivation therapy for up to six months before cryosurgery. The clinical story of one of these patients is presented in Physician's Note 13.

Physician's Note 13:

"Case Report of Long-Term Response to Cryosurgery." The patient above elected cryosurgery at a time when clinical trials were just beginning. He had extensively reviewed the medical literature regarding his treatment options and elected this treatment. He has done extremely well over the ensuing decade and has had no problems with incontinence.

At the age of 58, RJP was diagnosed with PC. His baseline PSA was 7.7, GS was (3,3) and clinical stage T2c. He was not sure of what treatment he wanted and elected to start ADT2 with Flutamide followed by Lupron one week later; this was begun on 5/14/91. ADT was stopped after 5 months at which time RJP elected to undergo cryosurgery in Pittsburgh with Dr. Jeffrey Cohen. The cryo procedure was done on 2/5/92 on an outpatient basis and totally without complications. At two years and eight months after cryosurgery, repeat biopsies involving six cores were negative for PC. The PSA has remained stable at approximately 1.5 with minor fluctuations for the last 10 years. RJP had no incontinence and all studies to evaluate disease have shown no evidence of PC recurrence.

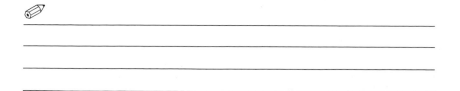

Radiation Therapy (RT)

Radiation therapy (RT) is an area of PC management that is complicated, even for a significant number of physicians intensely involved in treating PC patients. Therefore, it is understandable that most patients are confused about whether to select RT as primary therapy and if so, how to decide which of the many available types of RT to select. This confusion can be lessened and understanding will be enhanced if we take into account the rapid and momentous changes in technology and in our understanding of tumor biology that have occurred over the last 15 years.

First, it is important to realize that it is *radical prostatectomy* that has historically been the primary treatment for PC. RP is the oldest form of therapy for this disease. Urologists are the specialists who see most of the PC patients after diagnosis and therefore it is not surprising that RP has traditionally been by far the most widely used PC therapy. RT, on the other hand, has traditionally been a "second choice" therapy utilized for patients too old or too ill to undergo RP or for patients with obviously advanced PC who would not fare well with RP as initial therapy. Thus, the data defining the success rates of RT has been more limited than that of RP.

Moreover, during the last 15 years, the widespread use of PSA testing has led to earlier and earlier diagnoses of PC so that less advanced stages of PC are detected at the initial diagnosis. This *stage migration*, as it has been called,[73] has now resulted in the majority of patients in the United States having no palpable disease detected by DRE at the time of diagnosis, i.e. clinical stage T1c disease. (See Appendix G for descriptions and illustrations of the clinical stages of PC.)

Advances in RT

Within the same time frame as mentioned above, the technical aspects of RT have dramatically changed from standard or so-called "conventional" RT to highly advanced approaches directed at delivering higher amounts of RT to the appropriate targets (the prostate gland and an appropriate margin of tissue surrounding the gland) while at the same time sparing the nearby normal tissues of the rectum and the bladder. Since these normal tissues surrounding the prostate are also sensitive to these higher doses of RT, the *normal tissue complication probability* (NTCP) needed to be taken into consideration as this new technology developed.

Ironically, then, as more and more patients were diagnosed with lower clinical stage PC, and hence presented a smaller tumor burden, multiple publications in the medical literature pointed out the importance of higher and higher doses of RT necessary to heighten *tumor control probability* (TCP). This has led, in our opinion, to a situation where an entire industry has been focused on delivering higher and higher amounts of RT with rapidly evolving technological advances intended to optimize the ratio of TCP to NTCP while the presentation of patients has gone from that of a diagnosis with bulky tumor to one with non-palpable disease (T1c) as a result of the use of the PSA blood test.

With the above kept in mind, it is only to be expected that a reading of the RT literature on PC would be challenging, to say the least. Adding to this complexity are the variations on the theme of individual radiation oncologists and institutions, using different equipment, different doses, different selection criteria for treatment and different criteria for definition of success or failure of treatment. Many of these same factors complicate discussions of any aspect of the primary treatment of PC.

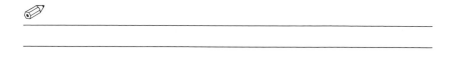

As a result, external beam radiation therapy (EBRT) that has been termed "conventional RT" has largely, but not totally, been replaced in the United States by one of the more technically advanced forms of EBRT, which are listed below. Conventional EBRT usually utilizes four treatment fields (anterior, posterior, and both lateral or side fields or ports), decides on a RT dose and then constructs lead blocks to shield tissues or structures that need to be avoided. Modern EBRT uses more technically advanced approaches to ensure that the radiation beams conform to the targeted tissues and not the nearby normal tissues such as the rectum and the bladder. The EBRT discussion that follows the brachytherapy discussion is therefore limited to just the newer forms of EBRT.

Overview

The goal of radiation therapy (RT) is the destruction of the cellular components of the target tissue by means of ionizing particles of energy. There are many forms of RT. These include:

- **Brachytherapy**
  - ○ Permanent seed implants using:
    - Iodine-125 isotope
    - Palladium-103 isotope
  - ○ Temporary wire implants called High Dose Rate (HDR) brachytherapy using Iridium-192 isotope

- **External Beam Radiation Therapy (EBRT)** which may be:
  - ○ "Conventional" RT
  - ○ 3D Conformal RT (3DCRT)
  - ○ Intensity Modulated RT (IMRT)
  - ○ Proton Beam RT (PBRT)
  - ○ Neutron Beam RT

In addition to all of the above, there are numerous combinations that couple a brachytherapy approach with one of the various types of EBRT that are in use as of 2002. These most commonly involve the use of either permanent seeds or HDR implants combined with either 3DCRT or IMRT.

Brachytherapy

The word "brachytherapy" comes from the Greek words "brachy" meaning "close by" (in this instance, referring to a radioactive source applied in or near the tumor) and "therapia", for therapy. Brachytherapy may be delivered in the form of *permanent* radioactive *seed* implants (traditional brachytherapy) or via the use of *temporary* radioactive wire implants (High Dose Rate or HDR brachytherapy).

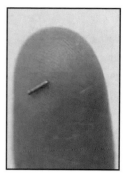

Figure 37: Seed used for implantation in comparison with the tip of the index finger. *The number of seeds implanted varies from 30-50 to as many as 150. This is dependent on the size of the prostate gland and the isotope used.*

Treatment by permanent seed implantation (SI) involves the introduction of radioactive seeds into the prostate gland. The seeds consist of radioactive material encased in a titanium shell smaller than a grain of rice. The radioactive material or isotope releases ionizing particles through the process of radioactive decay. This decay may either be relatively long, due to a longer half-life of the particular radiation particle, or it may be more rapid due to a shorter half-life of the isotopic particle. The two isotopes currently in use for permanent seed implants are iodine, with a half-life of two months, and palladium, with a half-life of two weeks. Your doctor will help make the determination as to which is most appropriate for your cancer and will calculate how many seeds are needed to adequately treat the size of your prostate gland. The smaller the gland size, the fewer the seeds needed to adequately treat the entire gland. An actual seed used in implantation is shown in Figure 37.

Technique of Seed Placement

This is usually "day surgery" or done as an outpatient procedure so it normally does not require an overnight hospital stay. Some doctors place seeds in areas outside the prostate such as the pericapsular tissue or the seminal vesicles if these areas are considered to be at risk for cancer spread. Frequently, external beam radiation therapy (EBRT) is used in addition to seeding to kill cancer thought to have escaped through the capsule but believed to be still contained within the pelvic area close to the prostate.

The seeds are inserted through hollow needles, under anesthesia, through the perineum (the space between the scrotum and the anus). Figure 38 shows a side view of the template through which many needles are guided into the prostate. The

94

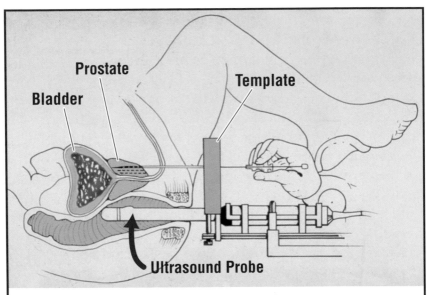

Figure 38: Seed Insertion into Prostate. *With the patient in a supine position, tiny hollow tubes or catheters are guided into the prostate via a template (see Fig. 36). The holes in the template have been specifically chosen for the patient, and they channel the catheters into the prostate or other target sites. Radioactive Iodine or Palladium seeds are pushed through these tubes to the desired location.*

patient is shown lying on his back. The rod within the rectum is the transrectal ultrasound probe (red arrow) that enables visualization of the prostate.

A major disadvantage of any form of radiation treatment (RT) is the inability to review pathologic material in order to microscopically determine whether the cancer has spread beyond the capsule to an area that the radiation cannot reach. *Optimal testing **prior** to the RT procedure is therefore very important.* **In addition, and most importantly, patients considering brachytherapy in any form, radical prostatectomy or cryosurgery need to refer to the Partin and Narayan Tables, Bluestein predictions and other predictive algorithms described in Chapter 3 to obtain a sense of risk for extracapsular extension as well as lymph node involvement.** A PAP should also be obtained for reasons cited in the PAP discussion in Chapter 3.

The Partin Tables

The Partin Tables were compiled by analyzing thousands of pathology specimens removed at the time of radical prostatectomy to determine the probability of organ-confined disease, capsular penetration, seminal vesicle and lymph node involvement. The Partin Tables (see Appendix C) are also available on the Internet and are part of a computer software application (Prostate Cancer Tools II) located on the PCRI Web site at www.prostate-cancer.org or www.pcri.org. PC Tools II is an

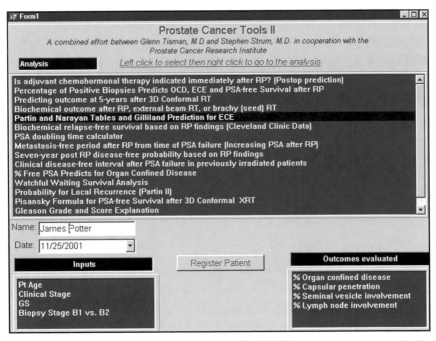

Figure 39: The Main Menu of Prostate Cancer Tools II. The computer user selects the analytical program of choice (in this case the Partin, Narayan and Gilliland analyses) and right clicks the mouse to open the desired program. The "Inputs" used in these analyses and the "Outcomes evaluated" are shown in the lower left and right, respectively.

analytical software suite based on peer-reviewed medical publications that analyze a patient's specific situation in regard to the extent of disease and prognosis with various treatment options, including surgery, external beam radiation therapy, seed implantation and combinations of the above, with and without androgen deprivation therapy (ADT). Figures 39-41 are computer screen shots using Prostate Cancer Tools II. These show how a user can apply Partin Table data to his case.

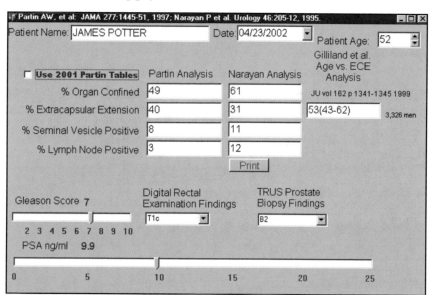

Partin AW, et al: JAMA 277:1445-51, 1997; Narayan P et al. Urology 46:205-12, 1995. _ □ X

Patient Name: JAMES POTTER	Date: 04/23/2002 ▾	Patient Age: 52

☐ Use 2001 Partin Tables	Partin Analysis	Narayan Analysis	Gilliland et al. Age vs. ECE Analysis
% Organ Confined	49	61	JU vol 162 p 1341-1345 1999
% Extracapsular Extension	40	31	53(43-62) 3,326 men
% Seminal Vesicle Positive	8	11	
% Lymph Node Positive	3	12	

Print

Gleason Score 7

2 3 4 5 6 7 8 9 10

PSA ng/ml 9.9

Digital Rectal Examination Findings T1c ▾

TRUS Prostate Biopsy Findings B2 ▾

0   5   10   15   20   25

Figure 40: The Partin, Narayan and Gilliland Analyses. _In this hypothetical example, James Potter, age 52, presents with a PSA of 9.9, validated Gleason score of 7, a T1c clinical stage and pathologic evidence of disease from both the right and left lobes ("B2" stage per Narayan[74]). His probabilities for disease found at RP based on the 1997 Partin and Narayan analyses are shown. Note that the "Use 2001 Partin Tables" has not been checked off. (See Fig. 41.)_

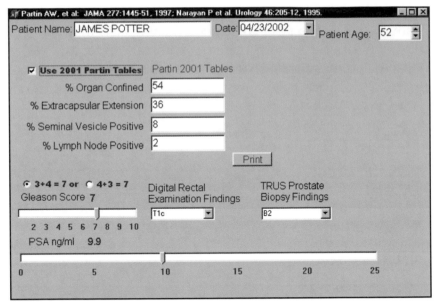

Figure 41: The 2001 Partin Tables. Clicking on the box for the 2001 Tables yields this modification of the Partin data. Note that the Gleason score of "7" can now be entered as either a (3,4) or a (4,3). These table shots can be printed or saved as a graphic file and should be a routine part of the patient's medical records. SnagIt 7.1.2 is a software program that can be used to capture computer monitor images and print them or save them to file. Information about this software is available at *http://www.techsmith.com*.

Potential Bowel and Urinary Problems

Treatment by seed implantation can result in bowel problems (*radiation proctitis*) and urinary problems (*radiation urethritis and/or cystitis*). Such problems are usually temporary and can be alleviated with medication and/or the passage of time. The biologic explanation of these problems is related to the anatomy of the prostate and its intimate association with the urethra, and the prostate's proximity to the bladder and to the anterior rectal wall (see Fig. 9).

As the urethra leaves the bladder, it traverses the prostate gland. The release of radioactivity from the implanted seeds or wires within the prostate causes the prostatic tissue to swell.

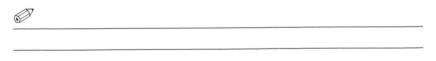

This compresses the urethra and can cause varying degrees of obstruction to urine flow. The urethral lining cells may also undergo swelling in response to radiation. In severe cases, a catheter may need to be inserted through the penis into the bladder to overcome obstructive difficulties in urination that arise as a result of brachytherapy, or for that matter, from any other type of therapy causing the same problem. Self-catheterization kits are available for home use if urinary retention problems persist for an extended period of time. **The selection of the treatment appropriate to the patient, the preparation of the patient, and the skill of the brachytherapist are paramount to the success of the procedure and in minimizing the frequency and severity of side-effects.** *If you want to know more about protection against radiation-induced side-effects, refer to Appendix B, Section 4.5.*

Additionally, the prostate gland volume is an important issue to consider in preventing radiation-induced side-effects. Patients with prostate gland volumes exceeding 35-40 cubic centimeters (cc) may experience more radiation injury to the rectum and to the bladder due to radiation scatter because of the larger area that needs to be radiated. In addition, more seeds are used for larger gland volumes and this too may increase the risk of radiation side-effects as well as increasing the cost of the procedure.

Brachytherapy has the theoretical advantage of being inherently nerve-sparing, which means that Viagra, or new medications that act similarly, will produce erections in approximately 75% of patients.[75-78] However, the incidence of at least partial impotence seems higher than usually disclosed, especially in patients 70 and older. Longer-term follow-up of patients having brachytherapy will clarify the true effect of brachytherapy on erectile function.

Brachytherapy, with either permanent seeds or temporary wires, is often used in combination with other treatments such

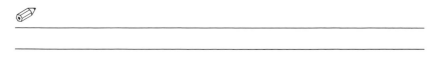

as androgen deprivation therapy and/or external beam radiation therapy. The selection of these combination therapies is theoretically tailored to the individual patient and depends upon the size of his prostate, the prostate cancer volume, the presence of a dominant cancer lesion within the prostate, the location of the PC, the presence of urinary symptoms, and other risk factors. An analysis of the existing literature on brachytherapy is challenging even to physicians well-read in the PC literature. It is impossible to imagine how daunting this must be to the PC patient trying to decide what to do to cure or control his disease.

Survival Results

The findings of a brachytherapy study involving a large number of patients treated at the Radiotherapy Clinics of Georgia (RCOG) with a uniform approach and having a significant follow-up period was published by Critz et al in 2000.[79] This study involved 689 men treated with ultrasound-guided transperineal [125]iodine permanent seed implants followed three weeks later by external beam RT. The average follow-up of patients in this study was four years (range 3-7). *Disease-free status was defined by the authors as the achievement and maintenance of a PSA nadir of 0.2 ng/ml or less.* As shown in Figure 42, the 5-year disease-free survival (DFS) according to baseline PSA was 94% (± 7) for PSA 0-4 ng/ml, 93% (± 3) for PSA > 4-10, 75% (± 8) for PSA > 10-20 and 69% (± 14) for PSA levels > 20 ng/ml. **An important part of this analysis is depicting the "men at risk" during each year of the analysis (shown in the lower portion of Figure 42). At five years, only the patients in the PSA group > 4-10 had a significant number of men at risk (n=128). It will be important to get updates of this data from the authors to ensure that the data is holding up.**

A study employing seed implantation alone using [103]Palladium in 230 men with clinical stage T1-2 disease was reported by Blasko et al from the Seattle Prostate Institute in 2000.[80] The median follow-up in this trial was 48.9 months. *Biochemical failure was defined in this study as two consecutive rises in PSA after seed implantation completion.* A PSA nadir to a particular level was not considered a mandatory criterion for a successful outcome. The median PSA decreased over time *after* seed implantation from 1.4 at one year, to 0.9 at two years, 0.7

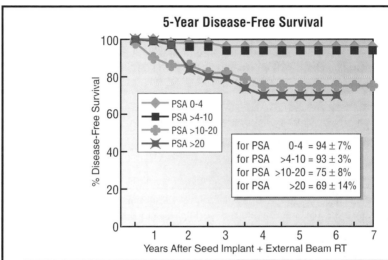

PSA Range	Men at Risk in Relation to Years After Seed Implant + External Beam RT							
	Years After SI + EBRT							
	0	1	2	3	4	5	6	7
PSA 0-4	50	50	48	46	29	12	6	1
PSA >4-10	451	447	422	401	243	128	61	13
PSA >10-20	144	142	124	103	60	31	17	3
PSA >20	44	43	37	32	20	9	4	—
Totals	689	682	651	582	352	180	88	17

Figure 42: Critz paper: Combined Seed Implantation (SI) + EBRT at RCOG. The importance of the baseline PSA in the outcome of combination SI + EBRT is shown. As the baseline PSA exceeds 10 ng/ml, the chance of PC confined to the field of radiation must be diminishing and/or the inability of the RT dose to eradicate too large a tumor volume must account for the decreasing biochemical disease-free survival as shown in the graph in the upper portion of this figure. In current times, patients diagnosed with PC have smaller tumor volumes, and coupled with technological advances in RT, would be expected to fare even better than those treated at the beginning of the time frame of this study. Modified after Critz et al.[79]

at three years, 0.5 at four years, and 0.2 at years 6-10. The percentage of patients achieving a PSA nadir of ≤ 0.5 ng/ml remained essentially constant from years 6-10 after seed implantation and was 75-78%. The 5-year biochemical progression-free rates with [103]Palladium implantation for pretreatment PSA levels of ≤ 4.0, > 4-10, > 10-20 and > 20 were 90%, 88%, 80%, and 67%, respectively. Although the end-points for defining success and the nature of the radiation employed in the Critz et al versus the Blasko et al studies were different, the results at five years are striking similar (Table 5). *If You Want to Know More about the Blasko et al study, see Appendix B, Section 4.6.*

PSA GROUP	RCOG (Critz et al)	Seattle (Blasko et al)
	5-Year Biochemical Disease-Free Survival (%)	
≤ 4-10	94	90
> 4-10	93	88
> 10-20	75	80
> 20	69	67

Table 5: Critz et al and Blasko et al 5-Year Biochemical Disease-Free Survival Comparisons.

This data contrasts the results of combination seed implantation using Iodine-125 + external beam RT (Critz et al) versus seed implantation alone using Palladium-103 (Blasko et al). These findings, reported from separate institutions, indicate a remarkable similarity in all ranges of pretreatment PSA groups despite differences in treatment strategy. Follow-up reports from these two centers will be very important.*

* **Definition of disease-free survival:**
  RCOG = achieve and maintain PSA nadir of ≤ 0.2 ng/ml
  Seattle = lack of two consecutive rises in PSA after seed implantation

PSA Bump

Approximately 35% of patients experience a temporary rise in PSA after first having a decline in PSA after completion of brachytherapy. This PSA "bump" or "bounce" has been defined as an increase of 0.1 ng/ml or greater above the preceding PSA level followed by a subsequent decrease below that level. The average time to PSA "bump" is 18-20 months. Figure 43 presents the basic information on PSA bump in the two largest studies published.

This phenomenon is believed to be the result of radiation-induced prostatitis and not due to PC. **A misdiagnosis of PSA**

Figure 43: PSA Bump Characteristics at the Seattle Prostate Institute (SPI) versus the Radiotherapy Clinics of Georgia (RCOG). These represent the two largest studies published on PSA Bump. The statistics from both groups are remarkably similar.

PSA Bump: SPI versus RCOG

Parameter	Seattle	Georgia
Patients Studied	534	779
Number with Bump	191 (35.8%)	273 (35%)
Median Follow-up	55.1 mos.	60 mos.
Type of Radiation	SI +/- EBRT	SI + EBRT
Definition of Bump	↓ and ↑ 0.2 or more	↓ and ↑ 0.1 or more
Time to Bump	20.4 mos. post Rx	18 mos. post SI

103

Figure 44: PSA Bump Statistics. Due to the variability in time to PSA bump, differences in both the lowest PSA reached prior to the "bump" and the peak PSA "bump" as well as occasionally prolonged "bump" durations, some type of differential testing is needed to differentiate "bump" from true PSA recurrence.

PSA Bump: SPI versus RCOG

Parameter	Seattle	Georgia
Longest time to PSA Bump	84 mos.	60 mos.
Pre-Bump PSA Nadir	0.5 median	0.7 (0.1–8.9)
PSA Bump Peak	1.1 median	0.4 median
PSA Bump Max (mos.)	16 (0.2–16)	15.8 (0.1–15.8)
PSA Bump Duration	a few mos. to 18 mos.	12 mos. or more in 36% / 18 mos. or more in 14%

recurrence and unnecessary treatment with ADT can be avoided if physicians and patients know that a rise in PSA after an initial drop in PSA following brachytherapy ± EBRT may not necessarily indicate a recurrence of the cancer, pending the timing of the PSA rise and the history of having received brachytherapy (Fig. 44).[81,82]

In both the Seattle Prostate Institute (SPI) and Radiotherapy Clinics of Georgia (RCOG) reports involving a combined total of 1,313 patients, the presence of a PSA bump was not correlated with an adverse outcome to seed implantation +/- external beam RT. On the contrary, when PSA bump was observed, progressive PC was seen in only 7% of the SPI patients and 10% of the RCOG patients. In contrast, in the absence of a PSA bump, progressive disease was about twice as common and seen in 14% of the SPI patients and 26% of the RCOG patients. Therefore, in these two studies, a better outcome after RT was associated with the occurrence of a PSA bump.

104

PSA bump (also called PSA bounce) has also been described in the setting of primary therapy with 3D Conformal RT (3DCRT), which did not involve the combined use of any type of brachytherapy. In the Fox Chase Cancer Center (FCCC) study, 95 of 306 (31%) patients treated only with 3DCRT experienced PSA bump.[83] However, the other conclusions from this study were significantly different from those of the SPI and RCOG. The median time after completion of RT to a PSA bump in the FCCC series was 35 months versus 20 and 18 months in the SPI and RCOG studies respectively. In the FCCC study, PSA bump had an adverse correlation in regard to freedom from PSA relapse. If PSA bump occurred, progressive PC was seen in 48% of patients (versus 7-10% in the other studies) whereas if it did not occur, progressive PC was seen in 31% of patients. *If you want to know more about PSA Bounce or Bump, refer to Appendix B, Section 4.7.*

"The PSA Bump Mimics PSA Recurrence." The PSA bump or bounce is an important differential diagnosis in men primarily treated with radiation therapy, especially brachytherapy. Understanding the characteristic features of the PSA bump may prevent a significant number of men from receiving unnecessary treatment for what appears to be PSA recurrence but actually is a PSA bump.

SB was 56 when he was diagnosed with PC. His baseline PSA was 9.3, his Gleason score read by an expert in PC pathology was (3,3), and his clinical stage was T2a. He had 1 of 9 cores positive for PC. An analysis of the Partin Tables indicated he had a 58% chance of organ-confined disease, a 37% chance of capsular penetration, a 4% chance of seminal vesicle involvement, and a 1% chance of lymph node involvement. He received three months of single agent Casodex followed by External Beam RT and then underwent permanent seed implantation in 6/98. His PSA dropped to 0.5 six months after seeding but then rose to 0.6 at 12 months and 1.3 at 17 months. At 19 months after seeding, a repeat PSA was down to 0.8 and his last PSA was 0.6 at 25.5 months after seed implantation.

Salvage Procedures: HDR, Cryosurgery, and Prostatectomy

In the setting of PSA recurrence after primary RT that indicates progressive PC, various treatment options can be discussed with the patient to determine which might be best suited to his particular circumstances. For example, High Dose Rate (HDR) temporary brachytherapy is now being used after permanent seed implant failure if recurrent disease is restricted to the confines of the gland or in the tissue surrounding the prostate.

Cryosurgery (freezing the prostate) is now being used by some as a salvage therapy after failure of primary radiation treatment. In a study by Ghafar et al, 38 men with recurrent PC after external beam RT underwent salvage cryosurgery. All men in the study had documented recurrent disease by virtue of a progressive PSA rise beyond that of the PSA nadir after RT, and a positive prostate biopsy showing PC. The response to

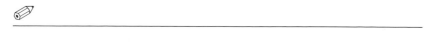

cryosurgery revealed a PSA nadir of ≤ 0.1 in 81.5% of the men treated. Biochemical recurrence-free survival was 86% at one year and 74% at two years. Complications reported included: rectal pain in 39.5%, urinary tract infection in 2.6%, incontinence in 7.9%, hematuria in 7.9%, and scrotal edema in 10.5%.[84]

In the setting of PC recurrence after primary RT, a salvage prostatectomy may be considered. This is not frequently performed because of the high incidence of severe complications. Many men prefer to avoid the increased risk of such complications and elect androgen deprivation therapy (ADT) or cryosurgery instead. The few publications on salvage prostatectomy that involve significant numbers of patients emanate from a handful of medical centers.[85,86] The common denominator in the successful outcome of patients subjected to this procedure is the finding of true organ-confined disease that was determined prior to RT and also confirmed to be still present prior to the salvage RP.

106

In one large series of 86 patients undergoing salvage prostatectomy from the Mayo Clinic in Rochester, Minnesota, the two most important prognostic factors obtained at the time of the salvage operation were the Gleason score and the ploidy status (DNA ploidy) of the tumor.[87] These findings correlated significantly with survival. In this series, no patients with a Gleason score of 6 or a diploid DNA died from PC. The mean follow-up after surgery was 5.8 years.

Local failure after permanent seeds or EBRT should not occur, however, if the patient has been properly selected and possibly prepared by first reducing both the gland volume and the tumor volume using ADT. It is also presumed that the radiation oncologist selected by the empowered patient is an artist with impeccable technique.

High Dose Rate (HDR) Brachytherapy

Unlike permanent seed implants, no "seeds" remain in the prostate after treatment using the HDR approach. This procedure usually involves an inpatient hospital stay of about two days. Tiny plastic catheters (hollow needles) measuring 1.9 millimeters in diameter are inserted into the prostate gland under transrectal ultrasound guidance using a template much like that used in permanent seed implants. Cystoscopy is performed to position the plastic needles just under the bladder mucosa to assure optimal coverage of the base of the prostate. The patient then undergoes a high-powered CT scan to aid in refining the position of the catheters within the prostate for a uniform distribution of radiation and to identify important anatomic landmarks such as the prostatic margin, rectum, bladder and urethra. **This post-implant CT scan is used as the basis for treatment planning after the needles are in place but before the radiation source is introduced into the needles or catheters.** Then, a computer-controlled machine pushes a radioactive iridium wire into the catheters one by one. The wires are left there for a few seconds, and then removed.

The computer controls the length of time a single wire remains in the catheter, thereby permitting precise dosages to different areas of the prostate and to sites clinically suspected to contain PC. Such sites can be treated with a higher dose of radiation while sparing healthy tissue and surrounding organs, thus minimizing bowel and bladder complications. Typically, HDR is multi-fractionated; that is, it is given in two to three separate treatments over a period of about forty hours. Review of the literature indicates HDR doses ranging from three fractions at 5.5 Gy for a total of 16.5 Gy to as much as two 15 Gy fractions for a total of 30 Gy.[88,89]

✐
_____

_____

_____

_____

_____

Patients report that urinary catheterization to relieve obstructive urinary symptoms is seldom necessary after HDR treatment. HDR is therefore a reasonable form of brachytherapy to use in patients requesting RT despite significant symptoms of obstructive urinary flow. HDR may be particularly indicated in those patients desiring seed implantation who clinically appear to have dominant PC lesions located in the apical region of the prostate. Due to the proximity of the urethra in the apex of the prostate (Fig. 14, Chapter 3), permanent seed implantation is more often associated with urinary obstructive symptoms, whereas the more precise targeting of HDR results in a relative radiation dose-sparing of the prostatic urethra.

The goal of HDR is to destroy the cancer quickly with higher radiation doses than those reached with permanently implanted seeds. HDR, in use since 1986,[90] is gaining acceptance as a highly effective alternative to permanent seed implants. The equipment and training are very expensive but the cost of treatment is competitive. Currently, HDR is most often combined with external beam radiation therapy. The rationale for such combination therapy is that (a) HDR would act as an intensified boost to dominant tumor locations within the prostate working synergistically with EBRT, while (b) EBRT would also act to eradicate PC that may be at the outer perimeter of the prostate gland or invading nearby regional tissue. However, there are now reports of significant efficacy of HDR used alone in patients with a high probability of organ-confined PC. Additionally, talented brachytherapists are able to implant disease that has penetrated the capsule and treat disease that is not organ confined but still regional. *If you want to know more about Experience with HDR, refer to Appendix B, Section 4.8.*

External Beam Radiation Therapy (EBRT)

Many radiation oncologists still effectively use EBRT without the more recent innovations in radiation therapy involving permanent or temporary implants. Studies of EBRT using an average dose of 6800 cGy (68 Gy) have shown 5-year PSA relapse-free rates that are almost identical to that achieved with RP (75% versus 76%, respectively) when patient characteristics such as PSA, Gleason score and clinical stage are equal in both treatment groups.[91] Radiation therapy and radical prostatectomy, therefore, appear to be equal in their success rates when patient treatment groups have clinical and pathological variables evenly matched. Today, a standard dose of EBRT would be at least 7200 cGy (cGy or centigray is a measurement of radiation dose). This can also be expressed as 72 Gy or Gray (1 Gy equals 100 cGy).

3D Conformal Radiation Therapy (3DCRT)

The goal of the radiation oncologist is to conform the radiation beam to the area of the tumor while sparing normal tissues. This level of conformality, therefore, must be optimal for the delivery of radiation to destroy the intended target while leaving nearby normal tissues unharmed. Since we are unable to detect with certainty all areas of involvement within the prostate gland, the standard targets of radiation are the entire gland, and part of the seminal vesicles. The rectum and the bladder are the normal tissues or innocent bystanders that we are trying not to injure. **Optimal conformality is the holy grail of the radiation oncologist.** A serious deficit of so-called "conventional EBRT" relates to not achieving a high level of conformality.

3DCRT is a major technologic advance in this regard. Computerized tomography (CT) using enhanced computer technology allows for the accurate identification of the target— the prostate gland. The calculation of radiation dose distributions in three dimensions using CT with three-dimensional planning programs combined with immobilization of the patient to minimize movement of the target are essential elements in the success of 3DCRT. This technology enables the radiation oncologist to accomplish the goal of hitting the entire target every day while including only 1 cm of surrounding normal tissue. Various other techniques are employed in modern external beam radiation treatment to control for such factors as the movement of the prostate and variations caused by fullness of the bladder or bowel (see discussion of the BAT in the IMRT section upcoming).

3DCRT may be administered as a single therapy, or in tandem with brachytherapy, with the latter being delivered as either permanent seeds or temporary wire implants (HDR). Brachytherapy acts as a boost to 3DCRT to achieve higher doses internally to the gland while 3DCRT also delivers RT to the area immediately surrounding the gland. When both modalities of radiation are employed, the radiation dose of each is lowered compared to the dose given when either brachytherapy or 3DCRT is administered alone. A typical radiation setup for 3DCRT is shown in Figure 45.

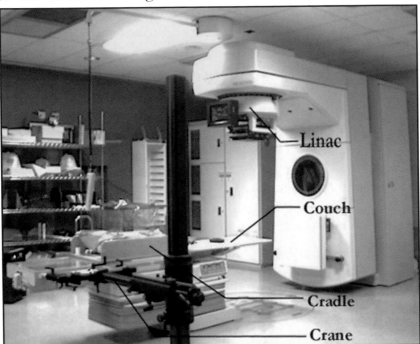

Figure 45: Radiation Therapy Setup. This is a fairly typical setup of what a patient can be expected to see going for RT. The "linac" is the linear accelerator that delivers the radiation. The table the patient lies on is called the "couch". It is shown here with an immobilization "cradle" to maintain the patient's position. The "crane" is equipment used with IMRT to adjust the table in concert with the linac.

Clinical Results Using 3D Conformal RT (3DCRT)

Hanks et al published results of 456 consecutive patients treated largely with 3DCRT prior to 1994. The patient population under study was heterogeneous and consisted of clinical stages ranging from T1 to T3, Gleason scores ranging from 2-10, a wide range of PSA levels and doses of RT that ranged from 66 to 79 Gy. The patient population consisted of 80 patients who received conventional RT and 376 patients treated with 3DCRT.

Despite this heterogeneous population, two noteworthy concepts relating to outcome resulted from this study. *First, treatment results were meaningfully related to the identification of patient subsets based on combining the pretreatment PSA with anatomic (clinical) stage, and Gleason score. Second, a meaningful definition of treatment success or failure was essential for outcome analysis.* These issues confuse much of the literature on the reporting of results involving all current therapies for PC.

In this study, the authors defined biochemical failure as a PSA of 1.5 ng/ml or higher and rising on two consecutive occasions. In a cohort of 259 patients limited to clinical stages T1 and T2a-b, Gleason scores of 6 or less and all PSA ranges, there were highly significant differences in outcome when the pretreatment PSA levels were sorted into three groups: < 10, 10–19.9, and ≥ 20 ng/ml. **The 5-year freedom from biochemical failure was 85% for patients in the PSA < 10 ng/ml group versus 66% when the pretreatment PSA was 10–19.9, and only 33% when the pretreatment PSA was 20 or higher.**

In the same study, the authors used the same analysis in patients with more clinically advanced PC who were staged T2c-T3. The respective results for the three PSA groups mentioned above were 70%, 44% and 21%.[92]

A highly important study of conformal RT employing the above concepts and involving 1,100 patients was reported by Zelefsky et al in 2001 (Table 6).[93] Patients were classified into 3 prognostic groups. *The most favorable prognostic group* involved patients with minimal indication of biological aggressiveness. These patients had a pretreatment PSA of 10 or less, a Gleason score of 6 or less, and a clinical stage of T1 or T2. The *intermediate prognostic group* had one negative prognostic factor such as a PSA > 10, a Gleason score > 6 or a clinical stage T3. The *least favorable prognostic group* had two negative prognostic factors. The authors defined biochemical failure as 3 consecutive rises in PSA after a post-treatment nadir was achieved.[94] Their average follow-up was 5 years with 339 patients (31%) followed 7 years or longer. The RT doses ranged from 64.8 Gy to 86.4 Gy (Table 7). The patients receiving 64.8 to 75.6 Gy all received 3DCRT while of those who received 81 to 86.4 Gy, 61 received 3DCRT and the rest received IMRT. (IMRT discussion follows this section.)

Table 6: RT Doses and Patient Numbers after Zelefsky et al.[93]			
Radiation Dose (Gy)	Radiation Type	Patient Number	Patient Percent
64.8	3DCRT	96	9
70.2	3DCRT	269	24
75.6	3DCRT	445	40
81	3DCRT (61) IMRT (189)	250	23
86.4	IMRT	40	4
Totals		1,100	100%

This is a significant trial insofar as the numbers of patients, the dose escalations employed, the analysis by prognostic group and the use of a biochemical end-point to assess treatment response.

The 5-year PSA biochemical relapse-free survival was associated with both the prognostic groups and radiation dose as shown in Table 7.

Table 7: 5-Year PSA Relapse-Free Survival (RFS). RFS at five years showed a significant improvement in all prognostic groups with RT doses 75.6 Gy or greater versus 70.2 Gy or less. After Zelefsky et al.[93]		
Prognostic Groups	**Radiation Dose (Gy)**	
	Low Dose (64.8 to 70.2)	**High Dose (75.6 to 86.4)**
	5-Year PSA Relapse-Free Survival	
Favorable	77%	90%
Intermediate	50%	70%
Unfavorable	21%	47%

Not detailed in Table 7 are the findings that within the "unfavorable prognostic group" there was a dose-response relationship. That is, the 5-year relapse-free survival was 21% for 64.8 to 70.2 Gy (median = 47%), 43% for 75.6 Gy and 67% for 81 Gy. The data presented in this landmark study therefore stress:

1) The value of using characteristics such as baseline PSA, Gleason score and clinical stage to identify prognostic risk groups.

2) The need for higher doses of RT to achieve end-points associated with successful outcome as defined by PSA trends and absolute values.

3) Improvement in the side-effect profile through the enhancements of IMRT technology.

This latter point will be discussed in the IMRT section that follows.

Intensity Modulated Radiation Therapy (IMRT)

IMRT is the newest major advance in treating PC that minimizes radiation damage to the normal tissues.[95] IMRT uses sophisticated computer planning that allows the radiation oncol-

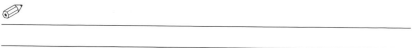

ogist to precisely designate how much RT he wants administered to the targeted tissue and how little RT he wants the adjacent normal tissues to receive (Fig. 46). The IMRT hardware allows the designated variation of the dose of RT while the equipment moves around the patient to fulfill the equation determined by the computer. This is a major advance in technology for all forms of external beam RT and should be the basis for all radiation in the near future. Download, print out and read the April 2000 vol. 3, no. 1 issue of the PCRI *Insights* newsletter (http://www.prostate-cancer.org/resource/insights.html) for an in-depth review of IMRT.

BAT (B-mode Acquisition and Targeting)

BAT is now being used in some centers in conjunction with IMRT. BAT is an ultrasound-based system (Fig. 47) that locates the prostate target on a daily basis prior to each daily radiation session. Since the BAT minimizes uncertainty in target organ lo-

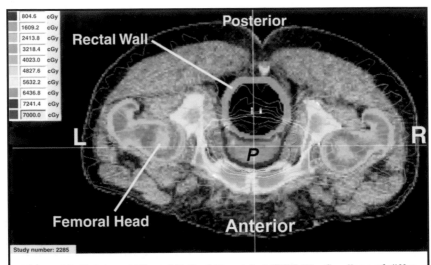

Figure 46: Treatment Plan of Patient Receiving IMRT. The fine lines of different colors in the center of this figure are the isodose contours that relate to the minimum dose of RT that is planned for the area they encompass. The color key for these contour lines is shown in the upper left. The prostate gland (P) in gold color with a heavy red border is circled by an isodose line of 72 Gy (7200 cGy). In this image, the anterior rectal wall would be receiving some radiation. The bladder and the dose of radiation it would receive are not shown in this view. Fig. 46 is from Teh BS, et al: Intensity Modulated RT (IMRT): A new promising technology in radiation oncology.[96] (Baylor College of Medicine) and is provided by courtesy of AlphaMed Press, publishers of The Oncologist. The original photo and the entire article can be found online at http://theoncologist.alphamedpress.org/cgi/content/full/4/6/433/F9.

cation, it helps spare sensitive healthy tissues from unnecessary radiation damage.[97,98] A PowerPoint presentation on the BAT is available for downloading off the PCRI Web site at **http://www.prostate-cancer.org/powerpoint/lectures.html**.

TomoTherapy Hi-Art System®

A new innovation in IMRT systems designed and manufactured by TomoTherapy Incorporated (**http://www.tomotherapy.com/**) is already in use in many centers in the U.S. and a few facilities in Europe. Called the TomoTherapy Hi-Art System®, this technology integrates treatment planning using 3-D images and special software, assures proper patient positioning using CT scans, and delivers a very sophisticated form of photon beam IMRT in a helical (or spiral) delivery pattern, all in one system.

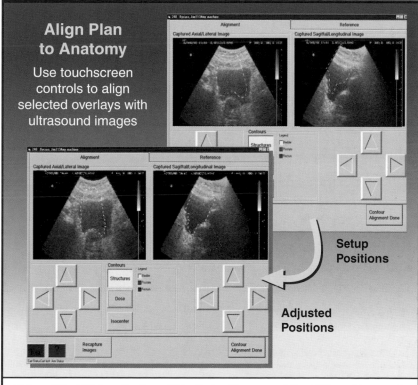

Figure 47: BAT Localization of Prostate. *The use of the BAT enables confirmation of the prostate location prior to each and every radiation treatment. The movements of the target seen in the upper ultrasound photos are adjusted on the BAT monitor by repositioning of the patient on the treatment couch using a mechanically integrated system. The corrected positioning of the patient is shown visually on the ultrasound in the bottom two ultrasound images.*

Radiation Toxicities

All types of radiation therapy may lead to injury to the bladder, rectum and urethra since part of these tissues lie within the radiation portals of treatment. Radiation induced side-effects are graded on a scale of 0-4 for both acute and chronic toxicity and separated into two broad categories: genitourinary and gastrointestinal toxicity. An example of the *chronic* gastrointestinal toxicity table is shown in Table 8. *If You Want to Know More about RT Toxicity Definitions see Appendix B, Section 4.9.*

In the Zelefsky et al study involving 1,200 patients treated either by 3DCRT (871 patients) or IMRT (229 patients), important

Table 8: Chronic Gastrointestinal (GI) Toxicity Radiation Therapy Oncology Group (RTOG) Grading System.

In the study by Zelefsky et al, GI toxicity was absent (Grade 0) in 807 of 1,100 patients (73%). Overall, 174 (16%) and 12 (1%) of patients had Grade 2 and 3 rectal toxicity, respectively. One patient with a history of inflammatory bowel disease who was treated with 64.8 Gy had Grade 4 toxicity.[93] See http://www.rtog.org/members/toxicity/ for the complete acute and chronic genitourinary and gastrointestinal toxicity tables.

GRADE:				
0	1	2	3	4
None	Mild diarrhea Mild cramping Bowel movement 5 times daily Slight rectal discharge or bleeding	Moderate diarrhea and colic Bowel movement > 5 times daily Excessive rectal mucus or intermittent bleeding	Obstruction or bleeding requiring surgery	Necrosis, Perforation or Fistula

findings became apparent in the 5-year actuarial analyses of Grade 2 rectal and genitourinary toxicity. With 3DCRT given to 365 men at RT doses of 64.8-70.2 Gy, **Grade 2 rectal toxicity was 5%. This contrasted with an almost 3-fold incidence (14%) in 506 men receiving 3DCRT at 75.6-81 Gy (p value < 0.001).** Grade 2 genitourinary toxicity was similarly dose-related for patients receiving 3DCRT with a **4% actuarial incidence in the lower RT doses versus 13% at the higher doses (p value < 0.001).** Of significance is that a comparison of 3DCRT and IMRT, both administered at 81 Gy, revealed a 3-year actuarial incidence of rectal toxicity of 14% for 3DCRT, but only 2% for IMRT (p value = 0.005). **Therefore, for the higher RT doses (75.6–81 Gy), which increase the probability of achieving biochemical freedom from PSA relapse, the rectal toxicity of IMRT is significantly less than that of 3DCRT.** At the highest IMRT dose level of 86.4 Gy, however, the preliminary data at an average of 31 months follow-up indicate that 8 of 40 patients (20%) have had Grade 2 genitourinary toxicity. Rectal toxicity remains low with only two of 40 patients (5%) having Grade 2 toxicity. No Grade 3 rectal toxicity was reported in that publication.

Finding the Proper RT Dose

In analyzing the data above, the take-home lessons would appear to be that in patients with favorable to intermediate risk PC based on pretreatment PSA, clinical stage and Gleason score, doses of RT should be in the 75.6 to 81 Gy range. Within this RT dose range, IMRT is associated with less Grade 2 chronic GI toxicity compared to 3DCRT—2% versus 14%, respectively. There is no significant benefit to IMRT in regard to GU toxicity. In patients within the unfavorable prognostic group, however, the 81 Gy dose gives superior biochemical freedom from relapse. Given the overall need to have at least 75.6 Gy administered, the lowest toxicity profile is currently attained with IMRT at a dose of 81 Gy. Doses of IMRT higher than 81 Gy may have unacceptable toxicity, especially involving the genitourinary system.

The real dilemma, however, appears to be the changing nature of the patients presenting with PC currently, as opposed to those in this and similar studies. As said earlier in this section, RT is a modality of treatment that is tumor-volume dependent. Given that the study by Zelefsky et al embraced treatment years from 1988 to 1999, one certainly has to speculate that the overwhelming majority of patients being treated currently have far less tumor volume at the time of diagnosis than those who were diagnosed in the 80s and early 90s. **The optimal balance in finding the RT dose necessary to achieve tumor kill while minimizing toxicity to the bladder and rectum requires further elucidation in light of the significantly lower tumor volumes now present at the time of diagnosis.** This entire discipline becomes more difficult to assess when ADT (androgen deprivation therapy) is used prior to and/or during RT. These

---

Physician's Note 15:

"Severe RT Side-Effects Can Occur." Despite the fact that MV received RT by recognized experts in the field of RT, his clinical course after completion of RT was characterized by much pain and suffering. His medical history of diabetes mellitus was probably a factor in his complicated course because small vessel disease, characteristic of diabetics, would make him more prone to tissue injury from RT. MV did show symptomatic relief with the use of superoxide dismutase (SOD), Vitamin E suppositories and Rowasa® but nevertheless experienced much distress for 18 months. On a positive note, his last PSA approximately three years after completing RT was 0.04.

Patient MV was diagnosed with PC on 5/21/98 with a bPSA of 11, and a GS of (2,3) read by David Bostwick, M.D. His clinical stage was T2b. An endorectal MRI in 9/98 disclosed possible extra-capsular extension at the left apex. While deciding what to do, MV began androgen deprivation therapy (ADT) on 9/21/98 with Casodex and Lupron and after three months his PSA was < 0.05. Proscar was added to his regimen in 1/99. 3DCRT was then given starting in 4/99 with 4500 cGy followed by Palladium-103 seed implants on 5/26/99. MV developed severe RT side-effects with rectal spasms and also hematuria. ADT was stopped on 6/2/99. He had marked dysuria, and a supra-pubic catheter was placed. After some improvement, the catheter was removed but urinary retention occurred and a transurethral resection of the bladder neck was performed. A year after completion of his RT, MV was improved but still symptomatic. Not until 1-1/2 years after the completion of RT did MV start to return to his normal self.

issues are not intended to confuse patients reading this, or to raise anxiety levels, but rather to stress again the evolving nature of the treatments of PC and how far we have come in such a short period of time.

Proton Beam RT (PBRT)

All forms of RT use particles from within the atom: electrons, neutrons, protons and subatomic particles such as alpha or beta particles or photons (x-rays or gamma rays). Particles carry excess energy that is intended to be deposited into the target tissue: either the prostate gland containing cancer, or nearby tissues with high risk of cancer spread. These energized particles interact with tissue in their path. In this interaction, electrons are displaced from their orbits within the atoms of a molecule causing a change in structure. This process is called "ionization" and the molecules that are the intended targets are the DNA of the tumor cell (Fig. 48). Therefore, the essence of

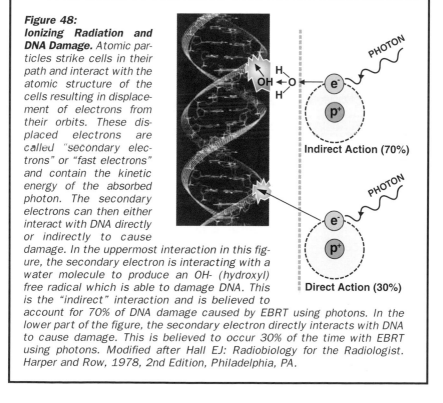

Figure 48:
Ionizing Radiation and DNA Damage. Atomic particles strike cells in their path and interact with the atomic structure of the cells resulting in displacement of electrons from their orbits. These displaced electrons are called "secondary electrons" or "fast electrons" and contain the kinetic energy of the absorbed photon. The secondary electrons can then either interact with DNA directly or indirectly to cause damage. In the uppermost interaction in this figure, the secondary electron is interacting with a water molecule to produce an OH- (hydroxyl) free radical which is able to damage DNA. This is the "indirect" interaction and is believed to account for 70% of DNA damage caused by EBRT using photons. In the lower part of the figure, the secondary electron directly interacts with DNA to cause damage. This is believed to occur 30% of the time with EBRT using photons. Modified after Hall EJ: Radiobiology for the Radiologist. Harper and Row, 1978, 2nd Edition, Philadelphia, PA.

RT is the delivery of excess energy via energized particles that alter atomic structure leading to ionization. Ionizing radiation, therefore, causes damage to DNA and leads to cell death. The intended target of this therapy is the tumor cell.

All conventional RT and most 3DCRT and IMRT use photons to deliver ionizing radiation. Electrons, protons and neutrons are other atomic particles that are also used in radiation therapy. Each particle has its own defined pattern for depositing the energy that is characteristic of that particle.

Photons have no charge, and no significant mass. The photon beam deposits energy as it encounters tissue and the power of the beam decreases exponentially as it penetrates the body. Photons begin to deposit energy as they enter the skin surface, but the depth at which the maximum energy is deposited depends on the energy of the *photons.* Deposition of maximal energy may therefore range from the skin surface to a depth of 4 cm. The deposition of energy falls off as the beam passes to the deeper structures, continues through the target volume, and exits the patient at the opposite side of the body. Again, each particle has its own defined pattern for depositing its energy which is characteristic of that particle.

Proton beam radiation therapy (PBRT) is a form of external beam radiation therapy that uses the proton rather than the photon to deliver ionizing radiation. PBRT was first used in the treatment of prostate cancer at the Massachusetts General Hospital (MGH) in Cambridge, Massachusetts in 1976. In 1991, Loma Linda Medical Center (LLMC) in Loma Linda, California joined MGH to be the second hospital facility to offer PBRT in the treatment of PC. The largest literature on PBRT has come from LLMC.

✐
_____
_____
_____
_____
_____

How Proton Beam RT Works

Protons have a positive charge and a mass 1836 times that of an electron. Whereas photons (x-rays) have a pattern of energy loss which is an exponential loss in relation to the thickness of the radiated tissue, a proton beam's dose of radiation decreases extremely rapidly to zero at the end of the proton range (in contrast to the dose from x-rays which continues to decrease exponentially). *The delivery of a radiation payload with protons versus photons relates to the different dose distributions that are the consequence of the physical characteristics by which protons lose energy.* Protons deposit only a small amount of their energy as they enter the body and approach the target volume. At this time they are traveling up to two-thirds the speed of light, a velocity at which less ionization occurs due to the short period of time the protons have to interact with any given electron.

The proton beam can be programmed to stop at a particular volume of depth. In this stopping region, ionization events increase rapidly so DNA damage results. The rapid increase in ionization is called the Bragg peak (Fig. 49). By varying the energy of the proton beam, the Bragg peak can be spread out to encompass the tumor volume. In essence, this is a focusing advantage of the

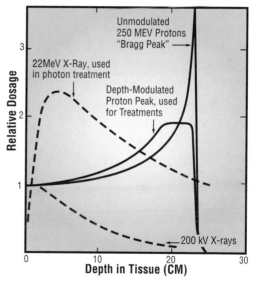

Figure 49: Rapid Increase in Ionization or Bragg Peak. *The Bragg peak relates to the point of energy release due to slowing down of the energized particle resulting in increased ionization and delivery of the "energy payload" used to irreparably damage DNA. Instead of the exponential drop-off in energy as seen with particles like photons, protons deposit their maximum energy at the end of their travel in tissue and do not deposit energy past that point. The creation of protons of varying energies (225-250 Mega electron-Volts or MeV) facilitates a depth-modulated proton peak used to treat PC, as shown in this figure.*

proton particle. In addition to their focusing advantage, protons, unlike conventional radiation, cause such a low number of injury events to **normal** cells that these cells are able to repair radiation damage. **Tumor** cells are less able to repair radiation damage. This differential in repair capability provides the selective cell destruction seen with these types of radiation. **By varying the energy, the technician can precisely shape the Bragg peak to deliver homogeneous doses of radiation to irregularly-shaped three-dimensional tumors.** *If you want to know more about Proton RT, refer to Appendix B, Section 4.10.*

Clinical Results Using Proton Beam RT (PBRT)

Clinical reports on the use of proton beam radiation therapy in the treatment of PC are few in number, reflecting that this therapy is being done only at two centers in the United States. The majority of patients with PC have been treated at LLMC. Slater et al, in a study published in 1998, reported their findings using proton beam radiation therapy for patients with PC clinical stages ranging from T1 to T3 who received 74-75 Gy using either proton beam radiation therapy alone or a combination of protons and photons.[99] The average follow-up period was 43 months (range 4-78 months). In a subset of patients who were followed for at least 24 months, Slater et al found a significant relationship between baseline PSA (bPSA) and biochemical disease-free survival or biochemical non-evidence of disease (bNED) at 4.5 years. Biochemical failure was defined as either three consecutive rises in PSA of greater than 10% or a single dramatic rise.[94] As shown in Table 9, patients with four different bPSA ranges had freedom from PSA relapse averaging 80.2%. The 4.5-year bNED rates were strongly influenced by the bPSA.

In the same study, a not surprising relationship was found between a lower baseline PSA (bPSA) and the ability to achieve a post-RT PSA nadir of ≤ 0.5 ng/ml. This likely relates to the fact that bPSA relates to the amount of PC present (the tumor volume) prior to treatment as well as the probability of the PC being within the radiation field (extent of disease). The smaller the volume of PC and the more likely the PC is within the radiation ports of therapy, the greater the chance that the PC will be controlled, if not cured. These findings are shown in Table 10.

Table 9: Effect of Baseline PSA (bPSA) on Freedom From PSA Relapse (bNED) in Clinical Stages T1-3 Treated with Proton Beam Radiation Therapy.

The baseline PSA heavily influenced the outcome of patients treated with either pure proton beam therapy or a combination of protons plus photons. These results need follow-up in light of ongoing biochemical relapses that may be seen over time. The use of predictive algorithms to select patients that would perhaps do even better than the excellent results shown below should be considered rather than simply using a single biological risk factor such as PSA.[99]

bPSA	Number of Patients	bNED at 4.5 Years Number (per cent)
≤ 4.0	49	49 (100%)
4.1–10.0	248	220 (89%)
10.1–20.0	144	104 (72%)
> 20.0	70	37 (53%)
Totals	511	410 (80.2%)

Table 10: The Ability to Achieve a Post-Treatment Nadir of ≤ 0.5 ng/ml Relates to the bPSA in Patients Treated with Proton Beam Radiation Therapy.

In the study by Slater et al, 58% of all patients achieved a PSA nadir of ≤ 0.5 ng/ml. The lower the baseline PSA, the greater the likelihood of achieving a post-treatment nadir of ≤ 0.5 ng/ml. For those patients achieving a post-RT nadir of ≤ 0.5ng/ml, the 5-year bNED was 91%. If the nadir was 0.51 to 1.0, the 5-year bNED decreased to 79% and if > 1.0, this decreased further to 40%. This data was based on a minimum follow-up of 24 months. Much longer follow-up is needed in assessing biochemical freedom from relapse.

Baseline PSA (bPSA)	Number of Patients	Post-RT nadir ≤ 0.5 ng/ml Number (per cent)
≤ 4.0	49	42 (86%)
4.1-10.0	248	159 (64%)
10.1-20.0	144	73 (51%)
> 20.0	70	24 (34%)
Totals	511	298 (58.3%)

Comparison studies of proton beam radiation therapy versus 3DCRT or IMRT have never been published; it is unlikely that they will, given the changing nature of all therapies and skills involved in the treatment of PC. *If you want to know more about Proton Beam studies, refer to Appendix B, Section 4.11.*

Neutron Beam RT

The basic effect of ionizing radiation is to destroy the ability of cells to divide and grow by damaging their DNA. For photon, electron and proton RT, the damage is caused primarily by activated radicals produced from interactions of the radiated particle with electrons orbiting the nucleus of the atom (Fig. 48). The term for these types of radiation is low linear energy transfer or low LET radiation.

Neutron beam RT uses neutrons to interact directly with the cell nucleus of the targeted molecules (Fig. 50). Neutrons are a form of high linear energy transfer (high LET) radiation because they deposit 20-100 times more energy-per-unit of traversed tissue than megavoltage photons. **High LET radiation such as neutron beam radiation therapy (NBRT) results in DNA damage to a tumor that is less reparable than to a tumor**

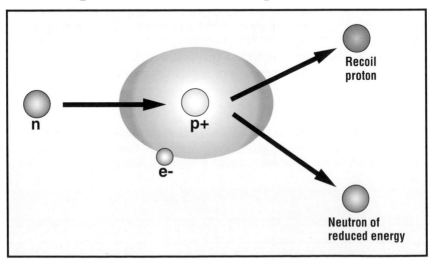

Figure 50: How Fast Neutrons Deposit Energy. *Fast neutrons (n) interact with hydrogen nuclei [containing one proton (p+) and one electron (e-)] in what is called a "knock on" reaction to produce recoil protons and neutrons of reduced energy. The recoil protons, in turn, produce a high density of ionization events as they pass through tissue.*

cell damaged by low LET radiation, which has a significant chance to repair itself and continue to grow.

Neutrons are created by sending 66 MeV (Mega electron-Volts) protons into a beryllium target (Fig. 51) to produce high-energy neutrons. The *relative biological effectiveness* (RBE) of neutrons is so high that the required tumor dose is approximately one-third the dose used with photons, electrons or protons. The basis for the higher RBE of neutron beam radiation appears to be related to their ability to cause double-stranded breaks in DNA, which are generally lethal to the cells that sustain them. Photons and protons predominantly cause a single-stranded break. Therefore, a full course of NBT is delivered in 10-12 treatments versus the 30-40 treatments used with the low LET forms of RT.

Large tumors have low levels of oxygen (hypoxic areas) in the center of the tumor and because of this they are not particularly sensitive to DNA damage through the indirect free-radical

STRUCTURE OF THE NUCLEUS
The nucleus is composed of protons and neutrons

	Symbol	Charge	Mass, kg	Mass, amu
electron	e^-	-1	9.10953×10^{-31}	0.000548
proton	p^+	+1	1.67265×10^{-27}	1.007276
neutron	n	0	1.67495×10^{-27}	1.008665

The 4 elements below show protons in pink & neutrons in gray

| hydrogen nucleus | helium nucleus | lithium nucleus | beryllium nucleus |

*Figure 51: Beryllium–Atomic Number and Atomic Mass. The atomic number of an element is the number of protons in its nucleus. Hydrogen, for example, has an atomic number of 1. The atomic mass equals the summed weight of protons, neutrons and electrons. Beryllium has an atomic number of 4 because it has 4 protons but an atomic mass of **approximately** 9 because it has 5 neutrons (and the mass of the electrons is relatively negligible).*

mediated form of cell killing (Fig. 48) that is characteristic of low LET radiation. Fast neutrons have the ability to eradicate bulky tumors because, unlike low LET radiation, neutrons do not depend on the presence of oxygen to kill the tumor. The biological effectiveness of neutrons is also independent of the phase of the cell's growth cycle, which is again different with low LET radiation. This aspect of NBRT becomes significant when patients develop androgen-independent PC (AIPC) and/or have bulky disease that cannot be reduced with ADT (androgen deprivation therapy). **In such a setting, NBRT would have a better chance of eradicating high volume tumors than would photon, proton or electron RT.** (See Physician's Note 16.)

Physician's Note 16:

"Neutron Beam RT: Update on Patient OG. (See Physician's Note 12.)"
OG presented with aggressive PC with a Gleason score of 9. His response to ADT (androgen deprivation therapy) was one of a mixed response with androgen-dependent PC (ADPC) in the bones showing complete resolution of activity per multiple bone scans but with progressive disease in lymph nodes apparently reflecting the androgen-independent PC (AIPC). His response to Neutron Beam RT directed at enlarged nodes was successful, suggesting that the patient's specific medical situation should bring into consideration an understanding of the scope as well as the limitations of what kind of RT is chosen for a patient. The choice of neutrons as the radiation particle most likely to penetrate bulky tumor appears to be validated by his successful outcome to date.

Patient OG presented with advanced PC indicating bone metastases at age 68 with a baseline PSA of 8.4 and a Gleason score of (5,4). Treatment with ADT using Casodex and Lupron resulted in a transient drop in PSA to < 0.05 for one month followed by a rise in PSA. A diagnosis of AIPC was made and different chemotherapeutic agents were given with no significant response. A CT scan of the pelvis revealed lymph nodes compressing the left ureter. In addition, the base of the bladder was involved by PC. Meanwhile, on ADT, repeat bone scanning studies showed resolution of the previously documented abnormalities. Neutron beam RT was elected at the FermiLab in Batavia, Illinois after discussion with the patient and radiation oncology consultants. Treatment was given in January of 2000. One year later, a repeat CT pelvis and abdomen showed no lymph node enlargement. A PSA was < 0.1, PAP was 1.0 and CEA was 2.7. However, a plasma CGA which was normal at 7.6 in 11/22/98 had risen to 67 in 10/01. The CEA as of 10/01 had increased to 4.2.

Clinical Results Using Neutron Beam RT (NBRT)

Neutrons have been used in the treatment of PC since 1977. In a Radiation Therapy Oncology Group (RTOG) clinical trial comparing a combination of neutrons plus photons versus photons alone for T_{3-4} N_{0-1} M_0 patients (see Appendix D for a detailed description of the TNM staging classification), superior outcomes at 10 years were seen for the patients receiving the mixed beam treatment.[100] This superiority was observed in overall survival, disease-specific survival, and freedom from clinical local tumor recurrence.

A subsequent study was done in locally advanced PC comparing external beam RT using photons at 70-72 Gy (prostate) and approximately 50 Gy (pelvic nodes) with external beam neutron irradiation at 20 Gy (prostate) and 13.6 Gy (pelvic nodes).[101] Eighty-five photon and 87 neutron patients were analyzed. At the time this study was published, the median follow-up was 68 months. **The 5-year actuarial clinical local-regional failure rate was 32% for photons but only 11% for neutron beam radiation therapy.** PSA values were elevated in 17% of neutron-treated patients and in 45% of photon-treated patients at five years ($p < 0.001$). Since this was a multi-institutional study involving four centers with differing equipment, toxicity data was difficult to interpret. Those hospitals with specialized equipment to shape and deliver the neutron beam, e.g. multileaf collimator and rotating gantry (see Glossary in Appendix D), had similar late toxicity effects as the hospitals administering photon beam RT.

3D conformal neutron therapy is currently in use at Wayne State University in Detroit, Michigan (telephone 313-745-2593) and also at the Midwest Institute for Neutron Therapy at FermiLab in Batavia, Illinois at **http://www-bd.fnal.gov/ntf/ntf home.html**. Outside of the United States, ¡Themba Labs in Somerset West, South Africa (**http://www.medrad.nac.ac.za/index.htm**) has both proton and neutron beam radiation treatment ability. We have had no patient or physician feedback regarding this center and welcome such input. *If you want to know more about Neutron Beam RT, refer to Appendix B, Section 4.12.*

Androgen Deprivation Therapy (ADT) or "Hormone Therapy"

A note from Dr. Strum: *Although it is the intent of the authors to be objective and unbiased in this book, it is virtually impossible if one of the authors has spent close to twenty years with a greater focus and experience on a particular topic. Therefore, it is important that I expressly state that I feel a need to share what I consider important observations and "truths" based my experiences in dealing with thousands of prostate cancer patients. I was privileged to be one of a handful of American investigators working with Dr. Fernand Labrie in the early eighties on ADT. In those years, the use of an anti-androgen such as Eulexin or of an LHRH agonist was considered investigational. The roles of these agents in the management of PC were questioned aggressively in those years, in stark comparison to their general acceptance now. ADT is being evaluated in a scientific fashion in multiple settings and many of the observations made during those early years are now being formalized in studies involving large numbers of patients. This section of The Primer on ADT is openly weighted more heavily than others in an attempt to share with the reader some of the insights on this topic that*

are now being discussed in seminars and published in the peer-reviewed literature.

ADT Overview

ADT is often described as a medical or chemical (as opposed to surgical) orchiectomy. Orchiectomy is a surgical procedure in which the testicles are removed from the scrotum surgically so that testosterone, normally derived from the testicles, is unavailable. This is an irreversible method of depriving the body of testosterone. It is sometimes done for reasons of economy because the drugs involved in "hormone therapy" are expensive.

Like surgical orchiectomy, ADT works by depriving prostatic tissue of testosterone (T) and its metabolite dihydrotestosterone (DHT), both of which are necessary growth factors for most prostate cancers. ADT also decreases blood vessel growth within the tumor by virtue of its anti-angiogenesis effects.[102-104]

Through these mechanisms, ADT results in cell death and/or growth arrest of both benign and malignant prostate tissue with a resultant reduction of both prostate gland and prostate tumor volume. This can, in certain cases, increase the effectiveness of RT or cryosurgery, potentially yielding a higher disease-free rate.

129

For men with advanced PC, indicated by widespread metastases, ADT is the only currently recognized effective treatment option. (See Physician's Note 17.) In patients where the PC is predominantly androgen dependent, such therapy can work for many years. Androgen-dependent PC (ADPC) depends on testosterone to nourish it, whereas androgen-independent PC (AIPC) grows even in the absence of testosterone. *Intermittent* androgen deprivation (IAD) therapy can have a positive impact on quality of life because during the "off therapy" months of the intermittent treatment cycle(s), patients are spared the side-effects of treatment, which are mainly due to

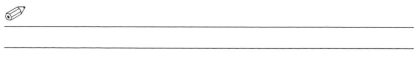

androgen deprivation.

ADT is often recommended for patients who are planning treatment with EBRT, brachytherapy or cryosurgery. This is most common in settings where the prostate gland volume is too large to be effectively treated without the risk of excessive radiation scatter to the bladder and/or rectum. The gland volume, therefore, needs to be reduced before these procedures can be optimally performed. For men with large prostates, ADT can make these local therapies more effective and reduce their side-effects by being able to dramatically reduce prostate gland volume over the course of six to eight months.

However, in addition to prostate gland volume, the cancer volume is also a critical factor that relates to the success of RT or

---

Physician's Note 17:

"Prostate Cancer is an Endocrine-Related Malignancy." Most patients with PC will show some response to ADT. The degree of response is related to the tumor cell population being either androgen-dependent PC (ADPC) or androgen-independent PC (AIPC) and whether or not the testosterone level has been reduced to levels below 20 ng/dl. The patient below was fortunate to have a highly responsive cancer suggesting a homogeneous population of ADPC. Most patients with advanced PC have mixtures of ADPC and AIPC.

One evening, while I was making hospital rounds, the family of CY asked me if I would see him in emergency consultation. CY had terrible bone pain due to widespread bone metastases from prostate cancer. He also was uremic due to kidney failure resulting from obstruction of his ureters. A review of his medical chart revealed that he had received no prior therapy for prostate cancer. My major recommendation to the family was to perform an emergency orchiectomy which was done by the attending urologist that evening. Within 24 hours of the orchiectomy, CY was essentially pain-free and needed no further narcotic analgesics. Within seven days of the orchiectomy, the kidney failure had resolved and the previously elevated BUN and creatinine blood levels had returned to normal. At his one year "anniversary" from the orchiectomy, the bone scan had reverted to completely normal. The following year, his PSA test result was 0.0 ng/ml. CY died at the age of 92 from a cerebral vascular accident without clinical or laboratory evidence of prostate cancer.

cryosurgical treatment modalities. **EBRT of any kind, brachytherapy and cryosurgery are all cancer-volume-dependent therapies. If the volume of the cancer and/or the gland is too great, these treatments will be less effective and in some cases completely ineffective.** ADT, therefore, is often used prior to and during these treatments.

Some patients initiate ADT in order to have time to research their options for treatment or because of other pressing life issues that prevent immediate treatment with the standard primary therapies of RP, RT or cryosurgery. **Patients should understand the rationale for the use of ADT prior to, during, and after such therapies.**

How ADT Works

The endocrinology of PC involves the important function of the pituitary gland, which, through its release of LH, stimulates the testicles to make testosterone (Fig. 52). Testosterone (T) drives prostate cell growth both directly and through its potent **131** metabolite dihydrotestosterone (DHT). The prostate cell itself has the enzymatic machinery (the enzyme 5-alpha reductase or 5-AR) to convert T to DHT.

ADT typically employs a drug called an LHRH agonist (luteinizing hormone-releasing hormone agonist or LHRH-A), which ultimately decreases the stimulation of the testicles. The mechanism of action of LHRH agonists is complex but essentially involves down-regulating (turning off) a pituitary hormone called luteinizing hormone (LH) that normally stimulates the testicles to make testosterone. LHRH agonists currently being used include leuprolide acetate (Lupron®), goserelin acetate (Zoladex®) or triptorelin pamoate (Trelstar LA®). Any one of these agents will have the effect of drastically decreasing the production of testosterone by the testes, thereby dramatically reducing the most significant growth factor involved in the proliferation of prostate cancer. Charles Huggins, M.D., of the University of Chicago, received the Nobel Prize in 1966 for his work that showed the importance of testosterone reduction in the treatment of PC (Fig. 53).

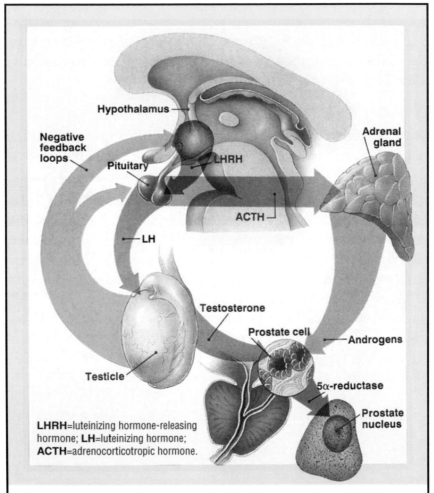

Figure 52: The Endocrine Pathways in PC. *The two major contributions to-wards male hormone production are from the pituitary release of LH, which stimulates the testicles to make T and from the stimulation of the adrenals to make the precursor androgens DHEA-S and Androstenedione. The latter two substances are converted within prostatic tissue to T and DHT. (Also see Fig. 54.) Art work reproduced with kind permission from Kevin Sommerville.*

A detailed discussion of ADT with illustrations was presented in the October 2000 and October 2001 issues of the PCRI *Insights* newsletter found at the PCRI Web site (www.pcri.org). *If you want to know more about hormone treatment, refer to Appendix B, Section 4.13.*

The pituitary also stimulates the adrenal glands to make the **androgen precursors** DHEA-S and androstenedione. These substances are converted *within the prostate cell* to T. As previously mentioned, the prostate cells contain 5-alpha reductase (5AR), an enzyme that converts T to the five times more potent DHT. Labrie has referred to this as the "Intracrinology" of PC. This relates to the intra-prostatic synthesis of androgens (Fig. 54).

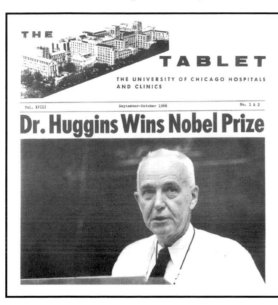

Figure 53: Charles Huggins, M.D. Dr. Huggins began work on the importance of testosterone and other androgens as far back as the 1940s. His group published landmark papers on the role of reduction of testosterone by orchiectomy as well as reduction of adrenal androgens by adrenalectomy. Papers on the role of removing the pituitary gland were also published by Huggins et al twenty years before the first LHRH-A was approved for the treatment of PC.[105]

A comprehensive listing of treatments used in the endocrine therapy of PC is shown in three tables, 11A-C. These treatments should be understood by visualizing their mode(s) of action or mechanism(s) in relationship to the anatomy of the endocrine axis. You should be asking yourself: "Does the treatment work by acting at the pituitary, testicular, or adrenal level, or does it work within the prostate cell itself? Are its actions, perhaps, through a combination of effects at different levels?"

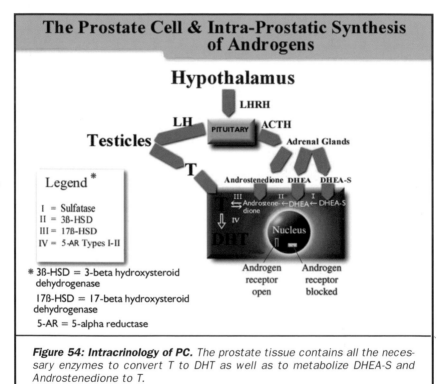

Figure 54: Intracrinology of PC. *The prostate tissue contains all the necessary enzymes to convert T to DHT as well as to metabolize DHEA-S and Androstenedione to T.*

Both orchiectomy and ADT using drug therapy are capable of reducing the testosterone to castrate levels (< 20 ng/dl or < 0.69 nM/L). The "thermostatic" or reflex response to both approaches is shown in the comments section of Table 11A. For example, removal of the testicles results in the body's attempt to compensate for a loss of androgen. The hypothalamus is stimulated to release LHRH, which in turn activates the release of LH, FSH (follicle stimulating hormone), and possibly ACTH (adrenocorticotrophic hormone). These findings are confirmed by laboratory test results.

The forms of ADT most often used to achieve chemical castration are single, double or triple androgen deprivation therapy

---

Table 11A: Endocrine Therapies Used in the Treatment of PC.

The essential mechanism involved in ADT (androgen deprivation therapy) is the prevention of access of androgen to the prostate cancer cell. This may involve actual decrease in available androgen (orchiectomy, LHRH-A or LHRH antagonist), interference with the ability of androgen to interact or make contact with the prostate cell receptor (anti-androgen) or an alteration in the androgen receptor. This table includes the major forms of ADT which work exclusively on androgen-dependent PC (ADPC).

Class of Therapy	Therapy Name	Mechanism(s)	Comments
Surgical removal of testicles	Orchiectomy	Removes testicular source of testosterone (T)	Reflex increases in LHRH, LH, FSH, and possibly ACTH leading to increase in adrenal androgens
LHRH agonists or LHRH-A	Lupron®, Zoladex® Trelstar LA®, Viadur® or Eligard®	Down-regulates LH to lower T; decreases FSH	Causes T surge lasting up 10-14 days; FSH rises after many months
LHRH antagonists	Abarelix™*or Cetrotide®	Blocks LHRH to lower T; decreases FSH	No T surge; No FSH increase after months of use
Anti-androgens	Eulexin®, Casodex®, Nilandron®, and Androcur® (CPA)	Blocks androgen receptor and prevents T and DHT from stimulating PC growth; CPA also lowers LH	Reflex increase in T with metabolism to estrogen can cause gynecomastia (breast enlargement and nipple sensitivity)

*Abarelix (Plenaxis™) has been approved by the FDA, as of November, 2003.

(ADT$_1$, ADT$_2$, or ADT$_3$, respectively). ADT$_1$ typically employs an LHRH agonist only, ADT$_2$ typically uses an LHRH agonist with an anti-androgen and ADT$_3$ uses three agents: an LHRH agonist, an anti-androgen and a 5-alpha reductase enzyme inhibitor, either finasteride or dutasteride. ADT$_3$ is the approach I have most commonly employed after 18 years of experience in treating and counseling thousands of men with PC. ADT is a management issue that continues to be hotly debated, and little agreement on the optimal form of ADT has been reached. The pros and cons for specific drugs to be used individually or

136

Table 11B: Endocrine Therapies Used in the Treatment of PC.

These approaches (estrogenic compounds and P450 enzyme inhibitors) are broader in activity because they have an anti-PC effect against both androgen-dependent PC (ADPC) and androgen-independent PC (AIPC). 5-AR inhibitors are gaining popularity in use and most often are combined with LHRH-A and anti-androgens or anti-androgens alone.

Class of Therapy	Therapy Name	Mechanism(s)	Comments
Estrogenic compounds	DES®, PC SPES™ ‡, Stilphosterol® Honvan®, Estradurin® Climara patch® Estraderm patch®	Lowers FSH, LH and lowers T; Direct cytotoxic effect on PC cell of androgen receptor	Increases sex binding hormone globulin which lowers free T; increases prolactin which increases sensitivity
P450 enzyme inhibitors	Nizoral® (HDK or Ketoconazole)	Decreases testicular T, decreases adrenal androgens, direct cytotoxic effect on PC cell	Synergistic with many chemotherapy agents; decreases MDR gene; causes reflex increase of LH if pituitary-testicular axis not blocked by LHRH-A or estrogen
5-alpha reductase (5-AR) inhibitors	Proscar® (finasteride) (Type 2 5-AR inhibitor) Avodart® (dutasteride) (Type I and Type 2 5-AR inhibitor)	Blocks conversion of testosterone to DHT DHT is 5 times more potent growth stimulator than T	Proscar®: reduces DHT in blood by 70% and by 80-90% in prostate Avodart®: reduces DHT in blood by 98%

‡ PC SPES™ is no longer being manufactured as of June 2002 due to detection of DES, Coumadin and Indocin in various lots of PC SPES™.

* Avodart® (dutasteride), manufactured by Glaxo, received FDA approval in November, 2001.

in combination need to be thoroughly discussed with your doctor. If you are a candidate for this therapy, it is recommended that you research all of your options very carefully. Important biological issues in understanding ADT are discussed and illustrated in the October 2001 issue of *Insights* on the PCRI Web site at www.prostate-cancer.org. Please read "Listening to the Biology of Prostate Cancer."

Table 11C: Endocrine Therapies Used in PC.
These forms of ADT work by decreasing the sensitivity of the androgen receptor or by decreasing adrenal androgens.

Class of Therapy	Therapy Name	Mechanism(s)	Comments
Steroids	Decadron or Hexadrol® Hydrocortisone, Prednisone	Decreases CRF and ACTH and diminishes adrenal androgens	Causes excessive bone loss unless bisphos-phonates and bone supplements are used
Selective blocker of adrenal androgens	Cytadren® (Aminoglutethimide)	Decreases adrenal androgens	Requires use of hydrocortisone
Prolactin Inhibitors	Dostinex® Bromocriptine®	Reduces sensitivity of the androgen receptor	Requires careful dose titration; nausea common, hypotension possible

_____

_____

_____

_____

_____

_____

_____

_____

Flare: Biochemical versus Clinical Flare

Before beginning a course of treatment with any LHRH agonist (Lupron®, Zoladex®, Trelstar LA®, Viadur®or Eligard®), it is important to initiate measures to prevent "flare." Flare results from an initial surge in testosterone production upon the initiation of the LHRH agonist (LHRH-A) caused by the release of LH. The LHRH-A will eventually down-regulate LH, but this may take up to 14 days. During this time, cell growth that is mediated by testosterone is increased. This means that prostate cells, benign or malignant, are being stimulated to grow for as much as the first two weeks of LHRH-A therapy if no measure to prevent flare or counter its effects has been initiated.

In most men currently initiating Lupron, Zoladex, Trelstar LA, Viadur or other LHRH agonist therapy, the effects of flare are

Two Different Types of Flare

Biochemical Flare

Initiation of LHRH-A always causes this **unless:**
• LH increase is blocked.
• Effect of LH on testicle (Leydig) cells is blocked.
• Effects of increased Testosterone and DHT are blocked.

In the setting of low volume disease, the effects of biochemical flare go undetected unless T and PSA levels are checked at 7–14 days.

Clinical Flare

This is seen in the setting of higher volume PC, at the initiation of LHRH-A therapy.

Occurs when the tumor burden location is at a critical site and the increased tumor volume resulting from flare causes symptoms.

Figure 55: Biochemical Flare. When LHRH agonists such as Lupron, Zoladex, Trelstar LA or Viadur are started (or restarted in those receiving intermittent ADT), the release of LH from the pituitary results in a rapid increase in testosterone (surge) that stimulates prostate growth of both malignant and benign prostate tissue. Unless LH or its downstream effects are blocked, biochemical flare MUST occur.

Figure 56: Clinical Flare. With clinical flare, the baseline **tumor burden** is larger than with biochemical flare and the flare increases or initiates clinical findings that were not present before LHRH agonist therapy was started. Also, the **tumor location** may be in a critical area and the increased tumor growth during flare turns an asymptomatic patient into one with major symptomatology which can permanently alter life.

only detected by measuring the testosterone and PSA levels and observing the testosterone surge followed by a rise in PSA. This is because most patients diagnosed with PC today have a small tumor volume and the effects of increased cancer growth go unnoticed. The effect of testosterone surge in this category of PC patients is called *biochemical flare* (Fig. 55) since it is unassociated with clinical manifestations of worsening PC. On careful questioning of men with biochemical flare, however, you will often hear them remark that they noticed an increased desire for sexual activity, which is an expression of testosterone surge.

In the presence of significant amounts of tumor, however, flare can result in the aggravation of clinical symptoms, i.e. clinical flare (Fig. 56). Such flare may involve growth of PC or normal prostate tissue within the prostate gland which may reduce the caliber of the urinary stream and possibly lead to complete obstruction of flow (urinary retention). Clinical flare can result in an increase in bone pain if bone metastases are present. In more serious circumstances, flare can result in spinal cord compression with possible paralysis if PC tissue near the spinal cord is stimulated to grow. Flare may result in kidney failure if lymph nodes near the the ureters—the drainage tubes from the kidneys—increase in size due to increased tumor growth and compress the ureters. (See Physician's Note 18.) Such occurrences are examples of clinical flare.

139

An anti-androgen such as flutamide (Eulexin®), bicalutamide (Casodex®) or nilutamide (Nilandron®) should be administered for seven days prior to the initiation of LHRH agonist. Otherwise, flare—manifested by a testosterone surge and an increase in PSA—will occur in all patients. The up-front use of the anti-androgen prevents both biochemical and clinical flare by saturating the docking sites (androgen receptors) for androgens within PC cells as well as benign prostate cells. This prevents testosterone and its potent metabolite DHT (dihydrotestosterone) from stimulating PC and benign prostate cell growth. Since it takes from 7 to 14 days for LH to be down-regulated after first starting Lupron®, Zoladex®, Trelstar LA®, Viadur® or Eligard®, **the patient is spared as much as two weeks of tumor growth by starting an anti-androgen seven days prior to LHRH agonist administration.**

Physician's Note 18:

"Flare: Tumor Growth That Can Be Avoided." Whether flare is apparent clinically or is silent, it is still reflective of tumor growth that has been caused by the very therapy that is intended to decrease tumor proliferation. There is no biological reason to stimulate cancer growth under any circumstance. Flare of any kind should be avoided.

Patient MF had elected a watchful waiting approach until his PSA rose to 31. At that time, his physicians administered a 3-month Lupron injection without any precautionary measure to prevent flare. Six days later, he developed severe back pain. Radiologic studies showed right hydronephrosis due to tumor obstruction of the right ureteral orifice at the junction with the bladder. Emergency surgery was performed to decompress the kidney, but because this was unsuccessful, a right ureteral stent had to be placed—this required five hours in the operating room. Forty-eight hours later, the patient experienced a massive heart attack. The patient's pain and suffering from the exacerbation of PC growth, the need for two emergency surgeries, and a massive heart attack could all have been avoided if measures relating to the prevention of flare had been undertaken.

The significance of biochemical flare on the outcome of patients treated with LHRH agonists who are not protected from the initial surge in testosterone is unknown. However, since testosterone promotes the growth of PC, it would seem prudent to prevent flare of any kind. A PowerPoint lecture on Flare can be downloaded from the PCRI Web site at www.pcri.org at no charge.

New Drug Prevents Flare

Abarelix (Plenaxis™), a new drug approved by the FDA in November, 2003, blocks LH by a different mechanism. This agent, an LHRH *antagonist*, immediately stops LH production without any testosterone surge and the associated increase in PSA. In contrast, the LHRH *agonists* currently in use (Lupron, Zoladex, Trelstar LA, Viadur and Eligard) cause an initial testosterone surge that leads to an initial increase in PSA before LH is down-regulated. In a study by McLeod et al,[106] 92 of 179 men (51%) achieved a testosterone level of ≤ 20 ng/dl by day 15 after Abarelix versus none of the 88 men who had received leuprolide acetate (Lupron®). The percent reduction in testosterone on day 15 after Abarelix was more than three times greater than that of Lupron (Fig. 57). In addition, LHRH antag-

141

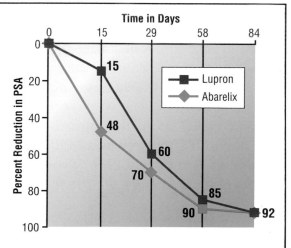

Figure 57: Percent Reduction in PSA Comparing Abarelix with Lupron.
The PSA-lowering effect of Abarelix is significantly greater than that of Lupron at days 15 and 29 after initiation of either drug (p < 0.001 and p = 0.001, respectively). There is no testosterone surge with Abarelix and no early rise in PSA as seen with conventional LHRH agonists. Since this increase in PSA usually occurs before day 15, the graph does not portray the actual increase in PSA resulting from testosterone surge since measurements of testosterone and PSA were not taken on days 4-10. Modified after McLeod et al.[106]

onists cause long-term suppression of follicle stimulating hormone (FSH).[107] FSH appears to be a growth factor for PC and FSH receptors have been detected on PC cells.[108] Current LHRH agonist drugs also decrease FSH initially, but after months of their use FSH starts to rise.

ADT and the Induction of Bone Loss

One of the most important and common side-effects of ADT is bone loss or resorption. This compromises the integrity of the bones and over time can result in fractures, bone pain, and shortening of height as the spinal vertebral bodies compress. **There are, however, effective treatments that can prevent these adverse effects of ADT and that can reverse osteoporosis or osteopenia induced by ADT and/or other causes. At the same time, these treatments have direct effects against the prostate cancer cell.** The operative theory here is based on the fact that the bone marrow is rich in growth factors that stimulate PC replication. In circumstances of excessive bone resorption, such growth factors are released and thus have detrimental side-effects to the man with PC.

Preventing bone resorption or correcting excessive bone resorption has become an important part of PC management. The mainstay of such therapy involves the use of a class of compounds called bisphosphonates (Table 12). These represent a major advance in the treatment of PC. We anticipate that they will become routine drugs in the everyday management of the man with PC and possibly play a major role in the prevention of PC. The PCRI Web site at www.pcri.org has a Web cast entitled "Bone Integrity Affects the Natural History of Prostate Cancer" from August 2001 as well as a PCRI *Insights* review of this subject published in January 1999. *If you want to know more about PC and Bone Loss, refer to Appendix B, Section 4.14.*

Table 12: Functions and Properties of Bisphosphonate Compounds.

Bisphosphonates (BPs) are one of the most important classes of compounds involved with integrative care of the cancer patient. At face value, these compounds appear to be only of importance in treating osteoporosis or osteopenia, but given the intimate relationship between the bone micro-environment and the growth and stimulation and possible causation of cancer, the BPs have tremendous possibilities in altering the natural history of prostate cancer as well as other malignancies.[109-114]

Function or *Property*	Fosamax®	Actonel®	Aredia®	Zometa®
Causes APOPTOSIS (programmed cell death) of osteoclast	+	+	+	+
Decreases SIGNALING to osteoclast precursor cells	+	+	+	+
Decreases osteoclast ATTACHMENT to bone matrix	+	+	+	+
Inhibits osteoblast-mediated osteoclast ACTIVATION	+	+	+	+
Causes APOPTOSIS of the PC cell	+	+	+	+
Interferes with ADHESION of tumor cell to bone matrix	+	+	+	+
Administered Orally	+	+	–	–
Administered Intravenously	–	–	+	+
Intravenous Administration 1.5–2 hours	–	–	+	–
Intravenous Administration 15 minutes	–	–	–	+
Can Cause an Acute Phase Response*	–	–	+	+

143

* An acute phase response (APR) may be seen within 24-36 hours after the first time an amino-bisphosphonate is given. It may be characterized by fever, chills, bone and muscle aches, malaise, and occasionally kidney injury. The risk of an APR is lessened by giving a smaller intravenous dose on the occasion of the first administration of the amino-bisphosphonate.[115] For Aredia, that first-time dose appears to be 30 mg. For Zometa, the recommended dose is 1 mg.

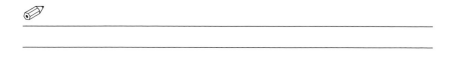

ADT as Primary Therapy for Earlier Stage PC

As described earlier, RP, RT, and cryosurgery are invasive procedures that have the <u>potential</u> to seriously affect a man's quality of life. Therefore, some men choose primary ADT because they are unwilling to undergo a more invasive treatment due to health issues, because of advanced age, because of fear of surgery or RT, or for other reasons. Other men, concerned over the likelihood that these standard forms of eradicating PC may cause *permanent* impotence, dry orgasms or other significant effects on their sexual performance, have elected ADT as a primary treatment for PC with the hope that the duration of such therapy would be limited or at the least intermittent. While ADT quickly results in decreased libido and impotence in almost all men, many men are using ADT as primary treatment with the idea that if the disease is brought under control with ADT, they may be able to stop ADT intermittently for long periods and still have an intact prostate and neurovascular bundles with preservation of potency.

144

Intermittent ADT Test Results

The above patient-driven factors led to a study, initiated in 1990 and published in 2000, of intermittent androgen deprivation (IAD) for a selected group of patients.[116] These were men who had achieved an <u>undetectable PSA defined as any value less than 0.05 ng/ml</u> while undergoing therapy with ADT_2 (LHRH-A and an anti-androgen) or ADT_3 (ADT_2 plus Proscar® or Avodart®). The hypothesis for this study was that ADT should be most beneficial in those patients who demonstrate the greatest drop in PSA, as this would indicate exquisite sensitivity of the targeted tumor cell population to androgen deprivation. In other words, ADT should be highly effective against predominantly homogeneous PC tumor populations that represent androgen-dependent PC (ADPC).

Why should patients with any significant amount of androgen-independent PC (AIPC) respond to ADT with a similar intense drop in PSA since ADT is meant to be directed against tumor cells that are *dependent* on androgen for their growth and vitality? If we were specialists in infectious disease administering an anti-bacterial therapy, we would expect it to show optimal results solely on a sensitive bacterial population and certainly not on a mixed infection consisting of bacteria and fungi. If some men diagnosed with PC have a mixed population of ADPC + AIPC at diagnosis, or anytime in the course of their disease, we can't expect a very selective therapy like conventional ADT to be effective across the board.

In fact, the preponderance of patients for whom conventional ADT has been used in the past are advanced PC patients with bone and/or lymph node metastases. This is the least favorable population to treat because these are the very patients with the highest probability that AIPC comprises a significant component of their tumor cell population.

Despite this obvious flaw in treatment strategy, conventional ADT has been used in many thousands of such patients, and conclusions based on the results of studies have been flawed because this critical point has not been given proper consideration.

Strum et al evaluated 255 patients previously untreated with androgen deprivation therapy. Of these, 216 (85%) achieved an UD-PSA (< 0.05 ng/ml) on either ADT_2 or ADT_3. Ninety-three (43%) of the 216 elected to stop ADT after maintaining a UD-PSA for an average of one year. Of these 93 patients, 52 were on ADT_2 and 41 were on ADT_3. During the "off-phase" of IAD, the PSA was checked periodically and patients were advised to restart ADT if the PSA reached 5.0 ng/ml for ADT_2 treated patients and 2.5 ng/ml for ADT_3 treated patients. The reason for restarting ADT_3 at a PSA of 2.5 ng/ml rather than 5.0

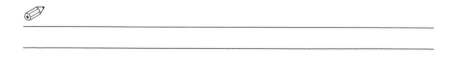

ng/ml as with ADT_2 was based on literature showing that Proscar routinely resulted in a 50% reduction in serum PSA values.[117] Since patients in the off-phase of ADT_3 were continued on Proscar® as compared to patients in the off-phase of ADT_2 who received no maintenance ADT, a different criterion was used to decide on when to restart a new cycle of ADT. The 52 ADT_2 patients were the basis for Strum et al's first report on IAD.[116] The researchers examined the group's time on ADT_2 versus the time off ADT_2 during the "intermittent" phase of this IAD approach. Overall, the average duration of the on-phase of IAD was 16 months.

The average off-phase duration for all ADT_2 patients in this study was 15.5 months with a range of 3.2 to 87+ months. In 28 patients who maintained a UD-PSA for at least one year, the average off-phase duration increased to 29 months (range 7.8

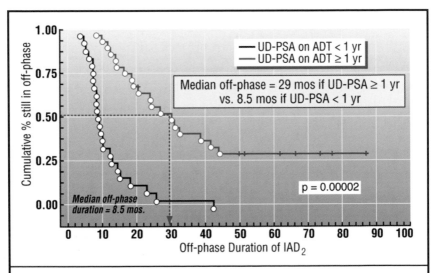

Figure 58: Intermittent Androgen Deprivation with ADT_2 (IAD_2)—Using Criteria of Undetectable PSA (UD-PSA). *Patients who achieved and maintained an UD-PSA for at least 12 months had a significantly longer time off ADT during their intermittent treatment approach compared to those who reached an UD-PSA but did not stay on ADT_2 for at least 12 months.*[116]

to 87+ months), with nine (32%) still off IAD after an average follow-up of over five years. In patients who did not maintain an UD-PSA for at least 12 months, the average off-phase duration was 8.5 months (Fig. 58).

For the ADT_3 patients who received finasteride (Proscar®) during their on-treatment period and also during their "off-phase" (maintenance period) of treatment, achieving and maintaining a UD-PSA for at least 12 months showed striking results. As shown in Figure 59, **these patients had an average time-off treatment duration of 44 months, during which time they were able to recover testosterone function and resolve many**

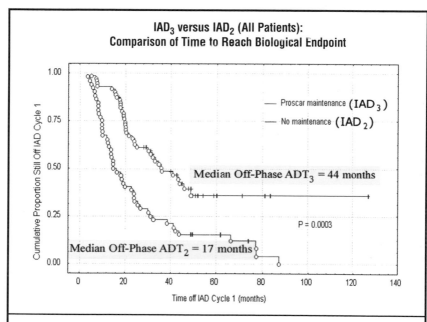

Figure 59: IAD_3—Using Proscar in Addition to ADT_2. *Patients who used 3-drug ADT (ADT_3) and who were eligible to go off treatment based on achieving and maintaining an UD-PSA for greater than one year (IAD_3) had an average time-off treatment duration of 44 months versus 17 months for patients on ADT_2 using a similar strategy for Intermittent Androgen Deprivation (IAD_2). In IAD_2 patients, the criterion for restarting ADT was a PSA that had increased to 5.0 ng/ml versus a 2.5 ng/ml end-point used for IAD_3 patients.*

if not all of their androgen deprivation signs and symptoms.

While this data is striking, it should be pointed out that the most impressive results were obtained in the subset of patients who had PSA recurrence (PSAR) after RP or RT or after both RP and RT and who selected IAD_3 as their next choice of therapy. The average time-off therapy for these patients has exceeded five years and still has not been reached (Fig. 60).

Using a somewhat different approach, Leibowitz et al achieved outstanding results in 110 consecutive patients with clinical stages T1-3 who refused any form of local therapy and who were treated with ADT_3. The average total treatment duration was 13 months and all patients had their PSA levels decline to ≤ 0.1 ng/ml. Eighty-four percent of the patients had T1c-T2a

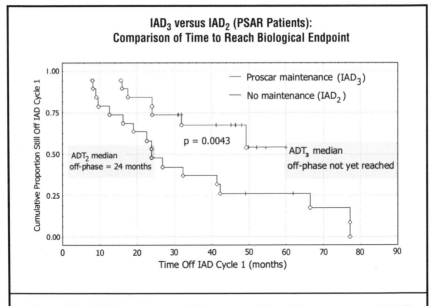

Figure 60: PSA Recurrence—IAD₃ versus IAD₂. *PSA recurrence (PSAR) patients electing IAD₃ do exceptionally well and have an average off-time that has exceeded 60 months. Even IAD₂ patients in this category do well with an average time-off treatment of two years.[118]*

disease. Fifty-one percent had a Gleason score of 4 to 6. With an average follow-up period of 36 months from the start of ADT$_3$, the mean PSA level was 1.3 ng/ml. Eighty-five of their 110 patients have been off ADT for ≥ 12 months with a mean PSA level of 1.6 ng/ml and have only received Proscar maintenance at 5 mg per day. As of May 2000, no patient in this series had required further treatment (personal communication from Dr. Leibowitz).

The major differences in the IAD approach of Strum et al versus Leibowitz et al are that (1) the former study required the achievement and maintenance of an undetectable PSA (UD-PSA) defined as less than 0.05 ng/ml to be part of the study, (2) the dose of Casodex employed was 50 mg per day rather than 150 mg per day, and (3) the induction and maintenance dose of Proscar was 5 mg twice a day rather than once a day. Certainly, both studies are provocative enough to warrant a large-scale trial of IAD$_3$ versus IAD$_2$, especially in the settings of clinically localized PC or PSA recurrence (PSAR) after RP, RT or cryosurgery.

149

Sequential Androgen Blockade (SAB)

Sequential Androgen Blockade (SAB) is a variation of ADT. It involves a two-medication approach intended to stop PC growth using androgen deprivation focused at the level of the tumor cell, **while at the same time maintaining normal serum testosterone levels so that sexual function will hopefully be preserved.**

Typically, the agents used are an anti-androgen (Eulexin or Casodex) and a 5-alpha reductase enzyme inhibitor (Proscar or Avodart). It is called "sequential androgen blockade" because (1) the anti-androgen blocks the androgen receptors on the prostate cancer cell, thus preventing testosterone and it's more potent metabolite DHT from binding to those receptors and stimulating PC growth, and (2) Proscar or Avodart reinforces

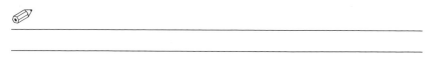

this anti-cancer activity by inhibiting the enzyme 5-alpha reductase which leads to a dramatic decrease in the conversion of testosterone to DHT (refer to Tables 11A and 11B).

Patients on SAB should be aware that high serum testosterone levels commonly achieved with this approach result in increased estrogen (estradiol) levels as a result of metabolic conversion of testosterone to estrogen by the enzyme "aromatase." These increased levels of estradiol cause hypersensitivity of the nipples and breast enlargement (gynecomastia). These hormonal effects of SAB may be prevented by prophylactic radiation of the breast tissue or blocked by the use of agents such as Arimidex® or Exemestane® that inhibit aromatase enzymes. Other possible treatment considerations could include the use of either Tamoxifen (Nolvadex®) or Raloxifene (Evista®) to block the estrogen receptors within breast tissue. If the patient and the physician are unaware of this side-effect of gynecomastia, psychological trauma with depression may occur due to the pain and embarrassment caused by breast pain and enlargement. Once a significant degree of gynecomastia has occurred, it does not respond well to treatment with radiation therapy nor does it significantly disappear when SAB or other forms of ADT are stopped. However, the breast and nipple pain associated with gynecomastia in such a setting may be dramatically relieved with the use of Nolvadex at doses of 10-30 mgs per day; the low dose of 10 mg was usually effective.[119]

Therefore, men who are considering any therapy that has the potential to induce significant gynecomastia should consider *prophylactic* RT to the breast tissue at a dose of 300-400 cGy a day for four days. Although aromatase inhibitors will block conversion of testosterone to estrogen, which in turn will prevent breast enlargement, it is important to point out that there is no data yet published on the effect these aromatase inhibitors may have on prostate cancer growth in the context of

SAB. In other words, it is possible that the estrogen produced in this setting, via the metabolism of testosterone by aromatase, may have inherent anti-cancer activity consistent with what we know about the anti-PC effects of estrogen.

Conventional ADT, unlike SAB, lowers serum testosterone. In fact, the goal of conventional ADT is to reduce serum testosterone to less than 20 ng/dl (0.69 nM/L). **Most of the adverse effects of conventional ADT administered over a relatively short term (less than two years) are typically reversible once the body naturally resumes testosterone production.** *If you want to know more about SAB, refer to Appendix B, Section 4.15.*

ADS: The Androgen Deprivation Syndrome

With the exception of hot flushes and impotency, the side-effects of ADT experienced by PC patients have until recently been discounted by most physicians and ascribed to signs of "old age." In 1998, we described a spectrum of clinical and laboratory abnormalities in PC patients that were associated with ADT. These men were physically active and in good general health. The authors termed this the "androgen deprivation syndrome" (ADS) and suggested that ADS represented a compressed, accelerated and exaggerated form of male menopause.[120] ADS is described in detail in the January 1999 issue of the PCRI newsletter *Insights.*

151

Since testosterone is a key substance affecting virtually every organ system in the male body, ADS can involve bone, blood, skin, hair, muscle, memory, and personality as well as sex drive and genitalia size. What was learned from careful observation and medical histories taken from patients undergoing ADT was that the spectrum of symptoms relating to androgen deprivation therapy was highly variable from patient to patient. Some patients seemed hardly bothered by castrate testosterone

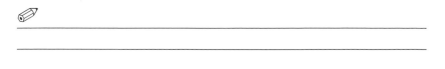

levels while others were overtly affected. As with all therapies for human maladies, successful treatment involves understanding the concept of therapeutic index (TI). Therapeutic index equates with the treatment benefits divided by the treatment side-effects.

$$\text{THERAPEUTIC INDEX} = \frac{\text{TREATMENT BENEFIT}}{\text{TREATMENT SIDE-EFFECTS}}$$

Improving the TI of ADT has involved the ability to achieve a testosterone level of less than 20 ng/dl (or < 0.69 nM/L) after starting ADT, while at the same time minimizing the treatment side-effects of ADT. In achieving both goals, we have learned a vast amount about prostate cancer and the myriad effects that testosterone has on the human male body. In achieving both goals, we have improved the quality and quantity of life of men with PC. Therefore, it is important to emphasize that learning about the possible side-effects of ADT should not dissuade the patient from embarking on a course of ADT but rather direct him to focus on what measures can be used to accentuate the positive aspects of ADT while minimizing the negative. For example, the aches and pains that *may* relate to the use of ADT dramatically disappear with the use of bisphosphonate compounds e.g. Fosamax®, Actonel®, Aredia® and Zometa®. At the same time, these very compounds benefit the patient in preventing osteopenia or osteoporosis while also having an anti-prostate cancer effect and apparently stabilizing the bone micro-environment to decrease the incidence of bone metastases. Treatment is available for most of the adverse effects that may be possibly encountered as part of ADS. Many, but not all, of these signs and symptoms can be prevented, corrected and/or reduced.

Few patients experience all of the possible side-effects of ADT. Younger patients who have a greater overall drop in testosterone resulting from ADT seem to be more sensitive to the side-effects of androgen deprivation, but this too is variable.

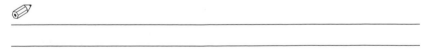

The PC patient must not be reluctant or embarrassed to speak freely to his physician about the occurrence of any new symptoms once ADT has been initiated.

To gain an appreciation of the incidence of ADS in men undergoing ADT, the data from 77 hormone naïve men with PC receiving combination LHRH agonist and anti-androgen are shown in Table 13.

Table 13: The Androgen Deprivation Syndrome or ADS in 77 Men During ADT. These were the seven most common signs or symptoms found in men undergoing ADT. If anything, these percentages are likely underestimates of the actual incidence due to the reticence of many male patients to discuss their symptoms. ADS was graded as absent (0), occasional (1), frequent/bothersome (2) or requiring drug treatment (3). After Strum et al.[120,121]

Signs and Symptoms	Onset (months)	Grade of Severity and Incidence Number patients (with ADS/total patients)		
		0–1	2-3	Totals
Mental/Emotional Changes	1-2+	2 (3%)	11 (14%)	13 (17%)
Bone and Joint Pain	2-6+	20 (26%)	3 (4%)	23 (30%)
Gynecomastia	>12	14 (18%)	15 (19%)	29 (38%)
Anemia	2-12	25 (32%)	10 (13%)	35 (45%)
Hot flushes	1-2	18 (23%)	19 (25%)	37 (48%)
Weakness	1-4+	39 (51%)	4 (5%)	43 (56%)
Hypercholesterolemia	4-6	14 (18%)	26 (34%)	44 (57%)

153

The recovery of natural testosterone production eventually restores normal testosterone blood levels. This resolves most of the adverse effects caused by androgen deprivation. This also presumes that the patient is not taking an anti-androgen or other medication that blocks interaction of testosterone and/or DHT with the androgen receptor. It should be mentioned that some men, highly sensitive to the effects of ADT, have very delayed recovery of their natural testosterone production and some haven't yet recovered this function despite four to five years of follow-up monitoring (Strum SB: personal communication). **Men who have received continuous ADT for longer than two years are those most prone to delayed recovery or possible non-recovery of normal testosterone production.**[122,123] The incidence, scope and treatment of ADS are now subjects of increasing interest and research effort.[124] *If you want to know more about ADT Side-effects, refer to Appendix B, Section 4.16.*

PC SPES™

PC SPES™ is an oral form of ADT comprised of seven Chinese herbs and one American herb. A major part of the anti-PC activity of PC SPES™ relates to its estrogenic activity. However, other mechanisms of action of PC SPES™ have been postulated.[125,126] PC SPES™ has typically been used in the setting of PC progression occurring during conventional ADT. An increasing number of patients are now using this as a treatment for earlier stage PC. Since PC progression during ADT most commonly represents androgen-independent PC, PC SPES™ is now accepted as an herbal therapy that demonstrates activity against androgen-independent PC as well as androgen-dependent PC.[127,128]

Since PC SPES™ is estrogenic, its side-effects include diminished libido and impotence due to the lowering of testosterone, as well as nipple sensitivity and breast enlargement. In about 5-7% of patients, PC SPES™ is associated with thrombotic or blood-clotting events such as deep vein thrombosis (DVT) of the lower extremities and pulmonary embolism. The thrombotic events induced by estrogenic compounds are due to an induced coagulation abnormality called antithrombin-III deficiency.[129]

The treatment of choice to prevent thrombotic events associated with antithrombin-III deficiency is Coumadin®. Although many physicians are using aspirin in place of Coumadin, aspirin has no effect against antithrombin-III deficiency. Therefore, aspirin will not abolish the abnormal coagulation findings in patients treated with PC SPES™ and other oral estrogenic compounds including DES® and Emcyt®.[130] A positive aspect of any estrogenic therapy of PC is that it does not cause the bone loss associated with standard ADT.[131]

At the time of publication of *A Primer on Prostate Cancer*, PC SPES™ was no longer being made available to men with PC due to the finding of Coumadin, and/or DES, and/or Indomethacin (Indocin®) within the product. There are positive lessons to be learned, however, from our experiences with PC SPES™ and the renewed interest in estrogens as effective agents against PC. Some of these lessons include:

- Estrogenic compounds have activity against androgen-dependent AND androgen-independent PC. They therefore have a broader spectrum of activity than the LHRH agonists.

- Estrogenic compounds administered to PC patients with less extensive disease are often associated with dramatic responses consistent with similarly impressive results obtained when other forms of ADT are used for localized rather than metastatic PC.

- Estrogenic compounds used against PC are not associated with bone loss and the attendant complications of bone resorption, e.g. osteoporosis, release of bone-derived growth factors having the potential to stimulate PC growth, acceleration of coronary artery disease and vascular calcifications, potential role in causation or aggravation of neurodegenerative diseases due to IL-6 release associated with bone loss.

- Understanding the mechanism of estrogen-induced venous thrombosis and the appropriate methods of anti-coagulation to prevent this side-effect of estrogenic compounds such as DES and estramustine phosphate (Emcyt®).

- Understanding that the route of administration of estrogens is important insofar as the incidence of thrombotic side-effects. The use of transdermal patches such as Estraderm® or Climara®, or the use of intramuscular or intravenous forms of estrogen all avoid the first-pass metabolism of estrogens through the liver, which occurs with oral administration of estrogens. It is the metabolism of estrogen within the liver that appears to be associated with the occurrence of the complication of venous thrombotic events.

Watchful Waiting or Objectified Observation

Some patients feel that they can preserve their quality of life by avoiding more aggressive treatment. Watchful waiting may be an option for patients if the PC is objectively documented to be slow growing and organ-confined. Such patients may require no treatment for prolonged periods of time, if ever.

Watchful waiting does not mean doing nothing. It implies that the patient is embarking on a regimen of diet and exercise best suited to his condition in consultation with his doctor. See Section IX in Appendix A on Preventive and Wholistic Approaches for specific information on what the experts recommend in this regard and what current research indicates. In addition, the July 1999 issue of the PCRI newsletter *Insights* has a review of nutritional aspects of PC. You can access this via the PCRI Web site. Most recently, in May of 2001, the PCRI has published a pamphlet entitled "What You Should Know About Prostate Cancer." This reviews additional literature on diet and vitamin supplements and discusses the early detection of PC.

Some patients on watchful waiting are using nutritional supplements (vitamins, minerals, herbs), meditation, exercise, prayer, humor and a variety of other methods in a concerted attempt to control the disease. Such patients initially should closely monitor the PC in order to ascertain the tempo of the disease and then periodically undergo laboratory and radiologic testing and physical examination to ensure the cancer has not become more aggressive or extensive. Such testing allows for interval assessments of disease volume and extent and enables the periodic calculation of PSA doubling time (PSADT) and PSA velocity (PSAV). These are essential steps to *initially* determine if watchful waiting is a realistic option as well as to monitor the course and status of patients who choose such an **157** approach.

Because watchful waiting mandates a sophisticated level of surveillance, we prefer the term "objectified observation" to the more passive term watchful waiting. The PCRI Web site at **www.prostate-cancer.org** has two software programs: **PC Tools I** (click on "Observation") and a **Tumor Volume Calculator** that can be used together to obtain a sense of the risk of spread of PC to the seminal vesicles and lymph nodes based on inputs of calculated PC volume and PSA doubling time (Figs. 61 and 62).

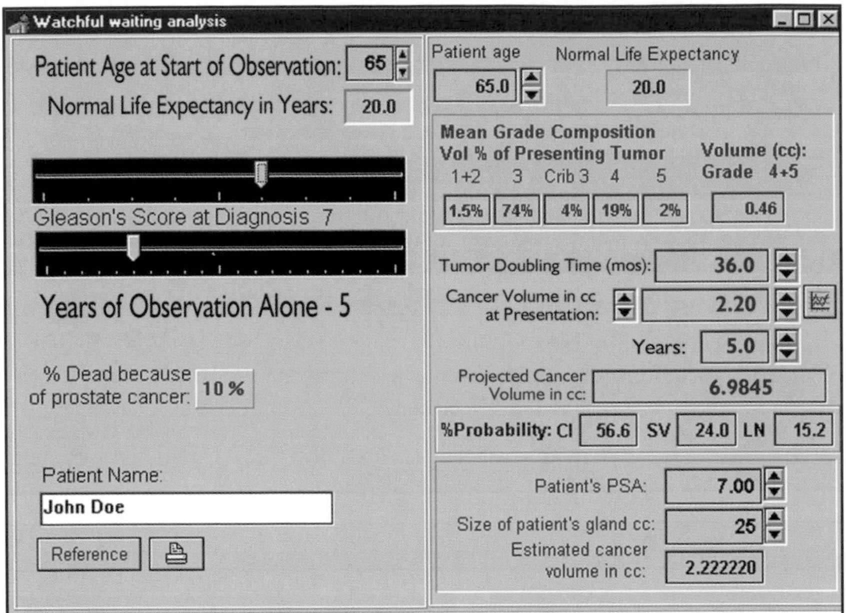

Figure 61: Two Computer Software Tools to Obtain Projected Outcome Using Watchful Waiting. *The program on the left side of this monitor screen-shot is based on work by Albertsen et al.[132] The program on the right necessitates first calculating tumor volume and PSA doubling times and then inserting those results into the program. Although there is a cancer volume calculator shown in the lower right portion of the figure, we have replaced this with another software program which more accurately calculates cancer volume. This is shown in Figure 62 and is also available at the PCRI Web site. In addition, the PSA doubling time calculator (tumor doubling time) can be found within the PC Tools II software suite. All of these programs can be downloaded without cost from the Web site.*

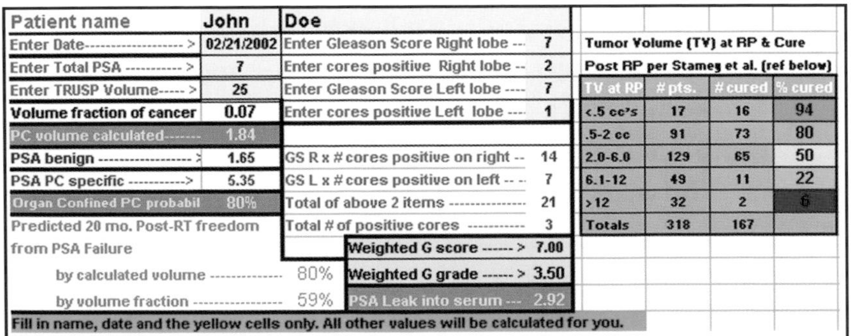

Figure 62: Tumor Volume Calculator. *This Excel software program is very easy to use. The inputs required are a validated Gleason score or scores, number of cores with PC from involved sides of the prostate gland, the total PSA and the gland volume determined by transrectal ultrasound of the prostate. These items of information needed to calculate tumor volume are highlighted in yellow within the program. This software has been created based on the peer-reviewed publications of Aihara et al, and D'Amico et al.[32,133,134]*

Chemotherapy of PC

Chemotherapy is used in the treatment of patients who have metastatic PC in the hope of slowing the growth of the cancer and prolonging life. Many patients with advanced disease face the issue of deciding when to begin chemotherapy. Some doctors prefer to attack PC with chemotherapy when the body is strong and the cancer is weak rather than waiting until the cancer is strong and the body is weak. These are decisions to be made by the doctor-patient partnership on a case-by-case basis.

If we are to learn how to optimally use chemotherapy against PC, we should use our experiences with breast cancer to guide us. Prostate and breast cancer are brother-sister diseases with striking similarities in their endocrine responsiveness as well as the active chemotherapeutic agents used in the treatment of both diseases. With breast cancer, we have made significant gains in prolonging life by the early administration of chemotherapy.

159

A listing of the major chemotherapy regimens active in the treatment of PC along with response rates, protocol details and references can be found in a compendium called "Disease Prevention and Treatment." This is part of an extensive chapter on prostate cancer co-authored by Stephen B. Strum and Jonathan E. McDermed. It is published by the Life Extension Foundation and can be ordered for a modest price (1-866-820-7457). Also available on the LEF Web site at **http://www.lef.org/protocols/prtcl-136.shtml.** The April 2000 issue of *Insights* also contains an extensive review of Taxotere, one of the most active agents in the chemotherapeutic treatment of PC. Taxotere was approved by the FDA in May 2004 for the treatment of advanced prostate cancer. The scope of this *Primer* does not allow for a full discourse on the chemotherapy of PC. A companion to *The Primer* on this topic has been proposed.

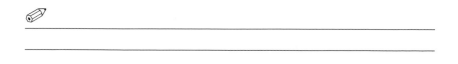

Treatments on the Horizon

There is currently no "magic bullet" to cure PC. However, research and clinical trials are proceeding to develop medications that will search out and destroy cancer cells in the body by various methods. In the future, some of these therapies will be approved by drug regulatory agencies such as the FDA and others and then will be made available to men with prostate cancer.

Aptosyn

Aptosyn® (Exisulind) is a drug that has been successfully used in clinical trials and is undergoing further testing. It directs precancerous and cancerous tissue to undergo programmed cell death (apoptosis) without harming healthy tissue. It does this by facilitating an enzymatic pathway that results in activation of a family of enzymes called caspases that are crucial to the process of apoptosis.[135] Aptosyn is manufactured by Cell Pathways, Inc. FDA approval of this agent is still pending.

Provenge

Also being tested are immunologic therapies that employ the body's own immune system to cause death of cancer cells. Therapies employing this mechanism are commonly called "vaccine" therapies. Dendritic cells (DC) are immune system cells that identify foreign proteins (antigens) and present them to other immune cells (T-cells) involved in cancer cell destruction. In current clinical trials involving PC patients, blood is removed from the patient and that portion containing DC is isolated. These immature dendritic cells are then incubated with proteins (PAP, or prostatic acid phosphatase, for example) outside of the patient's body to activate them. Dendreon Corporation is involved in two such trials where the DC are activated by a combination of PAP and GM-CSF (granulocyte macrophage-colony stimulating factor). These "turned-on" den-

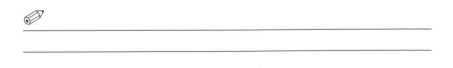

dritic cells (Provenge) are then infused back into the patient's body with the goal of destroying prostate cancer cells (Fig. 63).

The October 2001 issue of *Insights* contains two articles on dendritic cells. In a clinical trial of hormone-refractory PC patients by Small et al, all patients developed immune responses to the recombinant fusion protein used to prepare Provenge, and 38% developed immune responses to PAP. Three patients had a greater than 50% decline in PSA level, and another three patients had 25-49% decreases in PSA. The time to disease progression correlated with development of an immune response to PAP and with the dose of dendritic cells received.[136]

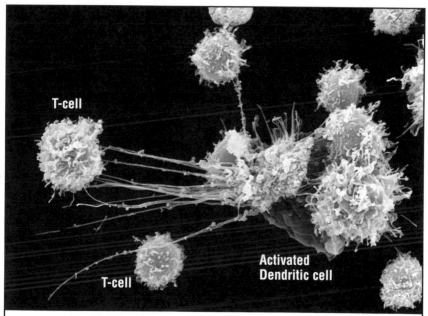

Figure 63: Dendritic Cell Activating T-cells. *The activated DC is in contact with T-cells. Long filamentous processes of the DC present a protein (antigen) to educate T-cells so they can recognize specific antigens on the surface of cancer cells and destroy them. T-cells, when activated, are the immune system's most potent defense against cancer. This activation of T-cells by DC is the essence of Provenge therapy. This is a photograph from a scanning electron microscope provided through the courtesy of Dendreon Corporation.*

Angiostatin and Endostatin

These are two of many anti-angiogenesis agents which are now under study in clinical trials. In order for tumors to develop, grow and metastasize, they need various nutrients that are delivered to them through a network of capillaries. The process by which a tumor is able to establish new vessel growth is called angiogenesis. It is controlled by various angiogenic factors, some of which are produced by the tumor cells themselves or by tumor-associated cells such as fibroblasts or macrophages. In prostate cancer, one of the most important of these angiogenic factors is called Vascular Endothelial Growth Factor or VEGF (pronounced veg-F). VEGF promotes the growth of cells that line the capillaries and plays an important role in capillary permeability and the metastatic process by which cancer spreads to other sites in the body. VEGF is synthesized within the prostate by normal ductal epithelial cells, prostate adenocarcinoma cells and by tumor-infiltrating lymphocytes.[137,138]

162

Of great importance is the fact that androgens stimulate the production of VEGF, whether the cancer cells are composed of androgen-dependent PC (ADPC) or androgen-independent PC (AIPC). ADT markedly decreases VEGF from as much as 50–90%. It is reasonable, therefore, to emphasize the importance of lowering testosterone to castrate levels defined as less than 20 ng/dl as well as the need to maintain testosterone suppression even when the PC is characterized as AIPC.[139] Studies are in progress combining ADT with other anti-angiogenic agents to kill both androgen-dependent and androgen-independent PC. Anti-angiogenesis agents such as Angiostatin and Endostatin may eventually be available to "turn off the switch" in molecules that signal blood vessels to develop and nourish tumors. Without such nutrients, the tumor shrinks. *If you want to know more about Angiogenic Factors and PC, refer to Appendix B, Section 4.17.*

Atrasentan: An Endothelin Receptor Antagonist

Endothelins are among the most potent substances to cause blood vessel narrowing or vasoconstriction. They are structurally peptides (a combination of amino acids) and are subclassified into endothelin types I, II or III. ET-1 is produced by normal prostate epithelial cells and the semen of the normal male ejaculate is very rich in ET-1. Some of the normal functions of ET-1 appear to be related to sperm activity and to the smooth muscle contraction within the prostate.

Excessive amounts of endothelin type I (ET-1) have been implicated in hypertension, heart disease, bronchoconstriction, kidney damage and brain injury. Prostate cancer research has shown that ET-1 also stimulates the growth of the osteoblast, a cell found within the bone that promotes bone formation. In PC patients, the *excessive* stimulation of osteoblasts results in the dense bone lesions or "osteoblastic" metastases that are characteristic of advanced PC. Such findings are usually clinically associated with blood elevations of the bone enzyme alkaline phosphatase and often elevations of serum PAP.[140] Studies of prostate cancer cell lines have indicated that ET-1 is produced by every PC cell line so far evaluated.[140]

Endothelin-1 (ET-1) is, therefore, a prostate cancer cell product that stimulates osteoblasts and also acts as a vasoconstrictor that may be responsible for bone pain in metastatic PC. ET-1 facilitates its action by interacting with the specific receptor of its intended target cells (Fig. 64). The receptor is a docking site to engage the chemical message of the amino acids that make up ET-1.

Recently, an ET receptor antagonist, i.e. an agent that blocks a specific ET receptor, has been studied in patients with either metastatic or non-metastatic androgen-independent PC. This agent is Atrasentan®. In 244 patients with androgen-independ-

163

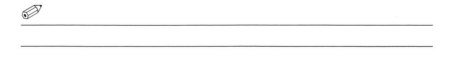

ent prostate cancer (AIPC) randomized to receive Atrasentan at either a 2.5 mg or 10 mg single daily oral dose, there was evidence that Atrasentan, compared to placebo, delayed the time to both clinical progression and to PSA progression. This occurred most significantly in those patients receiving the 10mg dose. With this dose, the median times for clinical progression of PC were 129 days for placebo group versus 196 days for the Atrasentan group. For PSA progression, the median times were 71 for the placebo group versus 155 days for the Atrasentan group. Atrasentan at both the 2.5 mg and 10 mg dose lessened the rise in other biologic markers of PC activity such as PAP, LDH, and alkaline phosphatase compared to placebo.[142]

In another report, involving 419 patients with AIPC, the results of Atrasentan at 2.5 mg and 10 mg doses were compared to

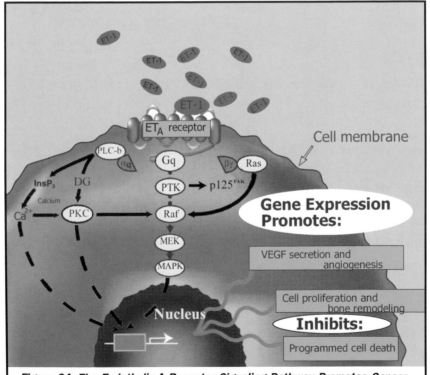

Figure 64: The Endothelin-A Receptor Signaling Pathway Promotes Cancer Cell Growth. *Binding of ET-1 to the ET_A receptor initiates signaling through the Ras and Raf pathways. This signaling terminates in gene expression which promotes various cell functions that include: bone remodeling, cell proliferation, secretion of VEGF, angiogenesis, and also the inhibition of programmed cell death (apoptosis). Modified after Bagnato et al.[141]*

those given a placebo. Atrasentan, in a dose-dependent fashion, was shown to prevent any increase in bone resorption markers such as Pyrilinks-D™ (Dpd) or Metra™ DPD and N-telopeptides.[143] Elevated bone resorption markers such as Dpd have been shown to be associated with distant metastases, even in men with apparent organ-confined PC.[144-146]

As of July 2002, there are two Atrasentan trials currently open to PC patients. Study 244 is a clinical trial using Atrasentan in men having AIPC (hormone refractory PC) without evidence of metastatic disease while study 211 focuses on patients with AIPC having evidence of metastatic disease. In both studies the patient is randomized to either receive either Atrasentan or placebo. If disease progression occurs, and if the patient had received placebo, he is then eligible to receive Atrasentan as part of an open-label extension study. Please call 1-866-626-5649 for more detailed information. Atrasentan is produced by Abbott Laboratories in Illinois, which has applied for FDA approval under the tentative brand name "Xinlay™". More details on the Atrasentan clinical trials can be found at:

165

http://abbott.com/innovation/innovation_center.html

Oncolytic Viruses

The objective of all anti-cancer therapy is to selectively destroy cancer cells while leaving the normal cell population intact and uninjured. At the present time, viruses have been employed in anti-cancer therapy using either of two approaches:

1) Viruses acting indirectly to restore or repair cancer cells to normal by carrying genetic information which is to be inserted into the defective cells.

2) Viruses acting directly to destroy the cancer cell by causing cancer cell death or lysis.

In the first scenario, the virus transports therapeutic genes into cancer cells in an attempt to confer new genetic information to correct the uncontrolled cell growth that is characteristic of

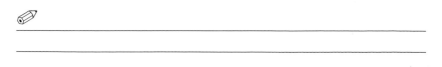

malignancy. In such approaches, the virus is acting as a vector or carrier. The second strategy, in contrast, uses specific viruses to selectively destroy or lyse cancer cells; these are called oncolytic viruses. Oncolytic viruses act directly on the tumor cell to induce their death (Fig. 65).

The use of oncolytic viruses as an anti-cancer therapy represents an approach where chances of attaining a high therapeutic index (benefit versus adverse-effects) are excellent and where the sacred quest of anti-cancer therapy may be realized. A number of oncolytic viruses that hold significant promise include Cell Genesys Viruses CG7060 and CG7870, VSV, Reolysin®, and ONYX-15, to name a few.

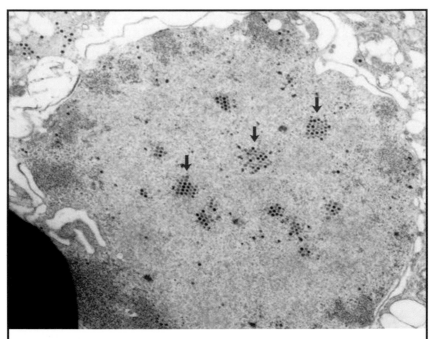

Figure 65: Adenovirus Within Prostate Cancer Cell. Packets of viruses looking like buckshot (arrows) are seen within a prostate cancer cell. Viruses are usually characterized as being either RNA or DNA viruses. A key advantage of oncolytic viruses is not only that they kill cells directly, but that they replicate and go on to infect other cancer cells.

Adenovirus Serotype 5 (Ad5) from Cell Genesys (CG7060, CG7870)

These adenoviruses were engineered to specifically seek out prostate cells that synthesize PSA. This was accomplished by removing a portion of the virus' genetic material (the viral replication promoters E1A and E1B), and inserting in its place genetic material that turns on viral replication, but only in cells that make PSA (Fig. 66). The genetic material that was inserted was the regulatory element of the PSA gene called PSE, or prostate tissue-specific enhancer. This newly created adenovirus grows only in cells expressing PSA. The original virus created by Calydon was called CN706. After Cell Genesys purchased Calydon in October 2001, this virus was renamed CG7060. This virus showed a therapeutic index ranging from 20:1 to 3,000:1. **In other words, from 20 to 3,000 prostate cancer cells were killed for each normal cell destroyed.[147] The therapeutic index for the most active chemotherapy agents ranges from 1:5 to 6:1.[148]**

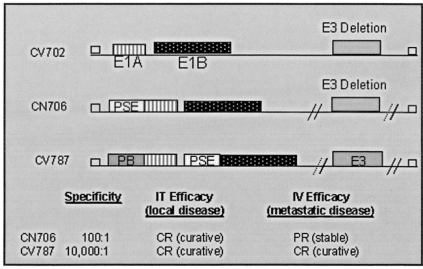

Figure 66: Viral Construction of the Cell Genesys Oncolytic Viruses. CV702 is a basic viral construct that does not include the prostate tissue-specific enhancer-promoter element called PSE, which is present in CN706 (CG7060). The most enhanced viral construction is CV787 (CG7870), which not only contains an additional prostate-specific promoter (rat probasin or PB) but also retains the E3 region that improves virus release and increases protection against the host immune response to the virus. CG7870 destroys PSA+ prostate cancer cells 10,000 times more efficiently than PSA negative cells and therefore the incorporation of the Ad5 E3 region significantly improves the target cell killing ability of CG7870.

In a Phase II study of 20 men with PSA-progressive disease after radiation therapy with evidence of local progression of disease, CG7060 was introduced into the prostate gland using a template similar to that employed during brachytherapy. An acceptable safety profile with both biochemical and histological evidence of anti-tumor activity was seen. The findings of this study[149] were:

- No significant adverse events in any of the 20 patients treated at the five dose levels.
- The PSA doubling time was prolonged in 18 of 20 patients (90%).
- Eleven patients showing the greatest antitumor response were all treated at one of the top two doses. Nine of these patients had a substantial decrease in PSA from baseline. Four of these 11 patients exhibited a PSA partial response, defined as a 50% or greater reduction in serum PSA for at least four weeks. In three of the patients, this partial response lasted for nine months or longer. The longest response duration was greater than 12 months.
- A study of post-treatment biopsy samples demonstrated that adenoviral replication—the therapeutic mechanism upon which CN706 has been designed to both target and kill prostate cancer cells—had occurred in patients.
- Sixty percent of post-treatment biopsies showed decreased PSA immunostaining.

CG7870 (formerly CN787) is currently being evaluated in a Phase I/II study involving men with metastatic PC. Patients receive only one intravenous administration of CG7870 at different dose levels. Six of 23 patients (26%) demonstrated stabilization of PSA levels for a median of four months. Three additional patients had PSA reductions of approximately 20% or greater from baseline. No serious or drug-related toxicities have been observed.

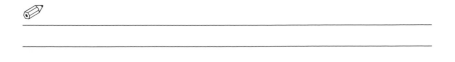

Most recently, studies of human prostate cancer cell lines have shown this oncolytic virus to have synergy with Taxane chemotherapy agents such as Taxotere or Taxol. *In vitro,* the combination of Taxane chemotherapy and CG7870 resulted in a significant increase in killing cells of the prostate cancer cell line LNCaP regardless of the timing of administration. The specificity of CG7870-based cytopathogenicity for prostate cancer cells versus normal cells was approximately 10,000 to 1 with the Taxanes. Wild-type (normal) p53 expression was also significantly elevated in the cells treated with CV7870 and Taxane. *In vivo,* using the PSA + LNCaP model of prostate cancer, a single intravenous dose of 1 x 10⁸ particles of CG7870 combined with Taxotere eliminated large preexistent distant tumors.

Moreover, toxicity studies show no synergistic increase of toxicity of this oncolytic virus when administered with either Taxotere or Taxol, but they do demonstrate a synergistic antitumor efficacy for CV7870 when combined with either of these Taxanes. The studies demonstrate an in vivo single-dose curative therapeutic index for CG7870 of over 1000:1.[150]

A phase I/II trial of CG7870 in combination with Taxotere is targeted for late 2002. In addition, trials are upcoming for CN7060, VSV, Reolysin®, ONYX-15, and other oncolytic viruses. Information about current and future clinical trials with these oncolytic viruses and other genetically engineered approaches to kill prostate cancer and other tumor types is available at:

http://www.cellgenesys.com/research/TrialEnrollment/
for Cell Genesys

http://www.onyx-pharm.com/
for Onyx Pharmaceuticals

http://www.oncolyticsbiotech.com/clinical.html
for Oncolytics.

Antisense Oligonucleotides (ASO)

The major threat to the man with prostate cancer is the emergence of Androgen-Independent PC (AIPC). **It is androgen-independent (AI) prostate cancer that most often results in advanced metastatic disease that becomes the life-taking event in this disease.** The therapies directed at the AI component of PC include agents such as estrogenic compounds (DES®, Stilphosterol®, Estraderm®, and Climara® patches), high-dose ketoconazole (HDK) + hydrocortisone (HC), as well as an assortment of chemotherapeutic drugs that include: 5-FU, Adriamycin®, Novantrone®, Velban®, Navelbine®, Etoposide®, Mitomycin-C, and most recently the taxanes such as Taxol® and Taxotere®. The patient that has AIPC or a mixture of AIPC with Androgen-Dependent PC (ADPC) may significantly benefit from any one of these treatments or a combination of these treatments if the physician is able to induce a partial or complete remission of the PC.

170 A treatment strategy that would inhibit or prevent the *emergence* of AIPC, rather than react to the development of established hormone-refractory disease would be a more rational approach to this problem. Pre-emptive or pro-active therapy, therefore, would be a superior strategy rather than reactive approaches to AIPC development. Recent advances in technology have opened new avenues to identify and target various genes involved in tumor growth and therapeutic resistance. The identification of dysfunctional genes that are expressed during AIPC progression and the investigation of their functional significance in this process has now been the focus of intense research across the world.

The chemical messages that are the expressions of gene activity and which take the form of sequences of amino acids, or more specifically nucleotides, are the most prevalent form of the cells' ability to communicate with each other. For the cancer cell population to grow and thrive, it too must be responsive to the laws of communication and balance. We can try to stop the cancer cell after its development by traditional methods of cell kill but a more clever approach would be to interfere with the life processes of the cancer cell by affecting its lines of communication. If we identify the chemical message that is maintaining a vital function for the cancer cell, and can affect this message, we can prevent cancer cell growth or affect cancer cell death.

A gene product, bcl-2, has emerged as a critical regulator of cell death and *functions to protect the cell <u>against</u> cell death (apoptosis)* in numerous tissues. Bcl-2 is part of a family of regulatory gene products, which function as either cell death antagonists (e.g. **bcl-2, Bcl-xL**) or death agonists (Bax, Bcl-Xs, Bad). The ratio of death antagonists to death agonists determines how a cell responds to an apoptotic signal. In cancer control, a desired goal is maintaining the ability of any treatment to induce apoptosis of the cancer cell. In other words, the desired communication is that of promoting death agonists and minimizing cancer cell death antagonists such as bcl-2 and Bcl-xL.

$$\frac{\text{Death Agonists}}{\text{Death Antagonists}} \cong \text{cancer cell death (apoptosis)}$$

In prostate cancer cells, bcl-2 is up-regulated within months after androgen deprivation and remains increased in AIPC tumors. Bcl-2 up-regulation after androgen deprivation serves as an adaptive mechanism to help some prostate cancer cells survive and subsequently progress to androgen independence. Bcl-2 also serves to protect the cancer cell by blocking pro-apoptotic signals by a variety of chemotherapy agents, and may contribute to multi-drug resistance which is characteristic of AIPC and other cancers.

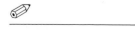

Antisense oligonucleotides (ASO) represent one such strategy to specifically target and inhibit genes involved in tumour progression and/or therapeutic resistance.[151] At a molecular level of cancer profiling, **an ASO is targeted to the messenger RNA (mRNA) of the protein responsible for cancer growth, drug resistance or whatever the pathologic process is that has given the cancer cell a survival advantage.** In a manner analogous to the principle of noise cancellation, an ASO targets a specific sequence of RNA to neutralize its biologic activity. This involves a process of *hybridization* of the complementary RNA sequence, which inhibits the expression of the disease-relevant protein (Fig. 67). Specifically, the ASO pairs up with specific nucleotide bases of mRNA. This results in inhibition of mRNA processing or translation by a variety of mechanisms including prevention of mRNA transport, splicing or translational arrest.[152] In essence, an ASO is stopping a chemical message that within the context of PC enhances our ability to kill the prostate cancer cell, prevent its growth, or affect some other vital function(s).

172

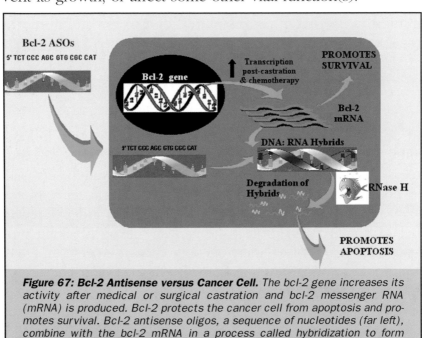

Figure 67: Bcl-2 Antisense versus Cancer Cell. *The bcl-2 gene increases its activity after medical or surgical castration and bcl-2 messenger RNA (mRNA) is produced. Bcl-2 protects the cancer cell from apoptosis and promotes survival. Bcl-2 antisense oligos, a sequence of nucleotides (far left), combine with the bcl-2 mRNA in a process called hybridization to form DNA:RNA hybrids which are broken down enzymatically by ribonuclease (RNase H). This blocks bcl-2 activity and promotes cell death (apoptosis) of the cancer cell.*

Induction of apoptotic cell death after androgen deprivation therapy or chemotherapy may be enhanced through functional inhibition of bcl-2. **ASO therapy directed against bcl-2 induces apoptosis and enhances chemosensitivity in numerous cancers.** Preclinical studies have shown that bcl-2 ASOs decreased bcl-2 protein and increased chemosensitivity in models of human melanoma[153] and prostate cancer.[154-156] In prostate cancer models, bcl-2 ASO following castration significantly delayed time to AI progression, and synergistically enhanced the activity of paclitaxel (Taxol®) in AI tumors. Synergistic activity between bcl-2 ASO and taxanes results from ASO-induced decreases in bcl-2 mRNA protein levels and taxane-induced bcl-2 phosphorylation which inhibits bcl-2 function.

Clinical Trials Using Bcl-2 Antisense

A dose escalation study of combined Genasense plus mitoxantrone (Novantrone®) was recently completed in Vancouver.[157] Twenty-six patients with AIPC were treated at seven dose levels of Genasense as a 14-day continuous intravenous (IV) infusion every 28 days with mitoxantrone given as an IV bolus on day 8. No dose limiting toxicities were observed. Hematologic toxicities were transient and included neutropenia, thrombocytopenia and lymphopenia. Two patients had > 50% reductions in PSA. Patient #1 received Genasense at 1.2 mg/kg/day and a low dose (4 mg/m2) of mitoxantrone and had symptomatic improvement in bone pain; he received a total of 6 cycles. Patient #2 also had measurable disease with a documented partial response and received 8 cycles. **Bcl-2 expression in peripheral blood lymphocytes decreased in all patients treated at the 5 mg/kg/day of Genasense.** Results from this trial suggest that biologically active doses of Genasense are well tolerated in combination with mitoxantrone without significant additional toxicity.

A Phase II trial is now underway in San Antonio and Vancouver to determine activity of combination docetaxel (Taxotere®) plus G3139 bcl-2 ASO in men with hormone refractory PC (HRPC, i.e. AIPC). Additional controlled multicenter trials in multiple myeloma, chronic lymphocytic leukemia (CLL), and lung cancer are ongoing.

Further Potential Targets For Antisense Therapy

Many ASOs are being evaluated preclinically while others are in early clinical trials in numerous cancers and other diseases. Two Phase I-II trials using ASO targeting the cell survival gene, Clusterin, will begin in Vancouver in September 2002 for men with AIPC. Additional genes currently validated as targets for antisense therapy in preclinical studies include growth factor receptor tyrosine kinases such as HER-2/*neu*, the epidermal and vascular endothelial growth factor receptors, angiogenesis factors such as VEGF, transcription factors involved in cell survival like NFκB, YB-1, and a myriad of protein kinases involved in cell cycle regulation. Specific examples include androgen receptor, Insulin Growth Factor Binding Protein 5 (IGFBP5), IGFBP2, Bcl-xL, and survivin. Although the available data are still preliminary, there is hope that some of these cancer-related targets will maintain their allure beyond preclinical testing.

This review of Antisense Oligonucleotides and the graphic in this section were contributed by Martin Gleave, M.D.

Clinical Trials

Drugs being tested and other experimental therapies are the subjects of clinical trials. Clinical trials are not usually a preferred primary treatment option. For patients who feel they have limited treatment options, clinical trials may be appropriate.

Clinical trials are done in phases, with Phase I being the most experimental. A Phase I trial is performed to ascertain proper *dosages and toxicity.* A Phase II study is conducted on a limited number of patients to establish *effectiveness*, once optimum dosage has been determined. Phase III trials *compare the effectiveness of the new treatment to current protocols* and require a widespread study population. Phase III trials precede the application for approval by the FDA (Food and Drug Administration) to make the drug or treatment available to the general public. The FDA is the United States government regulatory agency that oversees the safety and effectiveness of new drugs and medical treatments. Natural or herbal remedies are not subject to this agency's review; therefore, standards of quality of such substances vary widely in the marketplace.

If you are considering becoming involved in a clinical trial, you should research the proposed treatment thoroughly and ask questions. Do you meet the eligibility requirements of the study? Will you get the drug or will you be part of a double-blind study in which a control group does not get the medication or treatment, i.e. a placebo arm? What are the possible side-effects? Will you be able to leave the study at any time if you choose? Will you be eliminated from the trial under certain conditions? **Most importantly, are you giving up a treatment choice of known effectiveness for a new treatment where efficacy has not been determined at all?**

The costs of clinical trials are not covered by most insurance plans, but new legislation has resulted in changes in this policy for patients eligible for Medicare. This will make participation in clinical trials possible for more patients and thereby result in faster progress in bringing new medications and treatments to the general public. ∎

✔ The essence of any treatment option that employs local tumor removal (e.g. radical prostatectomy), or employs a method of treatment that destroys the tumor and surrounding local tissues (e.g. external beam RT in its various presentations, cryosurgery) is that the PC must be confined to such anatomic areas for any such treatment to be curative. If the PC has spread beyond such borders and is systemic, cure will not be achieved by such treatments.

✔ Major advances in our understanding of the nature of PC have been the result of our efforts to elaborate upon the above principle by correlating various biologic expressions of the cancer (clinical, pathological and radiologic features) with outcomes that relate to extent of disease or to response to therapy. This process creates the prognostic groups that are discussed in medical publications that relate to the success or failure of various treatment choices.

✔ The above is formalized in tens of thousands of careful observations—involving actual human life-events—manifested in correlative medical publications such as the Partin Tables, Kattan and D'Amico nomograms, Bluestein Table, and many others. Such studies use the patient's biology to teach us how to improve the outcomes of specific treatments.

✔ Just as we strive to be wholistic in our approach to the care of the patient, we must be more wholistic in learning how to identify patients most likely to succeed with our therapies or most likely to fail such treatments. We must adjust our strategy for each accordingly.

✔ If your probabilities for having organ-confined PC are high (greater than 75%), then your chance of cure with RP, RT or cryosurgery is accordingly high assuming that you have selected a physician(s) with outstanding technical skills to perform whatever curative procedure you have chosen.

✔ Incorporating the details of your unique medical profile into the selected medical and/or surgical therapies significantly minimizes treatment side-effects and increases your therapeutic index.

✔ Many of the potential adverse effects of every treatment for PC have a "work-around". The artistry and caring of your physicians should manifest itself in providing you with such fine adjustments. These involve, for the most part, preventing adverse outcomes of treatment and/or minimizing or resolving treatment side-effects as they occur.

✔ In regard to salvage RP or RT, the successful choice of a second treatment to control the cancer is significantly dependent upon: findings that relate to the risk assessment insofar as the probability of organ-confined disease (OCD) at the time of initial local therapy and the meticulous re-evaluation of the patient with the same concerns when a salvage procedure is being considered.

✔ Radiation therapy of PC has evolved through many rapid technical advances. At the same time, the extent and nature of PC at the time of diagnosis has changed with an earlier detection of disease and the associated smaller tumor volumes found in such fortunate patients. RT oncologists and patients must work together to determine the appropriate RT dose and extent of radiation treatment.

✔ The identification of a successful or non-successful outcome by carefully defined biologic end-points, although sounding like a simple issue, has only recently been addressed. The use of the PSA in such biologic end-point definitions is a major step forward in the ability to make an earlier and more accurate assessment of how well any therapy is working.

✔ Some studies use an absolute level of PSA drop—such as the PSA nadir—to define success while others may use changes in PSA levels over time which are expressions of PSA slope or trend. All of these approaches have a biologic basis and should provide a reasonable assessment of efficacy within the context of the patient's full medical situation to either reassure the patient or to caution the patient as regards his treatment outcome.

✔ All types of RT obviously have their best results in patients with the most favorable prognostic profiles. The major differences in deciding what type of RT to select relate to the toxicity profiles associated with the particular RT technique (EBRT versus Brachytherapy) and the nature of the ionizing particle (photon, proton, neutron, subatomic particles).

✔ After brachytherapy, with or without external beam RT, a PSA bump may occur in 1 of 3 patients. The results from two different centers, involving a total of 1,313 patients are remarkably alike and indicate a better prognosis for patients displaying a PSA bump. Therefore, carefully analyzing the patient's course of illness while understanding the clinical features of the PSA bump may prevent patients from undergoing unnecessary treatment for what is presumed to be PSA recurrence but what in reality is only a PSA bump.

✔ A major part of understanding ADT involves the realization that this approach assumes the PC cell population under treatment is relatively homogeneous and represents androgen-dependent PC (ADPC). It is unreasonable to expect ADT to effectively control PC when a significant component of the tumor is comprised of androgen-independent PC (AIPC).

✔ The mechanisms of ADT, and the reflex effects of each mechanism, are important to understand to optimize ADT results as well as to avoid the use of ADT therapies with redundant mechanisms of action. This can prevent months to years of treating PC patients with the wrong therapies due to a lack of understanding about what ADT can and cannot accomplish.

✔ The basic humanistic tenets of medicine involve treating the patient with therapies of known effectiveness and with those of possible effectiveness. Above all, it is mandatory that we **Do No Harm**. The avoidance of biochemical and/or clinical flare exemplifies that last tenet. The person that has the most to lose by ignoring the issue of "flare" is the patient. Anti-androgen therapy given for one week prior to starting LHRH agonist therapy or the use of an LHRH "antagonist" are major ways to prevent flare.

✔ Bisphosphonate compounds, and especially the aminobisphosphonates such as Fosamax®, Actonel®, Aredia®, and Zometa®, are highly important substances that can prevent bone breakdown, correct bone loss (osteopenia or osteoporosis), have a direct PC cell-killing effect and probably also alter the bone micro-environment to prevent the spread of PC to bone.

✔ In evaluating the immediate and long-term results of RP, RT, cryosurgery and ADT, the success of each therapy is mirrored in its effect on biological end-points. Currently, the most sensitive biological end-point (BEP) for over 95% of patients with PC is the PSA. Achieving and maintaining a PSA nadir after RP, RT or cryosurgery has been shown to equate with prolonged recurrence-free survival. The same principle is applicable to ADT in our ability to determine long-term response to ADT as well as to allow us to distinguish ADPC from AIPC.

Chapter

5

What You Should Have Learned
From This Primer

1. Your initial clinical, pathology, laboratory, and radiology findings, involving complicated sounding medical jargon, are merely pieces of information which you and your M.D. (medical detective) are able to use to define a tumor profile that is specific for your unique biology.

2. This tumor profile is, or should be, incorporated into peer-reviewed literature findings that involve tens of thousands of men with PC. This is done via the use of algorithms such as the Partin Tables, D'Amico algorithms, Kattan nomograms, and others. These outputs, based upon your tumor profile, establish multiple risk assessments, which again are more specific for your unique biologic manifestations.

3. These risk assessments provide an invaluable strategy to help you navigate through difficult decisions as to how to best treat your PC. Does the prostate cancer reflect a high probability of OCD (organ-confined disease), is there a significant risk of CP (capsular penetration), is there a risk of SV (seminal vesicle involvement) or LN (lymph node involvement)?

4. Your risk assessment at diagnosis also has pertinence if prostate cancer recurrence should occur after any primary therapy. If you had a low likelihood of OCD at diagnosis, this will not have changed if you are found to have recurrent disease. Don't make the same mistake twice.

5. In the context of risk assessment analyses where OCD probability is high (>75%) and CP, SV and LN are low (<15%, <10%, <4%, respectively), therapeutic approaches such as RP, RT, and cryosurgery are most likely to be successful in the attempt to cure prostate cancer.

6. The physician's goals should be to
   • honestly relate to patients their status and
   • inform them realistically of the chances of cure.
   Physicians should also relate to the patient that eradication of the primary tumor may have benefits even if the disease is not cured.

7. Local therapies can only cure OCD, or at best minimally invasive PC that is within the urologic surgeon's ability to excise, the cryosurgeon's ability to freeze, or the radiation oncologist's ability to irradiate. These approaches cannot cure systemic disease. Physicians must also focus their energies on attempts to determine if distant disease is present.

8. Any therapy, be it surgical or medical, must fit the needs of the patient. In addition, the patient must be prepared for such treatment to optimize the outcome. Large prostate gland volumes and lower urinary tract symptoms (LUTS), for example, must be taken into account and resolved to a significant degree before RT or cryosurgery is employed. Medical conditions such as diabetes, hypertension, immunologic disorders, osteoporosis and others may affect the patient's sensitivity to RT, surgery or ADT and should be factors in the overall treatment strategy that is developed.

9. Most importantly, the patient must be aware of the wide diversity of physician skills in all aspects of PC prevention, diagnosis, evaluation, local treatment, systemic therapy and supportive care. All physicians are not equal in their talents. The patients must network with each other to seek out the best-qualified doctors. Remember, this is your life and your choice of an artist most definitely im-

pacts on your quality and quantity of life. The squeaky wheel does get the grease.

10. ADT (androgen deprivation therapy), as most commonly employed, is a selective therapy; it does not work against androgen-independent PC (AIPC), but it is active against tumor cells that are dependent on androgen for their growth. The tumor profile referred to in Item 1, helps the discerning physician-patient team understand the biology of the malignant process and not waste months and months on a therapy that may not be applicable to the patient's situation. Listening to the biology of cancer is the essence of oncologic thinking that extends life.

11. If physicians are going to treat men with PC optimally, they must understand the endocrinology involved in PC management. Over 95% of the patients we evaluate have never had a serum testosterone level obtained as part of their evaluation while on a therapy that is defined as "androgen deprivation therapy." The serum testosterone must drop to below 20 ng/dl (0.69 nM/L) while on ADT to determine if ADT has been given a reasonable trial.

183

12. The endocrinologic treatments directed against PC reflect the many effects of testosterone on normal male functions as well as the many measures the body takes to maintain androgen balance. Understanding the mechanisms of such side-effects and the body's responses to hormonal manipulations can make the difference between success and failure of any of the therapies employed. Learn the biologic activities described in Tables 11A-11C. Optimize outcome by not forgetting preventive measures such as flare avoidance, prevention and treatment of the many manifestations of the Androgen Deprivation Syndrome (ADS) and the reflex thermostatic responses of the pituitary, adrenals and testicles.

13. The bisphosphonate compounds e.g. Fosamax, Actonel, Aredia, and Zometa, represent one of the most impor-

tant drug classes affecting PC. Evaluation of skeletal integrity with tests of bone resorption such as Pyrilinks-D™ (Dpd) or Metra™ DPD and bone mineral density with quantitative computerized tomography (QCT) bone densitometry, and initiation of therapy comprised of a bisphosphonate and a comprehensive bone supplement can change the internal milieu of the bone and affect the growth rate of PC and the metastatic events to the bone. Trials of such compounds after the diagnosis of PC are indicated, as are considerations for these drugs as chemoprevention against PC.

14. Every medical interaction with a patient is a two-edged sword that can either help or harm the patient. The essence of outstanding medical care is to accentuate the good that we do patients and minimize the harm that our actions may engender. This concept is embodied in the "Therapeutic Index."

15. The chemotherapy of PC is a rapidly evolving field. Chemotherapy is in much greater use today due to our ability to determine the presence of systemic disease earlier and to discern if such disease is androgen-independent PC. Those physicians using chemotherapy in PC must be intensely aware of the need for supportive care of the patient. Newer chemotherapeutic agents with well-tolerated drug scheduling should make the chemotherapy of PC very well accepted among the patient community. The proper use of such agents can extend life in the setting of quality time. Again, this involves artistry.

16. The future of PC treatment rests in an early diagnosis of this disease, when the tumor volume would be considered as "minimal tumor burden" and the use of a therapy that leaves the prostate intact has a real chance of being effective. Vaccines, gene therapies, oncolytic viruses, immunologic augmentations and other novel therapies may well provide the answer that has the patient having his cake and eating it too.

Afterword

You will change as a result of having prostate cancer touch your life. It's not ALL bad. You have opportunities, born of adversity, to change your life as well as the lives of others.

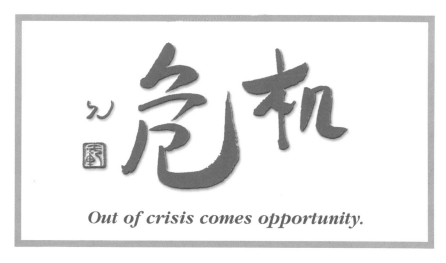

Out of crisis comes opportunity.

Many people report benefits of having been diagnosed with cancer as they progress down this road. For some, life becomes more precious, relationships improve, new joy is found in simple pleasures, spirituality is heightened, each new day is lived to the fullest, everything is appreciated more, a new intimacy with partners develops, sexuality is expressed at a more mature level, new friends are discovered as well as new attitudes formed, healthier lifestyles are adopted...the list goes on and on.

We hope the information contained in *A Primer on Prostate Cancer* has been helpful to you and that you will discover additional information through your further research. Your first task is to educate yourself about your own condition which then puts you in a position to educate other men and their families about prostate cancer as well.

Service

"It is so simple a remedy, merely service.

Not one ignoble thought or act is demanded of any or

of all men and women in the world to make fair the world.

The call is for nobility of thinking,

nobility of doing.

The call is for service,

and such is the wholesomeness of it.

He who serves all best serves

himself."

Jack London
1876-1916

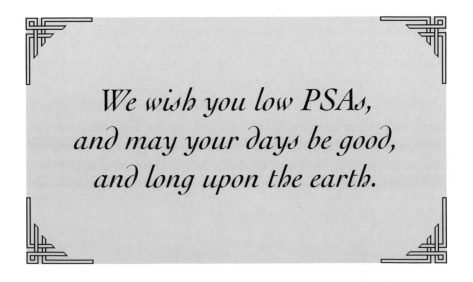

*We wish you low PSAs,
and may your days be good,
and long upon the earth.*

Acknowledgements

Compiled and written by:

Stephen B. Strum, M.D., medical oncologist specializing in prostate cancer, and Donna Pogliano, partner of a warrior in the battle against prostate cancer.

Published with support from Life Extension Foundation (www.lefprostate.org), and funded in part by the Prostate Cancer Research Institute (www.pcri.org).

Graphic design and layout courtesy of Diana J. Garnand, Visual Purple Graphics.

Special thanks to Georann Whitman and her family who provided the inspiration for this *Primer*.

Thanks also to the following men and women who reviewed the document, contributed material or provided moral support:

Joe Armon	Jim O'Hara
Charles Bader	Greg Oveson
Gail Betts	John Park
Don Cooley	Aubrey Pilgrim
Bill Donnelly	Harry Pinchot
Michael Dorso, M.D.	Rip Rinehart
Antonio Eiranova	Ann Salvato
Carl Frankel	Andrew M. Stevens
Ramon Henkel	Miwha Strum
Terry Herbert	Frank Teague
LaVonda Hurlbut	Howard Waage
Roy Huvala	Glenn D. Weaver
Esther Kutnick	Brad Wyatt
Jim Lamberth	Grayson S. Young
Linda Moore	Robert Vaughn Young

188

Appendix

Resources

This section is included to provide PC patients and those who love them with structured help as they search for information about prostate cancer. We have attempted to order these resources in a logical sequence that relates to how we believe most patients optimally obtain and process information. However, this is extremely difficult, if not close to impossible, due to the multi-faceted aspect of virtually all the resources that have been selected. To assist the reader, we have organized the material as shown below:

Resources for the PC Survivor

I.   To Educate You and Provide Guidance
II.   To Contribute to Your Knowledge Base
III.   To Communicate at a Higher Level with Your Medical Team
IV.   To Create a Personalized Assessment
V.   To Obtain Highly Focused Guidance
VI.   To Ask Your Doctors Questions
VII.   To Focus Further on Major Treatment Options
VIII. To Resolve and Prevent Treatment Side-Effects
IX.   To Employ Preventive and Wholistic Approaches
X.   To Further Your Assistance

This list in no way is intended to be all-inclusive and it certainly does not exhaust all the information available on any particular topic. In fact, the difficulty that an empowered patient and his family and friends encounter currently is the extensive amount of information now available via support groups, the

Internet and in printed form. Omission of any product, institution, person or other resource does not imply or constitute a negative endorsement.

I. To Educate You and Provide Guidance

These are only some of the major organizations offering substantial *foundational information and ongoing support.*

A. The Prostate Cancer Research Institute (PCRI) is a non-profit educational and research organization offering valuable information to PC survivors and physicians. PCRI staff interact by telephone, e-mail and/or fax with PC survivors and/or their family. The PCRI goal is to educate the patient and to interface with the patient's treating physician(s). The PCRI is a non-profit organization and is free to anyone in the world. The PCRI Helpline number is (310) 743-2110. The PCRI e-mail address is **pcri@pcri.org** and their Web site address is **www.pcri.org**.

A2   **B. *Us Too!*** is a not-for-profit organization providing information, counseling and educational meetings to assist men and their partners in making decisions about PC treatment. This international organization was started by PC survivors and continues to be governed by them. *Us Too!* groups offer fellowship, peer counseling, education about treatment options, and discussion of medical alternatives. The *Us Too!* telephone number is (630) 795-1002. Their support hotline number is (800) 808-7866 and the Web site address is **www.ustoo.com**. The Web site contains a list of support groups by state. There is an extensive resource list within the *Us Too!* Web site at: **http://www.ustoo.org/Resources.html**.

C. The American Cancer Society has a nationwide program involving support groups in many states called "Man to Man" where PC survivors offer support to the newly diagnosed. There is also an interactive section in which people can e-mail oncology nurses with questions and obtain referrals. The American Cancer Society's telephone number is 1-800-227-2345 and it's Web site address is **http://www.cancer.org**. Look for information on support groups in the "In My Community" section.

D. More on Support Groups.
Research has demonstrated that members of support groups survive longer than their peer survivors. You should definitely consider attending a formal "support group" meeting. Depending on the particular support group you attend, discussions of individual patient situations are often at a high level. Other group meetings combine personalized help with formal lectures by invited guest speakers, often physicians. The two largest PC support group organizations are "Us Too!" and "Man to Man." One of the most important values you will obtain is the chance to talk with other prostate cancer patients. Another list of support groups can be found at: http://www.cancerfacts.com/SupportGroups.asp?CB=14.

You can check with the National Prostate Cancer Coalition (NPCC) to see if your state has a "prostate cancer coalition" and also find out how you can become an advocate in the fight against prostate cancer. See the NPCC Web site at: http://www.pcacoalition.org/.

II. To Contribute to Your Knowledge Base
You and your circle of family and friends can work together and begin to *learn more about PC*. Later, you can share that information with someone else who is less knowledgeable than you are.

A. Internet Web Sites Created by Men with Prostate Cancer
"The Hypertext Guide to Prostate Cancer" by Bill Dyckes is an outstanding on-line resource of information about prostate cancer. The visitor to this site can choose to learn about PC in English, Spanish or Portuguese. See this Web site at: http://www.hypertext.org.

"Phoenix 5" is a Web site created by Robert Vaughn Young who died of PC in June, 2003. The contents are beautifully organized with excellent graphics. It is dedicated to helping men and their companions with the deeply personal issues related to prostate cancer. See this Web site at: http://www.phoenix5.org.

Virgil's Prostate On-line is an on-line guide to fighting prostate cancer. Virgil Simmons, diagnosed with prostate cancer at the age of 48, created this site for the purpose of providing a means to cope until there is a cure.
http://www.prostate-online.com/

B. Books

"Prostate and Cancer, A Family Guide to Diagnosis, Treatment and Survival" by Sheldon Marks, M.D., is a valuable book highly recommended for its organization, completeness and readability. Published in 1995. ISBN 1-55561-078-1.

"A Revolutionary Approach to Prostate Cancer", by prostate cancer survivor Aubrey Pilgrim, is a highly comprehensive book with many outstanding insights. There is also excellent coverage on areas relating to erectile dysfunction. It can also be read on-line at: http://www.prostatepointers.org/prostate/lay/apilgrim/. Published in 1998. ISBN 1-56315-0867.

"Smart Medicine for a Healthy Prostate" by Mark W. McClure, M.D. covers issues that relate to PC but also prostatitis and BPH. Published in 2001. ISBN 1-58333-113-1.

"Prostate Cancer Treatment Options, A Guide to the Basics" by Will Connell. This is a well-written book by a PC survivor. Published in 1999. ISBN 0-9673892-1-6.

"The ABCs of Prostate Cancer" by Joseph E. Oesterling, M.D. and Mark A. Moyad, M.P.H. is a comprehensive and highly illustrated book that is easy to read. Published in 1997. ISBN 1-56833-097-9.

"Prostate Cancer, What Every Man—and His Family—Needs to Know" (Revised Edition) by David G. Bostwick, M.D., Gregory T. MacLennan, M.D. and Thayne R. Larson, M.D. This is a good basic book available from the American Cancer Society published in 1999. ISBN 0-375-75319-2.

Go to http://www.phoenix5.org/books/books.html for a comprehensive listing of many of the books recommended within *The Primer*, as well as many others.

C. Prostate Cancer Newsletters Written by Physicians Focused on PC

PCRI Insights presents in-depth coverage of key scientific concepts and advances in prostate cancer. From October 1998 until July 2002, Stephen B. Strum, M.D. was the editor-in-chief of *Insights*. Dr. Strum continues to write the lead articles for Insights since leaving the PCRI in July 2002. *Insights* can be ordered, without charge, by calling the PCRI directly at (310) 743-2110. *Insights* is printed in full color with medical references and is written for the patient with intermediate to high levels of understanding about PC. However, for the less knowledgeable PC patient and/or family, there are multiple issues presenting foundational concepts that are essential to an understanding of PC. Past issues of *PCRI Insights* can be read or downloaded off the PCRI Web site at www.pcri.org by clicking on "Insights" on the main menu and then selecting a particular issue. All issues are chronologically arranged and a list of articles within each issue is provided.   **A5**

Prostate Forum is a newsletter written by Charles E. Myers, M.D. It contains comprehensive reviews of subjects of interest to the PC patient and to physicians. Dr. Myers is a medical oncologist who was formerly at the National Cancer Institute, was previously head of medical oncology at the University of Virginia and is now in private practice in Charlottesville, Virginia. The e-mail edition of *Prostate Forum* costs $36 per year and can be ordered by calling 1-800-305-2432. You can also order subscriptions and obtain back copies online via their Web site at www.prostateforum.com.

III. To Communicate at a Higher Level with Your Medical Team

You need to understand the terminology, or at least some of it, to communicate at a higher level with your medical team. It's not simply that the squeaky wheel gets the grease, but more that the empowered patient and his team are regarded more seriously by the health team. Thus, this kind of patient is more likely to have a better outcome.

The Glossary in Appendix D of this *Primer* is a substantial dictionary of PC related terms explained in more depth than many standard glossaries.

A "Glossary of PC-Related Terms" is an extensive glossary with hyperlinks and is online at the PCRI Web site at: **www.pcri.org/resource/glossary.html**.

A hard-copy version of the above Glossary was published in the August 2001 issue of *PCRI Insights*. You can download it by going to the PCRI Web site at **www.pcri.org** and clicking on "Insights" on the main menu to locate this particular issue.

An excellent glossary that may be viewed online and/or downloaded to your computer and used offline is available at the Phoenix5 Web site at: **http://www.phoenix5.org/glossary/glossary.html**.

IV. To Create a Personalized Assessment of Your Status

Using what you have learned about your unique biological findings, you can combine these different biologic expressions to obtain a sense of risk for yourself that leads you and your team to a more rational strategy.

A. The Partin Tables and Other Tools for Risk Assessment and Prognosis

The 2001 Partin Tables are reproduced in Appendix C of *The Primer*. The PCRI Web site contains software programs that include the Partin Tables along with multiple other software programs that allow for risk assessment as well as providing prognostic information. These are derived from the peer-reviewed medical literature, are presented in user-friendly format and include work by Narayan, Bluestein, Lerner, D'Amico, Kattan, and others. To access this software, go to the PCRI Web site at **www.pcri.org** and click on "Software" in the main menu. You can find a description of these software programs in the May 2001 issue of *PCRI Insights*.

B. Staging

A full narrative description of the TNM staging system is located within the glossary in Appendix D. Appendix G contains color illustrations of the clinical stages, concentrating on the T stage of PC, as based on the digital rectal examination. These illustrations have also been published in the April 2000 issue of *PCRI Insights*.

C. Biomarkers and other Tests

Information on biomarkers and other tests for prostate cancer can be found at:
http://www.prostate-help.org/camark.htm and
http://www.prostate-online.com/diagnostic.html

V. To Obtain Highly Focused Guidance

Interact with physicians to enhance a sophisticated understanding of your medical situation.

A. Patient to Physician (p2p) Mailing List

The purpose of the p2p mailing list is to provide the prostate cancer patient or other interested parties with information from physicians about the treatment of PC. This is a moderated list—without the high volume normally associated with mailing lists or the frequent off-topic questions. You can join p2p by addressing an e-mail to majordomo@prostatepointers.org, leaving the subject line blank, or show a dash (-) if required, and write, "subscribe p2p" in the body of the message. Within a few minutes, you should receive a welcome message from majordomo. Please follow the instructions "exactly" in order to activate your subscription. Every message sent to p2p must contain a Prostate Cancer Digest (PCD). Please see the next section for details.

B. Prostate Cancer Digest (PCD)

The PCD was created by Stephen B. Strum, M.D. as a way for PC patients to organize their PC medical history in a way that is more easily understood by physicians offering to help. The PCD is the required format of information presentation for those wishing to use the e-mail list called Patient to Physician (p2p). Instructions for preparing your digest were published in the premier issue of *PCRI Insights*, which can be read and/or downloaded in pdf format by going to http://www.pcri.org/resource/insights.html and scrolling down to the October 1998 issue. If you prefer, you can also get instructions at http://www.prostatepointers.org/p2p/pcd.html.

C. Prostate Cancer Research Institute (PCRI) Helpline

The PCRI interfaces with the PC patient and/or family to answer questions about various aspects of PC. They direct people to specific resources and Web sites, and provide software tools to analyze specific medical scenarios. The PCRI Helpline staff will mail out past issues of *Insights* and other papers relevant to your clinical situation.

VI. To Ask Your Doctor Questions

Once you are at a higher level you will feel comfortable interacting with your physician as a co-partner. Virgil Simmons' site, *Virgil's Prostate On-line* provides common questions and advice at: http://www.prostate-online.com/talking.html

VII. To Focus Further On Local Treatment Options

These are additional sources for those wishing to focus or "subspecialize" their knowledge about PC.

A. Radical Prostatectomy

"Man to Man: Surviving Prostate Cancer" by Michael Korda. This is a book specifically dealing with a patient's experience with surgery. People report that it frightened them, but they were glad they read it. Your library may also have this book on cassette tape. ISBN 0-679-44844-6.

The following two books were co-authored by one of the world's leading experts on prostate cancer. The 2001 book is written at a more detailed level than the 1995 book.

"The Prostate: A Guide for Men and the Women Who Love Them" by Patrick C. Walsh, M.D. and Janet Farrar Worthington. Pages 322. 1995. ISBN 0-8018-4989-6.

"Dr. Patrick Walsh's Guide to Surviving Prostate Cancer" also by Patrick C. Walsh, M.D. and Janet Farrar Worthington. Pages 462. 2001. ISBN 0-446-52640-1.

B. Brachytherapy—Permanent Seeds

"Seeds of Hope" by Michael Dorso, M.D. is a book available online and now available as a hardbound copy at the same site. This is a personal account by a doctor who had permanent seed implants (brachytherapy), hormone therapy and conformal beam radiation. The cost is $6 to obtain it online. It is also available by clicking on the title at: http://www.acornpublishing.com. ISBN 0-96788-016-5.

The American Brachytherapy Society Web site at www.americanbrachytherapy.org is devoted solely to brachytherapy information for patients and physicians.

C. Brachytherapy—High Dose Rate (HDR) Temporary Wires

There is good general information about HDR on the Web site of the manufacturer of the Nucletron afterloader at: http://www.nucletron.com.

The Cancer Treatment Centers of America at Tulsa (CTCA) Web site has an explanation of HDR as well as a link to the *Fortune* magazine article by Andy Grove (former CEO of Intel) which gives a personal account of his experience with HDR. The URL for this is http://www.brachytherapy.com/prost-brachy.html.

D. Cryosurgery

Good sources of information about Cryosurgery (freezing) are:
Endocare at http://www.ecare.org/ and
http://www.cryocarepca.org/ and
Galil Medical at http://www.galilmedical.com/.

VIII. To Resolve Treatment Side-Effects or Prevent Them

These are issues that need to be discussed with the idea of prevention or early correction.

A. Incontinence

An excellent resource for those needing help to regain urinary continence is the Web site for the National Association for Continence at http://www.nafc.org.

B. Erectile Dysfunction and Other Issues Dealing with Sexuality and Intimacy
"The Lovin' Ain't Over. The Couple's Guide to Better Sex after Prostate Disease" by Ralph and Barbara Alterowitz (ISBN 1-883257-02-6) is a forthright and clearly written guide written by a PC survivor and his wife that help men and their partners understand what affects sexual function and how to fix what is in need of repair.

IX. To Employ Preventive and Wholistic Approaches
Dietary and life-style approaches that are good for you in your journey with PC will also help you in virtually all other areas relating to maintaining your health and preventing other illness.

A. Diet

"The Prostate Cancer Protection Plan—The Food, Supplements, and Drugs that Could Save Your Life" by Dr. Bob Arnot is a book that includes nutritional and lifestyle recommendations for use in preventing and controlling prostate cancer. ISBN 0-31605-113-6.

"Eating Your Way to Better Health. The Prostate Forum Nutrition Guide." by Charles E. "Snuffy" Myers, Jr., M.D., Sara Sgarlat Steck, RT, and Rose Sgarlat Myers, PT, Ph.D. ISBN 0-9676129-0-X.

Dietary advice is available through the Prostate Cancer Foundation at http://www.prostatecancerfoundation.org under "Focus on Nutrition".

B. Integrative or Wholistic Approaches
The Life Extension Foundation (LEF) based in Ft. Lauderdale, Florida has pioneered in wholistic approaches to medicine, making contributions in this realm as far back as 1980. The May 2001 issue of *Insights* describes and illustrates these pioneering inroads from the Life Extension Foundation. LEF has a large staff of advisors who provide comprehensive information on a

wide spectrum of health and illness topics. Advisors are highly knowledgeable about vitamins, minerals and supplements. Advisors can be reached by calling the main LEF number at 1-866-820-7457 and specifically asking to speak to an advisor. LEF publishes an outstanding monthly magazine that presents the latest advances in medicine and also has published a book and CD ROM entitled *Disease Prevention and Treatment* that has an extensive chapter on prostate cancer written by Stephen B. Strum, M.D. and Jonathan McDermed, Pharm.D. The chapter is 64 pages long and has an extensive review of many PC treatments, including chemotherapy. The LEF Web site at www.lefprostate.org contains much of the above information as well as access to ordering LEF vitamins, minerals and other supplements. LEF has been a treasure to the PC patient in its long-term support of the efforts of Dr. Strum in the publication of the *PCRI Insights* as well as *A Primer on Prostate Cancer.*

"Choices in Healing: Integrating the Best of Conventional and Complementary Approaches to Cancer" is written by Michael Lerner. ISBN 0-26262-104-5. This book is also available online at http://www.commonweal.org/choicescontents.html.

"The Living Energy Universe" by Gary Schwartz, Ph.D. and Linda Russek, Ph.D., is a magnificent book that epitomizes the concepts of wholism. It is both a scientific and a philosophical treatise that joins science with medicine and mind with body. ISBN 1-57174-170-4.

X. To Further Your Assistance
A. E-mail Discussion Groups For PC Survivors
E-mail discussion groups (e-mail "lists") offer human interaction and support. They give technical information, share experiences and ask and answer questions. All are free of charge.

(1) Prostate Pointers
Prostate Pointers offers mailing lists specific to various treatment modalities. The Web page where patients and families can read descriptions of the lists and also subscribe is http://www.prostatepointers.org/mlist/mlist.html. The instructions on how to post messages to the specific list are

given in the "welcome" message after subscription has been activated.

There are currently 13 different lists available through Prostate Pointers that are used to ask questions relating to various aspects of the disease, treatment options, side-effects, supportive care and other issues. Some examples of these include: "Seedpods" for seed implantation, "RP" for radical prostatectomy, "IceBalls" for cryosurgery, "EBRT" for external beam radiation therapy, "CHB" for androgen deprivation therapy, "WW" for watchful waiting, and "The Circle" for support for PC survivors, their wives, family, friends and significant others.

(2) Prostate Problems Mailing List (PPML)

This online discussion group provides a forum for patients to exchange information and discuss all aspects of prostate cancer. Subscribe at http://www.acor.org/prostate.html.

View the archives at:

http://listserv.acor.org/archives/prostate.html.

B. Lists of Practitioners

Eventually, we need a consumer's union of PC patients that grades the physician and his staff in an objective manner. This is a beginning list to help the PC patient.

The Prostate Cancer Address Book (PCAB) on the PCRI Web site lists outstanding physicians in the world of prostate cancer. The input for this list has come from patient input and/or personal interactions with the physicians listed. Omission of any physician does not imply a negative endorsement. This list is evolving and does not presume to list every excellent physician in the world of PC. This list can be found at http://www.pcri.org/resource/name.html.

C. Help with Transportation

Free transportation by arrangement is available for cancer patients who need to travel for testing or treatment. Three to four weeks notice is recommended.

Volunteer Pilot's Association – Phone/FAX: (412) 221-4007 http://www.volunteerpilots.org/.

Corporate Angels – Phone: (914) 328-1313
http://www.corpangelnetwork.org/.

D. Help with Prescription Drugs

NeedyMeds.com: The Place to Learn About Pharmaceutical Manufacturer's Drug Assistance Programs.
http://www.needymeds.com/.

E. Help with Insurance

"A Consumer Guide for Getting and Keeping Health Insurance" contains specific information for each state and the District of Columbia—fifty-one in all. These guides are available at this Web site and are updated periodically as changes in federal and state policy warrant. This wealth of information is found at http://www.healthinsuranceinfo.net/.

F. Help for Patients with Hormone Refractory Prostate Cancer

A Web site and on-line support list managed, written and maintained by patients as a service to the men, the partners, and the caregivers who are fighting hormone-refractory prostate cancer. See it at http://www.hormonerefractorypca.org/index.html.

A14

Appendix

If You Want to Know More

This section is for those wanting to explore deeper into the issues raised in the main body of *The Primer*. It presents findings based on peer-reviewed publications with the relevant citations listed at the end of this appendix. The data presented here is sufficiently important or promising or perhaps controversial enough to be included separately in this section. The organization of Appendix B is based on the chapters of *The Primer*. Each chapter has its own Appendix B designation and each Appendix B section below relates to a particular chapter.

Chapter 2

2.1 **About Hereditary and Familial Prostate Cancer**

In the United States, approximately 75% of men diagnosed with PC have what is considered "sporadic" PC. The remainder, approximately one out of every four men diagnosed with PC, will demonstrate evidence of genetic clustering of PC. Of these men with genetic clustering, 19% are considered to be cases of hereditary prostate cancer (HPC) whereas 81% are designated as having familial PC or FPC[1] (Fig. 1). FPC is defined as simple clustering of the cancer in families.

HPC is characterized by a pattern of inheritance linked to a single gene that is transmitted from father to son, and from father to daughter and then to grandson i.e. an autosomal dominant gene. Due to the high penetrance of the gene, nearly half the male offspring will have PC and many of these will develop PC at an age younger than 55 years. Since the gene is also passed

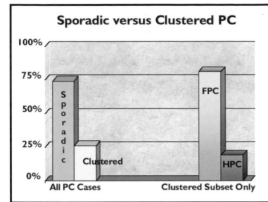

Figure B-1: Sporadic versus Clustered Prostate Cancer. *Of 100 men who present with PC, 74% will have sporadic PC while 26% will have clustered PC, i.e. evidence of genetic clustering. Of the 26% of men having clustered PC, 81% will have familial PC (FPC), and 19% will have hereditary PC (HPC). Adapted after Bastacky et al.[1]*

along via the female offspring, the family should be questioned about the maternal grandfather, maternal uncles and maternal cousins. HPC accounts for nearly 43% of PC diagnosed before the age of 55 years.[2-4] Extensive family studies of PC indicate that HPC shows a stronger familial aggregation than colon or breast cancer, but less than that of ovarian cancer.[5] These same investigators have shown that screening the first-degree relatives of men with HPC yields an eight-fold higher detection of PC than that found in the general population.[6]

Three criteria are required to designate a patient as having HPC.[2]

1. A family with three generations affected by PC.
2. Three first-degree relatives affected (brother(s), father).
3. Two relatives affected before the age of 55 years.

Men with FPC or HPC should be considered for more vigilant monitoring using such diagnostic measures as yearly PSA, DRE, free PSA percentage if the PSA rises to 2.0 or higher, neural net analysis, color Doppler ultrasound, endorectal MRI with spectroscopy and new promising techniques that may be available. Given the early age at diagnosis in many men with HPC, such monitoring should begin at age 35. Early nutritional intervention involving a low saturated fat diet, the use of supplements such as Vitamin E and selenium along with ample lycopenes, green tea, plenty of fresh fruit and vegetables, exercise, and attention to bone integrity are all important measures to prevent the emergence of PC and to detect it early. Table 1 details the key features of Hereditary as compared to those of Familial PC.

Table B-1: Hereditary Prostate Cancer (HPC) versus Familial Prostate Cancer (FPC). The major features of HPC versus FPC are shown in this table. These findings reinforce the concept that understanding the genetic aspects of PC should allow us to more vigorously approach earlier detection as well as prevention methods in such family members.

Feature	Hereditary PC (HPC)	Familial PC (FPC)	Reference number
Criteria	3 generations or 3 first degree relatives or 2 relatives with PC < 55 years of age	Clustering in families	2
Early Onset PC	Accounts for 43% of early onset PC		2-4
Number of 1st Degree Affected Relatives vs. Risk § 1 2 3 or more	Increased Risk (Odds Ratio) 2.2 4.9 10.9	95% Confidence Intervals 1.4–3.5 2.0–12.3 2.7–43.1	7
Number 1st or 2nd Degree Affected Relatives vs. Risk § 1 2 3 or more	Increased Risk (Odds Ratio) 1.5 2.3 3.6	95% Confidence Intervals 1.3–1.8 1.7–3.3 2.2–5.9	7

Type of Relative with PC vs. Risk of Getting PC
2nd degree:
  uncle or grandfather
1st degree:
  brother or father
1st & 2nd degree
	Increased Risk (Odds Ratio)
	1.7
	2.1
	2.0
	2.4
	8.8
		95% Confidence Intervals
		1.0 - 2.9
		0.8 - 5.7
		1.2 - 3.3
		1.3 - 4.5
		2.8 - 28.1
			7-8

Age of PC Onset in Patient vs. Risk for 1st degree relatives ‡ 50 60 70	No Additional Relatives Affected 1.9 (1.2–2.8) 1.4 (1.1–1.7) 1.0 (reference group)	1 or More 1st Degree Relatives Affected 7.1 (3.7–13.6) 5.2 (3.1–8.7) 3.8 (2.4–6.0)	2

§ This number does not include the patient

‡ This relates to risk for a first-degree relative(s) of a patient with PC.
  For example, a PC patient age 50 who has a father or brother(s) with PC would
  confer a 7.1 fold greater risk to any additional first-degree relative(s).

Chapter 3

3.1 About Prostatic Acid Phosphatase (PAP)

In a study from the Johns Hopkins Medical Institutions involving 1,681 men, PAP levels obtained prior to RP were predictive of patient outcome.[9] In this study spanning the years 1982 to 1998, the PAP methodology employed was based on an enzymatic assay described by Roy et al[10] in contrast to present-day methods which use immunoassays.[11] In the original paper by Roy, the mean PAP for normal healthy men was 0.28 ± 0.09 U/liter with a range from 0.11 to 0.60. In the Hopkins study, freedom from biochemical recurrence at five and 10 years after RP was 87% and 77% for those men with normal pre-RP PAP levels defined as < 0.4. However, this dropped to 79% and 65%, respectively, in men with preoperative PAPs of 0.4 to 0.5 U/liter and even further to 63% and 44% in those with baseline PAP levels of > 0.5 U/liter (Table B-2). This is now the third study to show that baseline PAP has major prognostic value.

B4

Table B-2: Preoperative PAP Levels Correlate with Outcome After RP.			
The baseline PAP using the methodology described by Roy et al significantly relates to a man's chances of remaining biochemically free of recurrence after having a radical prostatectomy. The definition of biochemical recurrence in this study was a PSA >0.2 ng/ml.			
Baseline PAP (Roy assay)	**Freedom From Biochemical Recurrence After RP**		
U/liter	At 5 Years	At 10 Years	p value
<0.4	87% (84-89)	77% (73-81)	p = 0.0001
0.4-0.5	79% (75-83)	65% (59-70)	p = 0.0001
>0.5	63% (52-72)	44% (30-57)	p = 0.0001

3.2 About Chromogranin A (CGA)

It must be emphasized that evaluating serum CGA levels is of relatively greater importance in a patient with a high Gleason score e.g. (4,3) and higher. As prostate cancer becomes more aggressive or anaplastic (i.e. more primitive in appearance or de-differentiated in appearance), its neuroendocrine differentiation increases.[12] The finding of progressively increasing CGA levels therefore indicates that an aggressive PC cell population is increasing. Most commonly, the growth of such cell clones reflects androgen-independent PC (AIPC) proliferation. In a study of AIPC patients, elevated serum CGA was detected in 10 of these 14 patients (71%) during treatment, and an early appearance of elevated serum CGA was found in six of 14 (43%) of these patients when serum PSA levels were less than 4.0 ng/ml.[13] Patients with PC who have low PSA levels and progressively increasing CGA levels appear to represent those with predominant AIPC. Such patients would be expected to have no significant response to ADT and, if not treated with therapies directed against AIPC, a poor survival.[14]

Lastly, it should be pointed out that serum CGA levels can be falsely elevated if kidney function is impaired. Those patients with abnormalities in kidney function manifested by elevated serum creatinine levels or abnormally low 24-hour urine creatinine clearance determinations should not be alarmed if an elevated serum CGA is found.[15] However, progressive CGA elevations in a setting of stable kidney function would be a cause for concern, and the patient should be treated with therapies directed against AIPC.

B5

3.3 About Transforming Growth Factor Beta 1 (TGF-ß$_1$)

An important study by Shariat et al involving 120 men undergoing radical prostatectomy (RP) for clinically localized PC (clinical stages T1-2), demonstrated that *plasma* levels of TGF-ß$_1$, *obtained preoperatively*, were highly correlated with PC progression after RP. Those patients with higher levels of TGF-ß$_1$ were found to have significantly higher rates of biochemical (PSA) recurrence or clinical recurrence during an average follow-up period of four years. When the preoperative TGF-ß$_1$ levels were stratified into < 4.9 ng/ml or > 4.9 ng/ml, the progression-free probabilities at three and five years after surgery were significantly different. **At five years, those men with baseline TGF-ß$_1$ values less than 4.9 ng/ml had a PSA progression-free probability of 93.4% (± 6.3%) compared to those with TGF-ß$_1$ values > 4.9 ng/ml whose progression-free probability was 74.8% (± 12.1%).** In other words, those with TGF-ß$_1$ levels < 4.9 had PSA progression 6.6% of the time ver-

Table B-3: Correlations of Preoperative Plasma TGF-ß₁ Levels with Postoperative Findings in 120 Men Undergoing RP for Clinical Stage T1-2 Prostate Cancer.*

Pathology Finding		Number Patients	TGF-ß$_1$ Level Median (ng/ml)	Range	p Value
Clinical Stage	T2	78	4.9	1.7-17.3	0.446
	T1	42	5.0	3.1-8.9	
Biopsy Gleason Score	7-10	40	4.9	3.4-17.3	0.176
	2-6	80	4.8	1.7-8.7	
Extraprostatic Extension	Present	33	5.4	3.3-8.9	**0.033**
	Absent	87	4.8	1.7-8.7	
Surgical Margins	Positive	16	4.9	3.7-8.9	0.383
	Negative	104	4.9	1.7-8.7	
Seminal Vesicle Involvement	Present	8	6.1	4.3-8.7	**0.042**
	Absent	112	4.8	1.7-8.9	
Lymph Node Involvement	Present	2	17.1	16.9-17.3	**<0.001**
	Absent	118	4.9	1.7-8.9	

Plasma TGF-ß₁ levels were significantly correlated with extraprostatic extension, seminal vesicle and especially lymph node involvement but not with clinical stage, biopsy Gleason score, or surgical margin status. *Adapted from Shariat et al.[16]

sus 25.2% of the time if TGF-ß₁ was > 4.9. **This represents almost a four-fold risk of recurrence based solely on the TGF-ß₁ level.** Other significant correlations were with ECE (extra-capsular extension) and seminal vesicle involvement (Table B-3).

Shariat et al also studied TGF-ß₁ levels in a separate group of PC patients with disease that had metastasized to regional lymph nodes (19 patients) or to bone (10 patients). They compared these findings with those of 44 healthy men who had no history of cancer of any kind. **These results, shown in Table B-4, showed even higher elevations in TGF-ß₁ levels in patients with metastasized disease in contrast to the healthy population.** It would therefore seem apparent that large-scale studies should be undertaken to evaluate plasma TGF-ß₁ levels in PC in various settings. Men with plasma TGF-ß₁ levels consistent with lymph node or bone metastases should have high-level staging studies to determine if their treatment strategy should be altered. These might include the ProstaScint-CT fusion study with or without PET scanning, the Pyrilinks-D™ or Metra™ DPD urine test, and serum biomarkers such as PAP, CGA, CEA and NSE.

Table B-4: High Levels of Plasma TGF-ß₁ Associated with Lymph Node and Bone Metastases versus Normal Controls.		
Patient Group	Number of Patients	TGF-ß₁ Median Level and (Range)
D1: Regional Lymph Nodes Involved	19	15.0 (80-192)
D2: Bone Metastases	10	15.2 (12.4-19.3)
Healthy Non-Cancer Controls	44	4.7 (1.0-6.6)

Plasma TGF-ß₁ is markedly elevated in patients with metastatic disease. The normal male control values of TGF-ß₁ are not significantly different from the values seen in patients without evidence of extraprostatic spread of disease at RP (see Table B-3). Adapted from Shariat et al.[16]

Chapter 4

4.1 About the Duke Study

A retrospective review was performed on all patients with stage D1 prostate cancer treated at Duke University Medical Center between 1975 and 1989. A total of 156 patients underwent a staging pelvic lymph-node dissection for clinically organ-confined prostate cancer (stage T1 or T2) but were found to have D1 disease (i.e. metastatic disease to the pelvic lymph nodes). Of this population, 42 patients also underwent radical prostatectomy (Group 1), leaving 114 who did not have their prostate removed (Group 2). The median cancer-specific survival was 11.2 years for Group 1 versus 5.8 years for Group 2 (p = 0.005). In patients with one or two positive lymph nodes the median cancer-specific survival was 10.2 years for Group 1 versus 5.9 years for Group 2 (p = 0.015). **There was no difference in survival if three or more lymph nodes were positive.**

Adjuvant treatment with immediate androgen deprivation and/or postoperative radiation therapy failed to improve the survival experience. The incidence of local problems, including stricture formation, bleeding, or re-growth of cancer that required dilation or surgical intervention (transurethral prostatectomy) averaged 9.5% in Group 1 and 24.6% in Group 2. **These data show that patients with limited node-positive disease selected for radical prostatectomy experience a survival advantage over those denied such therapy and that this advantage is independent of adjunctive therapy** (Table B-5).

Table B-5: Cancer-Specific Survival After Radical Prostatectomy (RP) versus Aborted RP in Men With Lymph Node Involvement At Time Of Surgery.

All Patients with D1 at Time of Surgery	Patient number	Cancer-specific Survival (mean)	p value
RP Performed- All patients	41	11.2 years	
Patients with 1-2 nodes involved	34	10.2 years	
RP Aborted- All patients	113	5.8 years	p = .005
Patients with 1-2 nodes involved	76	~ 5.9 years	p = .015

This landmark study indicated that performing a RP in a subset of patients with two or less nodes involved by PC conferred a meaningful survival advantage over a similar group of men who did not have their prostate gland removed. There was no difference in survival if three or more nodes showed PC involvement. Modified after Frazier et al.[17]

4.2 About Special Pathology Studies

B8 Special studies may be done on PC tissue obtained from either (1) the diagnostic biopsy specimen, or (2) from tumor specimens obtained at RP or at times when there is a recurrence of PC after a local therapy has failed. Some of these studies use antibodies to identify specific proteins such as p27, p21, p53, bcl-2, HER-2/*neu* and others. This involves an immunologic technique and is called "immunostaining." p27 and p21 are proteins involved with the regulation of cell growth and are associated with a better prognosis when levels are high. Loss of expression of p27 is an independent predictor of treatment failure of patients despite the lack of any evidence of lymph node involvement by PC at the time of RP.[18]

In treatments such as RT, cryosurgery, ADT, and chemotherapy, the desired goal is to kill the cancer cell via any mechanism available. One such mechanism occurring after DNA damage caused by RT is apoptosis or programmed cell death. Apoptosis is also a major mechanism of PC death or growth arrest with ADT. The cell has regulators, called oncogenes, which may either promote or inhibit apoptosis of tumor cells. The bcl-2 oncogene is one member of a family of genes involved in the regulation of apoptosis that can be identified in PC tissues by immunostaining. If bcl-2 is overexpressed in PC tissue, it blocks or inhibits apoptosis and cancer cells survive. In the same bcl-2 gene family, there are other *inhibitors* of apoptosis such as bcl-xL and mcl-1 as there also are other *promoters* of apoptosis, such as the Bax, Bcl-Xs and Bad genes.

In a study by Huang et al, patients with PC undergoing RT were evaluated to see if bcl-2 played any role in predicting success or failure with this treatment. Successful outcomes after RT were defined as a PSA ≤ 1.0 ng/ml that remained stable for three years along with a normal DRE. Tissue samples were obtained from both diagnostic pretreatment biopsy specimens as well as from available PC tissue from patients failing RT and immunostained for bcl-2 (and also mutated p53). Tissue samples were considered positive for bcl-2 if more than 10% of the cancer cells were bcl-2 positive (Fig. B-2).

In patients with no evidence of failure after RT, one of twelve (8%) had bcl-2 immunopositivity. In patients who failed RT, 17 of 43 (40%) with *diagnostic* biopsy material available for immunostaining for bcl-2 were positive. In 53 patients, pathology material was obtained after RT failure and 32 of the 53 (60%) showed bcl-2 immunopositivity. The differences in bcl-2 immunopositivity between patients with successful RT versus

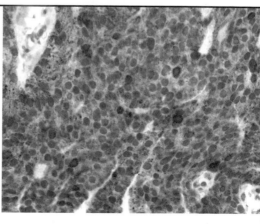

Figure B-2: Bcl-2 Immunostain in PC.
The brown staining within the cytoplasm of the PC cells represents bcl-2. The darker the stain, the stronger the immunoreactivity. The blue dots are the cell nuclei. Bcl-2, when present, is within the cytoplasm in contrast to mutated p53 which, when present, is within the nucleus. **Tissue blocks from either the biopsy or other PC tissue are required to do immunostaining for most of the proteins under study in PC.** Graphic courtesy of Bostwick Laboratories.

failed RT were significant ($p < 0.05$) when either pre-treatment biopsies or post-RT specimens from patients failing RT were examined (Table B-6).[19]

In 31 patients, both diagnostic biopsy material and post-RT material were available in the same patient. In this subset of patients, the diagnostic biopsy material was bcl-2 positive in 14/31 (45%) and the post-RT pathology material was positive in 18/31 (58%). Therefore, no significant increase in bcl-2 was demonstrated as a result of RT.

Table B-6: Bcl-2 Positive Immunostain Correlates with RT Failure.			
Treatment Group	Bcl-2 Immunostain Positive	Bcl-2 Positive (both pre-RT and post-RT pathology material available)	p53 Immunostain Positive
RT Successful n=12	1/12 (8%)	Not applicable	9/12 (75%)
RT Failure Diagnostic biopsies n=43	17/43 (40%)	14/31 (45%)	29/43 (67%)
Post-RT specimens n= 53	32/53 (60%)	18/31 (58%)	31/53 (58%)
Immunopositivity for bcl-2 appears to be a adverse risk factor insofar as identifying patients at higher risk for RT failure. In contrast, immunostaining for mutated p53 showed no significant correlation with RT success or failure. Table modified after Huang et al.[19]			

4.3 About Nerve Grafting

In their study of 12 men undergoing sural nerve grafting, Kim et al determined that six were able to achieve vaginal intercourse after radical prostatectomy. Of these six, four were able to do so without the use of Viagra® (sildenafil) although two of these four did experience a better quality of erection with Viagra. Five other men had partial erections after nerve grafting but were not able to achieve spontaneous medically unassisted erections sufficient for vaginal penetration. Of these five, two were able to have intercourse with the use of Viagra while the remaining three have had no response to date with a minimal follow-up period of 12 months; the mean follow-up was 16 months ± 4 months. Three remaining men had no erectile ability after sural nerve grafting and also no response to Viagra.

Twelve additional men acted as controls and underwent RP with both neurovascular bundles sacrificed at the time of RP. None of these 12 men had erectile ability after RP. No mention of their response to Viagra was made in this paper, but other authors have noted that a response to Viagra is dependent on the preservation of the cavernous nerves.[20]

While these are promising results, Walsh has written a convincing editorial citing evidence to support his contention that nerve grafts are rarely necessary in men undergoing a radical prostatectomy.[21] Walsh, the pioneer of the nerve-sparing RP, indicates that the neurovascular bundles (NVB) are located an average of 4.9 mm away from the prostate (range 3.2-9.5 mm) and that if organ-confined PC is found at RP, then there is no need for excision of either NVB. Moreover, when there is penetration of the capsule by PC, the growth of PC is only 1-2 mm away from the prostate and then further growth is directed upward toward the seminal vesicle (Fig. B-3). Walsh adds that in 75% of cases where capsular penetration is found, the amount of soft tissue extension is 2 mm. Therefore, the majority of men undergoing RP are amenable to a nerve-sparing procedure if their diagnosis is made in a timely fashion.

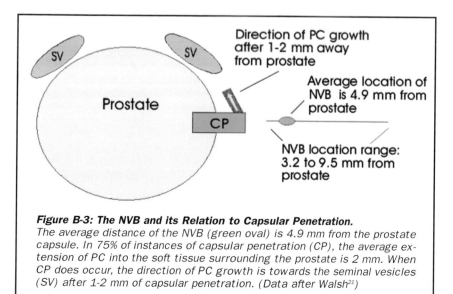

Figure B-3: The NVB and its Relation to Capsular Penetration.
The average distance of the NVB (green oval) is 4.9 mm from the prostate capsule. In 75% of instances of capsular penetration (CP), the average extension of PC into the soft tissue surrounding the prostate is 2 mm. When CP does occur, the direction of PC growth is towards the seminal vesicles (SV) after 1-2 mm of capsular penetration. (Data after Walsh[21])

In a contemporary series of 500 RP patients operated on by Dr. Walsh between August 1997 and January 2000 at Johns Hopkins, 73% presented with a *clinical* stage of T1c and 27% with T2c. At RP, the *pathological* stage was T2 in 78%, T3a in 18%, T3c in 3% and N1 in 1%. In this series, both neurovascular bundles were preserved in 86% of patients, and one NVB was preserved in 13%. In only two patients (0.4%) were both NVBs excised. Surgical margins that were positive in the region of the NVB were found in only 10 men, or 2% of the entire 500 men undergoing RP.

In this same series, with a follow-up of 12 months or more, 64% of men with one NVB preserved had sufficient sexual potency to have unassisted intercourse. Walsh et al found that sexual function was related to the age of the patient, extent of NVB preservation and the pathologic stage at RP. Table B-7 shows the inter-relationship of these important variables for men having one NVB preserved at the time of RP.

B12

Table B-7: Preservation of Potency with Unilateral Nerve-sparing at RP.		
Preservation of One NVB at RP and Potency		
Pathologic Stage (p Stage) at RP	**Potency Rates**	
	Men in their 50s	**Men in their 60s**
pT2	71%	62%
pT3a	47%	50%
pT3c	50%	16.7%

Most of the men in this series had a pathologic stage of pT2 at the time of RP. The overall rate of potency with one NVB spared was 64%. (Data after Walsh[21])

4.4 About Anastomotic Strictures

The occurrence of anastomotic strictures following RP in five large series of patients involving more than 3000 patients varied from 4.8% to 20.5% with an average rate of 14.9%.[22-26] In a recent series involving RPs performed between 1994 -1999, the stricture rate was 4.8%. The average time to stricture development was 4.22 months, and the stricture was detected within one year following RP in 97% of patients.

The development of anastomotic strictures correlated with

findings of excessive scar formation of the abdominal wound site from the RP operation. Those with scars wider than 10 mm were eight times more likely to have an anastomotic stricture than men with smaller scars. In other words, evidence of overly abundant scar formation present at the site of the abdominal incision was associated with similar excessive scar formation at the site of connection between the bladder outflow tract and the urethra. The authors of this study speculated that prior history of excessive scar formation may have implications in the adverse outcomes of other surgical procedures such as coronary bypass grafts, angioplasties, bile duct operations, etc.[22]

4.5 About Protection Against Radiation Side-Effects

A valuable study published by Sanchiz et al reported on the protective effects of Orgotein (SOD or superoxide dismutase) against the radiation-induced side-effects of cystitis and proctitis.[27] This study dealt with patients receiving RT for bladder cancer and not prostate cancer. The basic science, however, should be applicable to PC.

B13

The study was based on the publications that indicated that the anti-oxidant agent Cu/Zn superoxide dismutase is an effective drug in reducing acute and late radiation-induced tissue injury. At the Center of Radiotherapy and Oncology of Catalonia in Barcelona, Spain, a randomized prospective study to analyze the incidence and grade of side-effects in a group of bladder cancer patients was initiated in 1990.[27] After surgery, patients were randomly allocated to receive either: Radiotherapy (treatment A) or Radiotherapy plus SOD at a dose of eight milligrams per day as an intramuscular injection, given after each radiation treatment (treatment B). Between January 1990 and January 1995, a total of 448 patients were studied of whom 226 received treatment A and 222 received treatment B. **A highly significant incidence of radiation-induced acute and chronic cystitis and proctitis was detected in Treatment A patients who had not received SOD.** They concluded that SOD is effective in decreasing acute and chronic radiation-induced damage.

In his former PC practice, Dr. Strum has used *oral* SOD (Solgar brand SOD with catalase) at a dose of four tablets twice a day (taken on an empty stomach) to reduce symptoms of radiation cystitis and/or proctitis. This has been done in conjunction with the use of Rowasa® rectal suppositories inserted twice a day (AM and PM). This combination has significantly helped patients with severe RT-induced symptoms. Given the above, it would therefore be important to obtain follow-up information on the Barcelona study and, if no untoward findings have been noted, to initiate a clinical trial using this non-toxic and inexpensive natural anti-oxidant during RT in prostate cancer patients.

4.6 About the Blasko Study

The study by Blasko et al also analyzed their patient data by using a combination of variables and sorting the patients into three risk groups: low, intermediate and high. The Low Risk group required the clinical stage to be T1 or T2, the baseline PSA to be ≤ 10, and the Gleason score to be ≤ 6. The Intermediate Risk group also included clinical stage T1 and T2 patients, but either the PSA was > 10 or the Gleason score was > 6. The High Risk group were patients with both the PSA > 10 and the Gleason score > 6 as well as clinical stage T1 or T2 disease. The 5-year biochemical progression-free survival (PFS) by risk groups is shown in Table B-8.[28] Biochemical progression-free survival in this study was defined as the absence of two consecutive rises in PSA after completion of seed implantation.

It is our opinion that analyzing data using concepts such as risk groups based on multiple variable analysis (or based on a validated algorithm) make much more sense than using a single

Table B-8: 5-Year Biochemical Progression-Free Survival (PFS) Using Palladium-103 versus Risk Groups.			
Risk Group	Patient Number	Median follow-up	Biochemical PFS
Low	103	48.9 months	94%
Intermediate	107	39.5 months	82%
High	20	45.5 months	65%

Sorting patients into risk groups based on important biological variables such as baseline PSA, Gleason score and clinical stage is a highly significant concept that should be used in the analysis of any treatment option.[29]

variable for correlations with outcome. Since the Partin analysis is one such validated algorithm, we wonder why all studies involving treatment outcome do not employ such concepts. Moreover, given the observer disagreements in interpreting the Gleason score as well as evaluating the clinical stage based on DRE, we would suggest that such clinical trials utilize reference pathologists to test the validity of at least the Gleason scoring. Lastly, all reports on patient outcome should indicate the number of patients who actually have been analyzed for each year of follow-up rather then portray this as a line graph using an actuarial analysis. The latter may be terribly misleading.

4.7 About the PSA Bounce or Bump

An explanation for the differences in these series of patients treated by radiation therapy is not apparent. However, a few additional observations are pertinent to all of these studies.

PSA bounce or bump should be defined in the setting of RT of any kind as an initial fall in PSA as a result of RT, followed by a temporary rise. The PSA results should come from the same laboratory using the same PSA assay. The interval between PSA testing should be at least 30 days, at the minimum. **B15**

PSA bump should not be diagnosed in the setting of:

- Prostate manipulation by DRE,
- Vigorous exercise that may involve pressure on the prostate such as bicycle, motorcycle or horseback riding,
- Sexual activity involving ejaculation within 48 hours of PSA testing, or
- PSA testing within five weeks after transrectal ultrasound of the prostate, or Foley catheter insertion into the urethra, or other instrumentation of the prostate or nearby tissues.

4.8 About Experience with HDR

The Interdisciplinary Brachytherapy Center in Kiel, Germany has the longest experience with HDR. In a report of 144 patients with a median follow-up of eight years (range five to 14 years), Galalae et al indicate an overall disease-free survival rate of 82.6%. These patients received a combination of external beam RT to the prostate (40 Gy) and also to the pelvic nodes (50 Gy) as well as HDR with 15 Gy per fraction for two fractions to the peripheral zones of the prostate, while the entire gland received two fractions at 9 Gy. What is especially intriguing about this reported high survival rate is that 79.8% or 115 of the patients had clinical stage T2b or T3 disease. In addition, the PSA breakdown indicated that 54% of the patients had a baseline pretreatment PSA of 10 or higher.[30]

4.9 About RT Toxicity Tables from the Radiation Therapy Oncology Group (RTOG)

The RTOG grading system is an important concept in objectifying the true incidence of adverse events related to therapies directed against cancer. It is our opinion that patient consumer groups should be organized to contact patients and accurately record such events to maintain the most accurate accounting of what occurs after various treatments. This is true for surgical, radiation and medical therapies directed against PC. The toxicity table for chronic gastrointestinal toxicity was shown in Chapter 4. Following are the tables for chronic bladder (genito-urinary) toxicity (Table B-9) and also for acute bladder (Table B-10) and gastrointestinal toxicities (Table B-11).

Table B-9: Chronic Bladder Toxicity: RTOG Grading System.				
GRADE				
0	**1**	**2**	**3**	**4**
None	Slight epithelial atrophy Minor telangiectasia Microscopic hematuria	Moderate frequency Generalized telangiectasia Intermittent gross hematuria	Severe frequency and dysuria Severe generalized telangiectasia (often with petechiae) Frequent hematuria Reduction in bladder capacity (< 150 cc)	Necrosis Contracted bladder (capacity < 100 cc) Severe hemorrhagic cystitis

Table B-10: Acute Bladder Toxicity: RTOG Grading System.				
GRADE				
0	**1**	**2**	**3**	**4**
No change	Frequency of urination or nocturia twice pretreatment habit Dysuria, urgency not requiring medication	Frequency of urination or nocturia which is less frequent than every hour Dysuria, urgency, bladder spasm requiring local anesthetic (e.g., Pyridium®)	Frequency with urgency and nocturia hourly or more frequently Dysuria, pelvic pain or bladder spasm requiring regular, frequent narcotic Gross hematuria with or without clot passage	Hematuria requiring transfusion Acute bladder obstruction not secondary to clot passage, ulceration or necrosis

Table B-11: Acute Gastro-Intestinal Toxicity: RTOG Grading System.				
GRADE				
0	**1**	**2**	**3**	**4**
No change	Increased frequency or change in quality of bowel habits not requiring medication Rectal discomfort not requiring analgesics	Diarrhea requiring parasympatholytic drugs (e.g., Lomotil®) Mucous discharge not necessitating sanitary pads Rectal or abdominal pain requiring analgesics	Diarrhea requiring parenteral support Severe mucous or blood discharge necessitating sanitary pads Abdominal distention (flat plate radiograph demonstrates distended bowel loops)	Acute or subacute obstruction, fistula or perforation GI bleeding requiring transfusion Abdominal pain or tenesmus requiring tube decompression or bowel diversion

4.10 About Proton RT

Protons are low LET (linear energy transfer) particles. (Neutrons, in comparison, are high LET particles). This means that the energy loss along the proton's proximal path by means of ionizing and exciting atoms/molecules is small and is comparable to that of photons. At the end of the range, however, there is a rapid loss of energy with protons that produces a limited zone of high LET (dense ionization). This results in the Bragg peak—a small region of steeply increased dose. By the use of a modulated proton energy beam with a range of proton energies, one can use the Bragg peak characteristic to achieve a spread of energy to the target tissues.

4.11 About Proton Beam Studies

In a subset analysis of the 511 patients described in Chapter 4, Slater et al evaluated 319 patients who presented with baseline PSA values (bPSA) of 15 ng/ml or less and clinical stages T1 or T2b, and who were treated with PBRT or PBRT plus photons. The results of PBRT or PBRT/Photon combination therapy on biochemical freedom from relapse (bNED) are shown in Table B-12.[31] Overall, 89% of these patients remained free of biochemical relapse.

A further analysis of 288 patients who had achieved a nadir or who had been followed for at least 24 months was then performed. Of these 288 patients, 187 patients or 65% achieved a post-radiation PSA nadir of ≤ 0.5 ng/ml (Table B-13).

Table B-12: Subset Analysis of Patients Presenting with bPSA of ≤ 15 ng/ml versus Freedom from Biochemical Relapse (bNED) at Five Years.		
bPSA	**Number of Patients**	**bNED @ 5 Years Number (per cent)**
≤ 4.0	39	39 (100%)
4.1-10.0	220	202 (92%)
10.1-15.0	60	44 (73%)
Totals	319	285 (89%)

Risk assessment and selection of patients with a greater chance of organ-confined disease and a smaller tumor burden results in an overall 89% chance of freedom from biochemical relapse using PBRT or PBRT with Photons. Table modified after Slater et al.[31]

Table B-13: Achievement of a Post-RT Nadir Using PBRT or PBRT + Photons.		
bPSA	**Number of Patients**	**Post-RT nadir ≤ 0.5 ng/ml Number (per cent)**
≤ 4.0	39	32 (83%)
4.1-10.0	200	132 (66%)
10.1-15.0	49	23 (48%)
Totals	288	187 (65%)

The lower the bPSA, the higher the probability of achieving a nadir of ≤ 0.5 ng/ml. Table modified after Slater et al.[31]

Achieving a *post*-RT PSA nadir of 0.5 ng/ml or less resulted in freedom from biochemical relapse 98% of the time; this compared to 88% for achieving a PSA nadir of 0.51–1.0, and 41% for achieving a nadir of > 1.0 ng/ml. These figures represent an actuarial analysis that is not a substitute for actually observed biochemical freedom from relapse. Therefore, given that this paper was published in 1999 and the patients within the study were treated between 1990 and 1995, there now should be sufficient patients with significantly mature data to provide a more accurate 5-year follow-up.

4.12 About Neutron Beam RT

A simple representation of the atom is that of a nucleus with electrons orbiting around it—similar to the planets orbiting around the sun. Within the nucleus is the mass of the atom consisting of protons and neutrons. Protons have a positive charge while neutrons have no charge. The proton number is called the atomic number. The number of electrons in a neutral atom equals the number of protons in order that their charges balance. The atomic mass is comprised of protons plus neutrons plus electrons. Since electrons have almost a negligible weight, the atomic mass is essentially that of the number of protons plus neutrons.

4.13 About Androgen Deprivation Therapy (ADT)

The critical hormone involved in the hypothalamic-pituitary axis is gonadotrophin-releasing hormone (GnRH), which is also known as luteinizing hormone-releasing hormone or LHRH. LHRH travels from the hypothalamus to the pituitary gland via a vascular pathway called the portal system. LHRH normally binds to the LHRH receptors in the pituitary and forms a natural complex. This is essentially a "sandwich" made up of a ligand (LHRH), and its receptor (LHRH receptor). This complex is broken down by a chemical reaction involving a peptidase enzyme, which then frees the receptor for more LHRH. This interaction results in a pulsatile production of LH as well as FSH (follicle stimulating hormone). FSH is now implicated as an additional factor in the growth of PC. Receptors for FSH have been shown to be present on prostate cancer cells.

The synthetic LHRH analogs (LHRH agonists or LHRH-A) bind to the receptor and are more resistant to enzymatic degradation by peptidase. This results in the decreased production of LH. Another hypothesis is that the continuous exposure of the LHRH receptor to synthetic LHRH-A results in a down-regulation of the peptidase enzyme.

Men who are receiving LHRH-A therapy for time periods in excess of two years may have difficulty in returning to a state of normal testosterone production despite discontinuation of the LHRH-A. This is related to pathological events in the pituitary; it is not the result of atrophy of the testicles due to the LHRH-A therapy. If the pituitary had recovered its function but testicular malfunction was operative, then very high levels of LH would be found. This is not the case. What appears to be occurring is that prolonged binding of the LHRH-A to the LHRH receptor results in a tight complex that prevents any remaining peptidase action that could liberate LH, or, that peptidase is simply depleted from the system and takes a prolonged time to recover—or perhaps never does recover.

Men who have been on prolonged ADT can have the LHRH-A discontinued and have their testosterone levels or LH levels monitored. This could result in savings of millions of health-care dollars and possibly also allow eventual recovery of the LHRH-A≈LHRH receptor≈Peptidase complex.

In women, LH and FSH (these are called gonadotrophins) act sequentially on the ovary. LH triggers the production of progesterone and androgens, and FSH stimulates production and secretion of estradiol.

4.14 About PC and Bone Loss

The bone tissues are an important micro-environment. Bone is not a static tissue but a dynamic one that undergoes constant formation and resorption. When bone breakdown or resorption is in excess of formation, bone loss occurs. If this contin-

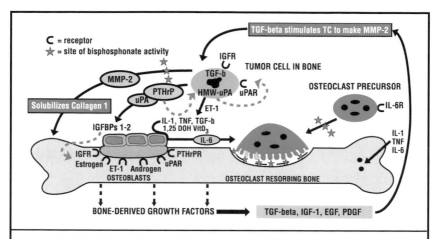

Fig. B-4: The Vicious Cycle of Bone Loss and PC Growth. *The vicious cycle of bone loss and release of bone-derived growth factors appears to bc operative in PC. Growth factors such as IGF-1, EGF, and TGF-ß₁ appear to correlate with more aggressive and extensive PC. The use of bisphosphonate compounds to shut off bone resorption also reduces PSA levels.*[33]

ues unabated, osteopenia and eventually osteoporosis develops. Excessive bone resorption appears to be operative in **B21** prostate cancer even without the contributing factor of bone loss induced by androgen deprivation therapies. Osteopenia represents a decreased bone mineral density of more than one standard deviation and up to 2.4 standard deviations (SD) below that which occurs in normal subjects at age 25. If the bone density drops to 2.5 or more standard deviations below normal, the patient then is considered to have osteoporosis. This measurement is reflected in the T-score shown on bone mineral density reports. Therefore, a T-score within the range of -1.0 to -2.4 SD represents osteopenia, and a T-score of -2.5 or more indicates osteoporosis.

The most common technique used to evaluate bone mineral density is the DEXA scan. However, the DEXA scan is falsely "improved" by arthritis and calcium deposits in blood vessels close to the bones being studied. In a report studying both DEXA bone density and quantitative CT (QCT) bone mineral density in the same population of men with PC who had not been treated with ADT, Smith et al found osteopenia in 32% and osteoporosis in 63% using QCT technology. Only 5% of patients who were studied with QCT had normal bone density. With DEXA, in contrast, osteopenia was detected in 12/41 (29%) and osteoporosis in 2/41 (5%) of men in the same study population.[32]

The cycle of bone loss and formation therefore may play a crucial role in the natural history of the genesis and progression of PC. Assessing the bone mineral density in men, however, is currently a neglected aspect in general medical practice. Preventing further bone loss and advising the patient on how to restore bone mineral density seems logical while saving billions of dollars in health care expenses. In-depth discussions of bone integrity can be found within the January 1999, May 1999 and December 1999 issues of PCRI *Insights*. These issues can be printed off of the PCRI website at **www.pcri.org** (go to "Insights") or requested from the PCRI by calling 310-743-2110. The vicious cycle of bone loss stimulating PC growth is depicted in Figure B-4.

4.15 About SAB

Androgen deprivation therapy (ADT), as it is used in the vast majority of PC patients, involves a testosterone-lowering strategy. However, some patients are using testosterone-preserving ADT comprised of a combination of finasteride (Proscar®) or dutasteride (Avodart®) and flutamide (Eulexin®) or bicalutamide (Casodex®). This has been called *Sequential Androgen Blockade (SAB)*. This combination blocks DHT production by means of finasteride or dutasteride, and it also utilizes androgen receptor blockade of testosterone and any remaining DHT by means of flutamide or bicalutamide (Fig. B-5). The goal is to maintain sexual function yet stop PC growth by providing adequate androgen deprivation at the tumor cell level. This strategy may diminish many of the typical side-effects of conventional ADT and allow preservation of sexual function.

In a pilot study of SAB, Brufsky et al used Eulexin or Casodex as the initial treatment to see how low the PSA would drop. After achieving a nadir level, they added Proscar at 5 mg per day and again evaluated the patient for a new PSA nadir. There was a statistically significant drop in the PSA from the nadir with Eulexin

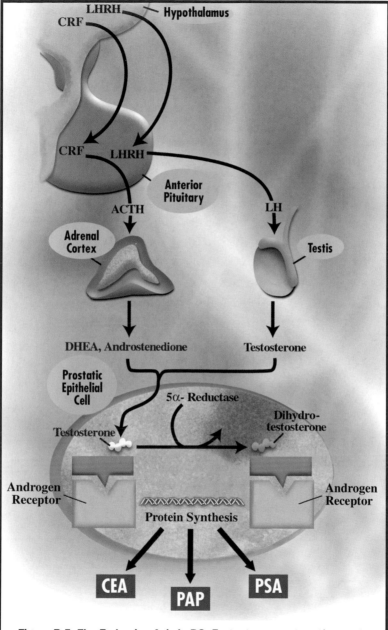

Figure B-5: The Endocrine Axis in PC. *Testosterone enters the prostatic epithelial cells where it interacts with androgen receptors to stimulate DNA production and the eventual secretion of multiple proteins. PSA is one such example. Most importantly, T is converted by the 5a-reductase enzyme to DHT, which has more avidity for the androgen receptor than does T. Blocking DHT to reduce intra-cellular levels is therefore an important part of androgen deprivation therapy.[34]*

or Casodex compared to that achieved with the addition of Proscar. After Proscar had been added, DHT levels fell by a mean of approximately 35% ± 5%. The average PSA nadirs after Eulexin or Casodex were 7.8 ng/ml. After the addition of Proscar the PSA nadir dropped further to 4.7 ng/ml. Potency preservation was seen in six of 11 (55%) of men. In this study, the patients who were treated either had PSA recurrence after RT (13 patients) or were asymptomatic with D1-D2 disease (seven patients). These PSA responses are not impressive compared to other forms of ADT. Possible contributing factors to this less exuberant PSA decline include the high baseline PSA levels (94.7 ± 38.2 ng/ml), the structure of the treatment plan, and the overall short duration of therapy which averaged 16.9 months. This approach using SAB may be valid in men who are intolerant to testosterone deprivation and who refuse to have conventional local therapy. More work on the use of SAB is being done.[35]

B24 A larger multi-institutional study reported by Wheeler et al involved 64 patients randomized to either LHRH-A plus flutamide versus finasteride plus flutamide. These regimens were compared in the setting of preparation of patients with apparent organ-confined PC for definitive local therapies with the goals of reduction in gland volume and tumor burden. This therefore represents patients in more favorable prognostic risk groups than those in the study cited above. Moreover, it must be remembered that patients with earlier stage disease are less likely to have PC that has mutated to androgen-independent PC and therefore are more likely to respond to ADT.

Table B-14: Randomized Trial of Sequential Androgen Blockade (SAB) versus Conventional ADT Using LHRH-A + Flutamide.				
Treatment Group	Baseline PSA	Nadir Average	Days to Reach Nadir	Net Change in PSA
Flutamide-LHRH-A n = 29	9.3	0.45	59.83	8.85
Flutamide-Finasteride n = 35	10.95	0.59	60.06	10.36
In this trial of patients with apparently organ-confined PC, the PSA nadirs and average time to reach nadir was not significantly different between the two treatment arms studied.				

The stopping point in the Wheeler study for either regimen was a PSA reduction to less than 2 ng/ml at which point patients were scheduled to undergo treatments including radical prostatectomy, brachytherapy, EBRT, combination RT or cryosurgery. The baseline PSA, the average nadir and time to reach nadir, and days to nadir are shown in Table B-14.

Follow-up on the above study regarding a comparison of side-effects and response to treatment is forthcoming.[36]

4.16 About ADT Side-Effects

These are additional findings relating to the data presented in Table 13 in Chapter 4. In the category of "bone and joint pain", grade 2 to 3 bone pain occurred more often in patients receiving ADT for more than 15 months as contrasted to less than 15 months. **Bone and joint pain was highly responsive to treatment with bisphosphonate compounds such as Fosamax, Actonel, Aredia, and Zometa.** These compounds were taken in combination with a bone supplement containing calcium, magnesium, boron and other trace elements. Synthetic vitamin D (Rocaltrol®) was also routinely administered as part of this bone stabilizing and restorative regimen. Grade 2-3 weight gain was more common in patients of up to 70 years of age than in older patients (p < 0.01). Weight control was improved with dietary fat restriction and exercise. Memory difficulties of grade 2-3 severity were more common if ADT was given for more than 15 months. Grade 2-3 anemia was more common in patients receiving flutamide than in those receiving bicalutamide (p < 0.005), yet this anemia was highly responsive to Procrit®, even at doses as low as 4,000 units every one to two weeks.[37]

4.17 About VEGF

In a clinical study of plasma VEGF in 80 men with prostate cancer and 26 normal men, the median levels of plasma VEGF were 0.0 for controls, 7.0 pg/ml for localized PC and 28.5 pg/ml for metastatic PC. Statistical analysis established that a VEGF level of 18 pg/ml was the optimal cutoff for differentiating between malignant and localized PC. Patients with a plasma VEGF of > 18 pg/ml were 10 times more likely to have metastases. Plasma VEGF may therefore be a useful marker of non-organ-confined PC.[38]

B25

References

1. Bastacky SI, Wojno KJ, Walsh PC, et al: Pathological features of hereditary prostate cancer. J Urol 153:987-92, 1995.

2. Carter BS, Bova GS, Beaty TH, et al: Hereditary prostate cancer: epidemiologic and clinical features. J Urol 150:797-802, 1993.

3. Carter BS, Steinberg GD, Beaty TH, et al: Familial risk factors for prostate cancer. Cancer Surv 11:5-13, 1991.

4. Carter BS, Beaty TH, Steinberg GD, et al: Mendelian inheritance of familial prostate cancer. Proc Natl Acad Sci U S A 89:3367-71, 1992.

5. Cannon L, Bishop DT, Skolnick M, et al: Genetic epidemiology of prostate cancer in the Utah Mormon Genealogy. Cancer Surv 1:47-69, 1982.

6. McWhorter WP, Hernandez AD, Meikle AW, et al: A screening study of prostate cancer in high risk families. J Urol 148:826-8, 1992.

7. Steinberg GD, Carter BS, Beaty TH, et al: Family history and the risk of prostate cancer. Prostate 17:337-47, 1990.

8. Spitz MR, Currier RD, Fueger JJ, et al: Familial patterns of prostate cancer: a case-control analysis. J Urol 146:1305-7, 1991.

9. Han M, Piantadosi S, Zahurak ML, et al: Serum acid phosphatase level and biochemical recurrence following radical prostatectomy for men with clinically localized prostate cancer. Urology 57:707-11, 2001.

10. Roy AV, Brower ME, Hayden JE: Sodium thymolphthalein monophosphate: A new acid phosphatase substrate with greater specificity for the prostatic enzyme in serum. Clin Chem 17:1093-1102, 1971.

11. Moul JW, Connelly RR, Perahia B, et al: The contemporary value of pretreatment prostatic acid phosphatase to predict pathological stage and recurrence in radical prostatectomy cases. J Urol 159:935-40, 1998.

12. Abrahamsson PA, Falkmer S, Falt K, et al: The course of neuroendocrine differentiation in prostatic carcinomas. An immunohistochemical study testing chromogranin A as an "endocrine marker". Pathol Res Pract 185:373-80, 1989.

13. Wu JT, Astill ME, Liu GH, et al: Serum chromogranin A: early detection of hormonal resistance in prostate cancer patients. J Clin Lab Anal 12:20-5, 1998.

14. Isshiki S, Akakura K, Komiya A, et al: Chromogranin a concentration as a serum marker to predict prognosis after endocrine therapy for prostate cancer. J Urol 167:512-5, 2002.

15. Hsiao RJ, Mezger MS, O'Connor DT: Chromogranin A in uremia: progressive retention of immunoreactive fragments. Kidney Int 37:955-64, 1990.

16. Shariat SF, Shalev M, Menesses-Diaz A, et al: Preoperative plasma levels of transforming growth factor beta(1) (TGF-beta(1)) strongly predict progression in patients undergoing radical prostatectomy. J Clin Oncol 19:2856-64, 2001.

17. Frazier HA, 2nd, Robertson JE, Paulson DF: Does radical prostatectomy in the presence of positive pelvic lymph nodes enhance survival? World J Urol 12:308-12, 1994.

18. Tsihlias J, Kapusta LR, DeBoer G, et al: Loss of cyclin-dependent kinase inhibitor p27Kip1 is a novel prognostic factor in localized human prostate adenocarcinoma. Cancer Res 58:542-8, 1998.

19. Huang A, Gandour-Edwards R, Rosenthal SA, et al: p53 and bcl-2 immunohistochemical alterations in prostate cancer treated with radiation therapy. Urology 51:346-51, 1998.

20. Kim ED, Nath R, Kadmon D, et al: Bilateral nerve graft during radical retropubic prostatectomy: 1-year followup. J Urol 165:1950-6, 2001.

21. Walsh PC: Nerve grafts are rarely necessary and are unlikely to improve sexual function in men undergoing anatomic radical prostatectomy. Urology 57:1020-4, 2001.

22. Park R, Martin S, Goldberg JD, et al: Anastomotic strictures following radical prostatectomy: insights into incidence, effectiveness of intervention, effect on continence, and factors predisposing to occurrence. Urology 57:742-6, 2001.

23. Fowler FJ, Jr., Barry MJ, Lu-Yao G, et al: Patient-reported complications and follow-up treatment after radical prostatectomy. The National Medicare Experience: 1988-1990 (updated June 1993). Urology 42:622-9, 1993.

24. Kao TC, Cruess DF, Garner D, et al: Multicenter patient self-reporting questionnaire on impotence, incontinence and stricture after radical prostatectomy. J Urol 163:858-64, 2000.

25. Geary ES, Dendinger TE, Freiha FS, et al: Incontinence and vesical neck strictures following radical retropubic prostatectomy. Urology 45:1000-6, 1995.

26. Surya BV, Provet J, Johanson KE, et al: Anastomotic strictures following radical prostatectomy: risk factors and management. J Urol 143:755-8, 1990.

27. Sanchiz F, Milla A, Artola N, et al: Prevention of radioinduced cystitis by orgotein: a randomized study. Anticancer Res 16:2025-8, 1996.

28. Blasko JC, Grimm PD, Sylvester JE, et al: Palladium-103 brachytherapy for prostate carcinoma. Int J Radiat Oncol Biol Phys 46:839-50, 2000.

29. Zelefsky MJ, Leibel SA, Gaudin PB, et al: Dose escalation with three-dimensional conformal radiation therapy affects the outcome in prostate cancer. Int J Radiat Oncol Biol Phys 41:491-500, 1998.

30. Galalae RM, Kovacs G, Schultze J, et al: Long-term outcome after elective irradiation of the pelvic lymphatics and local dose escalation using high dose rate brachytherapy for locally advanced prostate cancer. Int J Radiat Oncol Biol Phys 52:81-90, 2002.

31. Slater JD, Yonemoto LT, Rossi CJ, Jr., et al: Conformal proton therapy for prostate carcinoma. Int J Radiat Oncol Biol Phys 42:299-304, 1998.

32. Smith MR, McGovern FJ, Fallon MA, et al: Low bone mineral density in hormone-naive men with prostate carcinoma. Cancer 91:2238-45, 2001.

33. Coleman RE, Vinholes J, Purohit OP, et al: Effect of pamidronate on tumour marker levels in breast and prostate cancer-correlation with clinical and biochemical response. Proc Am Soc Clin Oncol 16:330a, 1997.

34. Scholz MC, Strum SB, McDermed JE: Intermittent androgen deprivation (IAD) with finasteride (F) during induction and maintenance permits prolonged time off IAD in localized prostate cancer (LPC). J Urol 161:156, 1999.

35. Brufsky A, Fontaine-Rothe P, Berlane K, et al: finasteride and flutamide as potency-sparing androgen-ablative therapy for advanced adenocarcinoma of the prostate. Urology 49:913-20, 1997.

36. Wheeler RE, Yun S, Vukovich J, et al: Randomized comparison of neoadjuvant treatment arms in organ confined prostate cancer using PSA nadir as the end point. Manuscript in preparation, 2002.

37. Strum SB, McDermed JE, Scholz MC, et al: Anemia associated with androgen deprivation (AAAD) due to combination hormone blockade (CHB) responds to recombinant human erythropoietin (r hu-EPO). J Urol 157:232A, 1997.

38. Duque JL, Loughlin KR, Adam RM, et al: Plasma levels of vascular endothelial growth factor are increased in patients with metastatic prostate cancer. Urology 54:523-7, 1999.

Appendix

The Partin Tables

It is often emphasized that medicine is an **art**, not a **science**. An *art* involves skill that is attained by study, practice, or observation whereas *science* is more formal and involves a system of knowledge covering general truths or the operation of general laws as obtained and tested through the scientific method and concerned with the physical world and its phenomena. In the world of prostate cancer, medicine tries to become more scientific by learning from the experiences of tens of thousands of human lives. It does this with greater validity **C1** through the use of tools like the Partin Tables.

The Partin Tables look at information such as the clinical stage as determined by the digital rectal exam (DRE), the Gleason score obtained at the time of diagnostic biopsy, and the PSA result obtained prior to the diagnostic biopsy, and the tables correlate such *inputs* with various findings or outputs obtained as a result of a radical retropubic prostatectomy. The *outputs* for the "new" Partin Tables (2001), shown in this appendix, involve the findings of (1) organ-confined disease, (2) established capsular penetration, (3) seminal vesicle involvement, and (4) lymph node involvement.

The original Partin Tables[1] were published in 1993 and involved 1,058 men undergoing retropubic radical prostatectomy (RRP) between the years 1982 and 1991 at a single medical center, the Johns Hopkins Hospital, with all surgery performed by one urologist, Patrick Walsh, M.D. An "update" of the Partin Tables[2] was published in 1997 and involved combining data on a total of 4,133 men with PC operated on at three medical centers: the Johns Hopkins Hospital (3,116 patients), Baylor College of Medicine (782 patients) and the University of Michigan (235 patients).

The 2001 Partin Tables[3] use more contemporary data inputs from 5,079 men with PC between the years 1994 and 2000. These tables represent only Johns Hopkins Hospital patients with all surgery again performed by Dr. Walsh.

The basis for these new Tables is the changing nature of prostate cancer, which reflects an earlier diagnosis of PC due to the advent of the PSA.[4] The clinical stage, which is essentially based on the DRE, is now T1c in the vast majority of patients. Again, this almost certainly reflects an earlier diagnosis of PC because of the use of PSA testing. In centers or specialized laboratories where the Gleason score is reviewed by a dedicated PC pathologist(s), the Gleason score is most often in the range of 5-7, and scores of 2-4 obtained from diagnostic biopsies are seldom, if ever given.[5]

The Partin Tables presented here, and many of the other similar "tools" that relate to prognostic outcomes in PC (tables, nomograms, algorithms, neural network analyses) are simply tools. **Their value relates to the ability of the medical team to fine-tune treatment strategy by evaluating the patient's unique biology and arriving at a sense of risk for organ-confined PC versus non-organ-confined PC.** In scenarios with a substantial risk of non-organ-confined PC (e.g. greater than 20%), the medical team can obtain additional laboratory, radiology or pathology assessments, the purpose of which are to confirm or refute the existence of non-organ-confined disease. Obviously, the "truth" is out there, and physicians should optimize their strategies with their patients by seeking such biological realities.

The limitation in accuracy of tools such as the Partin Tables, and other similar aids, relates to the validity of the biological data inputted from the patient. Using the Partin Tables, for example, implies that the clinical stage (as determined by the DRE) and the Gleason score (at biopsy) is on the same level of accuracy as that performed by physicians at Johns Hopkins Hospital. We know from our experiences obtaining second opinions on the Gleason score that validation of the Gleason score by an expert in PC pathology is critical to our understanding of PC and the use of more scientific approaches to this disease.[6]

The Partin Tables, and similar assessments help us profile patients with PC and focuses our attention on prognostic groups.

Such medical "subsets" involving clinical data, pathology, and radiology findings can enable us to stratify patients into differing categories of risk as low, intermediate or high, or into prognostic categories such as favorable, intermediate or unfavorable.

Such approaches clarify winning or losing strategies. The landmark papers cited within *The Primer* have employed such thinking.

2001 Partin Tables

The 2001 Partin Tables shown in this Appendix are used to obtain probabilities for specific pathologic findings in men considering a radical prostatectomy (RP). Those pathologic findings include:

- Organ-confined disease (OC)
- Capsular penetration—established (CP)
- Seminal vesicle involvement (SV+)
- Lymph node involvement (LN+)   C3

The inputs used include the PSA, Gleason score (G) and clinical stage. The PSA value used is the maximal PSA obtained *prior to any treatment* and preceding the RP. The Gleason score is based on the diagnostic biopsy and should have been initially read by a pathologist with expertise in PC pathology. If this has not been done, then a second opinion should be rendered by a pathologist of such caliber for the Partin Tables to have significant value. The clinical stage (see Appendix G) is solely based on the findings of the digital rectal examination (DRE).

To use these tables, find the table with the PSA range relating to your baseline PSA and next find your Gleason score (G) within the listings shown in the left column. Then move across the columns until you locate your clinical stage (T1c, T2a, T2b or T2c) and note the predictions for OC, CP, SV, and LN. The numbers in parentheses are 95% confidence intervals, i.e. you have a 95% chance of having the finding within the range indicated. For example, if you have a baseline PSA of 2.3, a Gleason score of 6, and a clinical stage of T1c, you would have the following probabilities (Partin Predictions) for OC, CP, SV and LN: 90, 9, 0 and 0, respectively.

PSA 0 – 2.5 ng/ml

G Score	Path Stage	Clinical Stage							
		T1c		T2a		T2b		T2c	
2-4	OC	95	(89-99)	91	(79-98)	88	(73-97)	86	(71-97)
	CP	5	(1-11)	9	(2-21)	12	(3-27)	14	(3-29)
	SV+	0	(0-0)	0	(0-0)	0	(0-0)	0	(0-0)
	LN+	0	(0-0)	0	(0-0)	0	(0-0)	0	(0-0)
5-6	OC	90	(88-93)	81	(77-85)	75	(69-81)	73	(63-81)
	CP	9	(7-12)	17	(13-21)	22	(17-28)	24	(17-33)
	SV+	0	(0-1)	1	(0-2)	2	(0-3)	1	(0-4)
	LN+	0	(0-0)	0	(0-1)	1	(0-2)	1	(0-4)
3+4=7	OC	79	(74-85)	64	(56-71)	54	(46-63)	51	(38-63)
	CP	17	(13-23)	29	(23-36)	35	(28-43)	36	(26-48)
	SV+	2	(1-5)	5	(1-9)	6	(2-12)	5	(1-13)
	LN+	1	(0-2)	2	(0-5)	4	(0-10)	6	(0-18)
4+3=7	OC	71	(62-79)	53	(43-63)	43	(33-54)	39	(26-54)
	CP	25	(18-34)	40	(30-49)	45	(35-56)	45	(32-59)
	SV+	2	(1-5)	4	(1-9)	5	(1-11)	5	(1-12)
	LN+	1	(0-4)	3	(0-8)	6	(0-14)	9	(0-26)
8-10	OC	66	(54-76)	47	(35-59)	37	(26-49)	34	(21-48)
	CP	28	(20-38)	42	(32-53)	46	(35-58)	47	(33-61)
	SV+	4	(1-10)	7	(2-16)	9	(2-20)	8	(2-19)
	LN+	1	(0-4)	3	(0-9)	6	(0-16)	10	(0-27)

PSA 2.6 – 4 ng/ml

G Score	Path Stage	Clinical Stage							
		T1c		T2a		T2b		T2c	
2-4	OC	92	(82-98)	85	(69-96)	80	(61-95)	78	(58-94)
	CP	8	(2-18)	15	(4-31)	20	(5-39)	22	(6-42)
	SV+	0	(0-0)	0	(0-0)	0	(0-0)	0	(0-0)
	LN+	0	(0-0)	0	(0-0)	0	(0-0)	0	(0-0)
5-6	OC	84	(81-86)	71	(66-75)	63	(57-69)	61	(50-70)
	CP	15	(13-18)	27	(23-31)	34	(28-40)	36	(27-45)
	SV+	1	(0-1)	2	(1-3)	2	(1-4)	2	(1-5)
	LN+	0	(0-0)	0	(0-1)	1	(0-2)	1	(0-4)
3+4=7	OC	68	(62-74)	50	(43-57)	41	(33-48)	38	(27-50)
	CP	27	(22-33)	41	(35-48)	47	(40-55)	48	(37-59)
	SV+	4	(2-7)	7	(3-12)	9	(4-15)	8	(2-17)
	LN+	1	(0-2)	2	(0-4)	3	(0-8)	5	(0-15)
4+3=7	OC	58	(48-67)	39	(30-48)	30	(22-39)	27	(18-40)
	CP	37	(29-46)	52	(43-61)	57	(47-67)	57	(44-70)
	SV+	4	(1-7)	6	(2-12)	7	(3-14)	6	(2-16)
	LN+	1	(0-3)	2	(0-6)	4	(0-12)	7	(0-21)
8-10	OC	52	(41-63)	33	(24-44)	25	(17-34)	23	(14-34)
	CP	40	(31-50)	53	(44-63)	57	(46-68)	57	(44-70)
	SV+	6	(3-12)	10	(4-18)	12	(5-22)	10	(3-22)
	LN+	1	(0-4)	3	(0-8)	5	(0-14)	8	(0-22)

PSA 4.1 – 6 ng/ml

G Score	Path Stage	Clinical Stage							
		T1c		T2a		T2b		T2c	
2-4	OC	90	(78-98)	81	(63-95)	75	(55-93)	73	(52-93)
	CP	10	(2-22)	19	(5-37)	25	(7-45)	27	(7-48)
	SV+	0	(0-0)	0	(0-0)	0	(0-0)	0	(0-0)
	LN+	0	(0-0)	0	(0-0)	0	(0-0)	0	(0-0)
5-6	OC	80	(78-83)	66	(62-70)	57	(52-63)	55	(44-64)
	CP	19	(16-21)	32	(28-36)	39	(33-44)	40	(32-50)
	SV+	1	(0-1)	1	(1-2)	2	(1-3)	2	(1-4)
	LN+	0	(0-1)	1	(0-2)	2	(1-3)	3	(1-7)
3+4=7	OC	63	(58-68)	44	(39-50)	35	(29-40)	31	(23-41)
	CP	32	(27-36)	46	(40-52)	51	(44-57)	50	(40-60)
	SV+	3	(2-5)	5	(3-8)	7	(4-11)	6	(2-11)
	LN+	2	(1-3)	4	(2-7)	7	(4-13)	12	(5-23)
4+3=7	OC	52	(43-60)	33	(25-41)	25	(18-32)	21	(14-31)
	CP	42	(35-50)	56	(48-64)	60	(50-68)	57	(43-68)
	SV+	3	(1-6)	5	(2-8)	5	(3-9)	4	(1-10)
	LN+	3	(1-5)	6	(3-11)	10	(5-18)	16	(6-32)
8-10	OC	46	(36-56)	28	(20-37)	21	(14-29)	18	(11-28)
	CP	45	(36-54)	58	(49-66)	59	(49-69)	57	(43-70)
	SV+	5	(3-9)	8	(4-13)	9	(4-16)	7	(2-15)
	LN+	3	(1-6)	6	(2-12)	10	(4-20)	16	(6-33)

C5

PSA 6.1 – 10 ng/ml

G Score	Path Stage	Clinical Stage							
		T1c		T2a		T2b		T2c	
2-4	OC	87	(73-97)	76	(56-94)	69	(47-91)	67	(45-91)
	CP	13	(3-27)	24	(6-44)	31	(9-53)	33	(9-55)
	SV+	0	(0-0)	0	(0-0)	0	(0-0)	0	(0-0)
	LN+	0	(0-0)	0	(0-0)	0	(0-0)	0	(0-0)
5-6	OC	75	(72-77)	58	(54-61)	49	(43-54)	46	(36-56)
	CP	23	(21-25)	37	(34-41)	44	(39-49)	46	(37-55)
	SV+	2	(2-3)	4	(3-5)	5	(3-8)	5	(2-9)
	LN+	0	(0-1)	1	(0-2)	2	(1-3)	3	(1-6)
3+4=7	OC	54	(49-59)	35	(30-40)	26	(22-31)	24	(17-32)
	CP	36	(32-40)	49	(43-54)	52	(46-58)	52	(42-61)
	SV+	8	(6-11)	13	(9-18)	16	(10-22)	13	(6-23)
	LN+	2	(1-3)	3	(2-6)	6	(4-10)	10	(5-18)
4+3=7	OC	43	(35-51)	25	(19-32)	19	(14-25)	16	(10-24)
	CP	47	(40-54)	58	(51-66)	60	(52-68)	58	(46-69)
	SV+	8	(4-12)	11	(6-17)	13	(7-20)	11	(4-21)
	LN+	2	(1-4)	5	(2-8)	8	(5-14)	13	(6-25)
8-10	OC	37	(28-46)	21	(15-28)	15	(10-21)	13	(8-20)
	CP	48	(39-57)	57	(48-65)	57	(48-67)	56	(43-69)
	SV+	13	(8-19)	17	(11-26)	19	(11-29)	16	(6-29)
	LN+	3	(1-5)	5	(2-10)	8	(4-16)	13	(5-26)

		PSA > 10 ng/ml						
G	Path	Clinical Stage						
Score	Stage	T1c		T2a		T2b		T2c
2-4	OC	80	(61-95)	65	(43-89)	57	(35-86)	54 (32-85)
	CP	20	(5-39)	35	(11-57)	43	(14-65)	46 (15-68)
	SV+	0	(0-0)	0	(0-0)	0	(0-0)	0 (0-0)
	LN+	0	(0-0)	0	(0-0)	0	(0-0)	0 (0-0)
5-6	OC	62	(58-64)	42	(38-46)	33	(28-38)	30 (21-38)
	CP	33	(30-36)	47	(43-52)	52	(46-56)	51 (42-60)
	SV+	4	(3-5)	6	(4-8)	8	(5-11)	6 (2-12)
	LN+	2	(1-3)	4	(3-7)	8	(5-12)	13 (6-22)
3+4=7	OC	37	(32-42)	20	(17-24)	14	(11-17)	11 (7-17)
	CP	43	(38-48)	49	(43-55)	47	(40-53)	42 (30-55)
	SV+	12	(9-17)	16	(11-22)	17	(12-24)	13 (6-24)
	LN+	8	(5-11)	14	(9-21)	22	(15-30)	33 (18-49)
4+3=7	OC	27	(21-34)	14	(10-18)	9	(6-13)	7 (4-12)
	CP	51	(44-59)	55	(46-64)	50	(40-60)	43 (29-59)
	SV+	11	(6-17)	13	(7-20)	13	(8-21)	10 (3-20)
	LN+	10	(5-17)	18	(10-27)	27	(16-39)	38 (20-58)
8-10	OC	22	(16-30)	11	(7-15)	7	(4-10)	6 (3-10)
	CP	50	(42-59)	52	(41-62)	46	(36-59)	41 (27-57)
	SV+	17	(10-25)	19	(12-29)	19	(12-29)	15 (5-28)
	LN+	11	(5-18)	17	(9-29)	27	(14-40)	38 (20-59)

References

1. Partin AW, Yoo J, Carter HB, et al: The use of prostate specific antigen, clinical stage and Gleason score to predict pathological stage in men with localized prostate cancer. J Urol 150:110-4, 1993.

2. Partin AW, Kattan MW, Subong EN, et al: Combination of prostate-specific antigen, clinical stage, and Gleason score to predict pathological stage of localized prostate cancer. A multi-institutional update. Jama 277:1445-51, 1997.

3. Partin AW, Mangold LA, Lamm DM, et al: Contemporary update of prostate cancer staging nomograms (Partin Tables) for the new millennium. Urology 58:843-8, 2001.

4. Noldus J, Graefen M, Haese A, et al: Stage migration in clinically localized prostate cancer. Eur Urol 38:74-8, 2000.

5. Epstein JI: Gleason score 2-4 adenocarcinoma of the prostate on needle biopsy: a diagnosis that should not be made. Am J Surg Pathol 24:477-8, 2000.

6. Carlson GD, Calvanese CB, Kahane H, et al: Accuracy of biopsy Gleason scores from a large uropathology laboratory: use of a diagnostic protocol to minimize observer variability. Urology 51:525-9, 1998.

Appendix

Glossary of Terms

> A symbol that means "greater than".

≥ A symbol that means "greater than or equal to".

< A symbol that means "less than".

≤ A symbol that means "less than or equal to".

3DCRT (3-Dimensional Conformal Radiation Therapy): An approach to treatment planning that focuses on directing the radiation energy to the tumor target while sparing the surrounding normal tissues; see CONFORMAL THERAPY.

5-AR: 5-alpha reductase; the enzyme that converts testosterone to dihydrotestosterone (DHT).

ADS (ANDROGEN DEPRIVATION SYNDROME): A constellation of findings associated with low levels of androgen associated with ADT.

ABDOMEN: The part of the body below the ribs and above the pelvic bone that contains organs like the intestines, the liver, the kidneys, and the stomach.

ABLATION: Relating to the removal or destruction of tissue or a system; androgen ablation refers to blocking the effects of androgens by surgical or medical means.

ACT: Alpha-1 chymotrypsin; a protein that binds PSA to create complexed PSA or CPSA that is associated with prostate cancer; compare to free PSA that is associated with benign conditions.

ACTH: Adrenal corticotrophic hormone or adrenocorticotrophic hormone. A pituitary hormone that stimulates the outer portion of the adrenal glands to secrete various hormones including cortisol, DHEA and androstenedione.

ADENOCARCINOMA: A form of cancer that develops from a

malignant abnormality in the cells lining a glandular organ such as the prostate. Almost all prostate cancers are adenocarcinomas.

ADPC (ANDROGEN-DEPENDENT PC): PC cells that depend on androgens for continued cell growth and vitality.

ADRENALECTOMY: The removal of the adrenal glands, usually accomplished by surgery.

ADS: An abbreviation for Androgen Deprivation Syndrome. See ANDROGEN DEPRIVATION SYNDROME.

ADT: See ANDROGEN DEPRIVATION THERAPY.

AGONIST: A chemical substance (as a drug) capable of combining with a receptor on a cell and initiating a reaction or activity; in PC, the LHRH agonist is also called LHRH-A. The most commonly used LHRH-A are Lupron and Zoladex. Either of these agents interact with the LHRH receptor and form a complex that over a period of two weeks results in a decrease in release of LH and hence a lowering in serum testosterone.

AIPC (ANDROGEN-INDEPENDENT PC): PC cells that do not depend on androgen for growth.

D2

ALGORITHM: A step-by-step problem-solving procedure clearly defined for obtaining the solution to a general type of problem. Algorithms often involve mathematical formulas and are computational in nature. Algorithm is named after the 9th-century Persian mathematician al-Khowarizimi.

AMU: Atomic mass unit.

ANASTOMOSIS: A connection, usually a physical connection between anatomical structures. When the prostate is surgically removed, an anastomosis is made that connects the bladder neck with the remaining urethra.

ANASTOMOTIC STRICTURE: A narrowing at the junction of two tissues or structures that have been connected. After RP, an anastomotic stricture may occur at the site of anastomosis between the bladder neck and urethra.

ANDROGEN: A hormone (e.g., testosterone) which is responsible for male characteristics and the development and function of male sexual organs produced mainly by the testicles but also in the cortex of the adrenal glands. Androgens have far reaching effects on blood formation, muscle and bone mass, cognitive function, emotional stability, skin and hair, etc.

ANDROGEN-DEPENDENT PC (ADPC): PC cells that depend on androgens for continued cell growth and vitality.

ANDROGEN DEPRIVATION SYNDROME (ADS): A constellation of findings associated with low levels of androgen associated with ADT.

ANDROGEN DEPRIVATION THERAPY (ADT): A prostate cancer treatment that is based on blocking the amount or availability of androgen to the PC cell. Includes diverse mechanisms such as surgical or medical castration, anti-androgens, 5-AR inhibitors, estrogenic compounds, agents that interfere with adrenal androgen production, agents that decrease sensitivity of the androgen receptor (AR). It also includes monotherapy, ADT with two drugs (ADT$_2$), triple therapy (ADT$_3$) or more.

ANDROGEN-INDEPENDENT PROSTATE CANCER (AIPC): PC cells that do not depend on androgen for growth.

ANDROGEN RECEPTOR (AR): A structural entity that is the site of interaction of a chemical substance called a ligand, in this case androgen; the receptor is essentially a docking site for the ligand and the interaction of the two is responsible for turning on the cell's DNA machinery.

ANDROSTENEDIONE: One of the two major adrenal androgen precursors (the other being DHEA-S); androstenedione is metabolized to testosterone within the prostate cell; see DHEA-S.

ANEUPLOID: Having an abnormal number of sets of chromosomes; for example, tetraploid means having two paired sets of chromosomes, which is twice as many as normal. Aneuploid cancer cells tend not to respond well to androgen deprivation therapy. Aneuploidy refers to the state of being aneuploid; see DIPLOID.

ANGIOGENESIS: Relating to the formation of blood vessels.

ANTAGONIST: A chemical that acts within the body to reduce the physiological activity of another chemical substance.

ANTI-ANDROGEN: A substance that intereferes with the biochemical effect of an androgen by blocking the site of interaction of an androgen with its receptor. Eulexin® and Casodex®, the most commonly used anti-androgens in the treatment of prostate cancer, bind to the androgen receptor. This prevents both testosterone and dihydrotestosterone (see DHT) from interacting with the receptor, thus halting DNA synthesis and stopping tumor growth.

ANTIGEN: A substance that elicits a cellular-level immune response or causes the formation of an antibody; "foreign" material introduced into the body (a virus or bacterium, for example) or other material which the immune system considers to be "foreign" because it is not part of the body's normal biology (e.g. prostate cancer cells).

ANTITHROMBIN-III DEFICIENCY: A deficiency of a substance in the coagulation system of the body that leads to a tendency to form blood clots. The mechanism, or at least the main mechanism, by which estrogens and estrogenic compounds cause blood clots in the legs or lungs.

APOPTOSIS: Programmed cell death due to an alteration in a critical substance or chemical necessary for cell viability; the lack of male hormones causes apoptosis of androgen-dependent PC.

ARM: Androgen receptor mutation; a change in the androgen receptor that leads to the receptor utilizing an anti-androgen as if it were an androgen. In the face of a castrate testosterone level and a rising PSA, an ARM must be excluded by stopping any use of an anti-androgen.

AROMATASE: An enzyme that converts testosterone to estrogen (estradiol or estrone).

AUA SCORE (AUA SYMPTOM SCORE): American Urologic Association grading system that quantitates a man's urinary function.

AUS: Artificial Urinary Sphincter; a surgical implant used in the treatment of incontinence.

BASELINE PSA (bPSA): The PSA level before a new treatment has begun; used to establish efficacy of a therapy based on response of the PSA to the treatment. Can also be used in principle with any other marker, radiologic imaging study or any finding that indicates the patient's status prior to starting a new treatment; in essence, a parameter to gauge success or failure of treatment.

BAT: B-mode acquisition and targeting. An ultrasound evaluation of the prostate localizing it prior to each and every RT therapy treatment. Currently used in conjunction with IMRT and mechanically integrated into the treatment program.

BC: Breast cancer.

BENIGN: Relatively harmless; not cancerous; not malignant.

BENIGN PROSTATIC HYPERPLASIA or HYPERTROPHY (BPH): A noncancerous condition of the prostate that results in the growth of both glandular and stromal (supporting connective) tissue, enlarging the prostate and obstructing urination.

BID (bid): A Latin abbreviation for "Bis In Die" meaning "twice a day". This is used in designating frequency of medication or treatment, as in "Flomax 0.4 mg bid".

BILATERAL: Both sides; for example, a bilateral orchiectomy is an orchiectomy in which both testicles are removed and a bilateral adrenalectomy is an operation in which both adrenal glands are removed.

BIOLOGY: The study of living organisms, of life forms and all their vital processes including their structure, function, growth, origin, and evolution.

BIOMARKER: An indicator of biological activity of cells or tissues that can be used as a means to monitor a state of health or disease; most often a laboratory test used to mark the response to treatment (e.g. PSA) but can also be a physical finding (e.g. prostate size and texture) or an expression of function of the living organism (e.g. AUA score). Biomarkers are important parameters to judge the status of a patient's health.

BIOPSY: Sampling of tissue from a particular part of the body (e.g., the prostate) in order to check for abnormalities such as cancer. In the case of prostate cancer, biopsies are usually carried out under ultrasound guidance using a specially designed device known as a prostate biopsy gun. Removed tissue is routinely examined microscopically by a pathologist in order to make a precise diagnosis of the patient's condition. Biopsy is the only current method of positively diagnosing PC at the present time and of obtaining tissue to evaluate the aggressiveness of the cancer. Negative biopsies are inconclusive for PC and are not a guarantee that no cancer exists.

BISPHOSPHONATES (BPs, ABPs): A class of compounds that stop bone loss (resorption) by actions directed against the osteoclast—the cell that is implemented in bone resorption. Examples of bisphosphonates include Fosamax®, Actonel®, Aredia® and Zometa®.

BLADDER: The hollow organ in which urine is collected and stored in the body.

bNED: Biologically with No Evidence of Disease. One example would be using a biological end-point such as PSA of <0.2 for a definition of bNED for successful brachytherap .

BONE SCAN: A technique that uses a radioactive agent (isotope) to identify abnormal or cancerous growths within bone. In the case of prostate cancer, a bone scan is used to identify bone metastases. Metastases appear in the scan as "hot spots" due to increased uptake of the isotope in bone, however the absence of hot spots does not prove the absence of tiny metastases.

BPH: See BENIGN PROSTATIC HYPERPLASIA.

bPSA: See BASELINE PSA.

BRACHYTHERAPY: A form of radiation therapy in which radioactive seeds or wires which emit radiation are implanted within the prostate in order to destroy PC; subcategorized into permanent seed implants versus temporary wire implants. See HDR BRACHYTHERAPY.

BRAGG PEAK: The point of energy release due to slowing down of the energized particle resulting in increased ionization and delivery of the "energy payload" used to irreparably damage DNA.

BUN: Blood urea nitrogen, a laboratory test that relates to kidney function as well as to the state of hydration of the patient; a normal BUN level is usually less than 20.

CANCER: The growth of abnormal cells in the body in an uncontrolled manner. Unlike benign tumors, these tend to invade surrounding tissues and spread to distant sites of the body via the blood stream and lymphatic system.

CARCINOGENESIS: Cancer development.

CARCINOMA: A form of cancer that originates in tissues that line or cover a particular organ; see ADENOCARCINOMA.

CASODEX®: Brand or trade name of bicalutamide in the USA. An anti-androgen that blocks the androgen receptor and prevents natural androgens from stimulating cell growth.

CASTRATE: A level associated with what occurs after castration; traditionally surgical removal of the testicles. A castrate testosterone is defined by most physicians as less than 20 ng/ml (or less than 0.69 nM/L).

CASTRATION: The use of surgical or medical techniques to eliminate testosterone produced by the testes.

CAT SCAN (CT or COMPUTERIZED AXIAL TOMOGRAPHY): A method of combining images from multiple x-rays under the control of a computer to produce cross-sectional or three-dimensional pictures of the internal organs which can be used to identify abnormalities. The CAT scan can identify prostate enlargement but is not always effective for assessing the stage of prostate cancer. For evaluating metastases of the lymph nodes or more distant soft tissue sites, the CAT scan is associated with a high degree of insensitivity—it misses a great deal of the disease that really is present unless there is bulky tumor present.

CBC: Complete blood count; includes the white blood count (WBC), hematocrit (HCT) and the platelet count (PLT).

CC: Cubic centimeter or cc; a measure of volume used in assessing the prostate gland or the amount of prostate cancer. Cubic centimeters (cc) are equivalent to grams in determinations of the prostate gland volume.

CEA: Carcinoembryonic antigen; a fetal antigen or protein that may be expressed by PC that is aggressive and often androgen-independent.

CGA: Chromogranin A; a substance produced by the neuroendocrine cells that are associated with androgen-independent PC. A progressive increase in serum CGA indicates an aggressive clone of PC cells that has an increased tendency to metastasize to lymph nodes, liver and lungs.

cGy (centigray): A unit for radiation absorbed dose (rad) in any material. When the International System SD (skin dose), was adopted, the unit for radiation absorbed dose became the Gray (Gy) instead of the rad. One Gy = 100 rads = 100 cGy. One centigray (cGy) = 1 rad. Use of the term cGy is not restricted to x- or gamma radiation, but can be used for all forms of ionizing radiation.

CHB (COMBINED HORMONE BLOCKADE): Also referred to as CHT, MAB, TAB; the preferred term is ADT (androgen deprivation therapy) with number attached to show number of agents, e.g. ADT_3 (Flutamide, Lupron®, Proscar®) or ADT_3 (FLP). The use of more than one hormone in therapy; especially the use of LHRH analogs (e.g., Lupron®, Zoladex®) to block the production of testosterone by the testes, plus anti-androgens (e.g., Casodex® (bicalutamide), Eulexin® (flutamide), Anandron® or Nilandron® (nilutamide), and Androcur® (cyproterone acetate) to compete with DHT and with T (testosterone) for cell sites thereby depriving cancer cells of DHT and T needed for growth. May involve other agents such as Proscar® or prolactin inhibitors such as Dostinex®.

CHEMOTHERAPY: The use of pharmaceuticals or other chemicals to kill cancer cells. In many cases chemotherapeutic agents kill not only cancer cells but also other cells in the body, which makes such agents potentially very dangerous.

CHT (COMBINED HORMONAL THERAPY): See CHB.

CIALIS®: Brand name for tadalafil, an oral phosphodiesterase type 5 (PDE5) inhibitor used in the treatment of impotence.

CLINICAL TRIAL: A carefully planned experiment to evaluate a treatment or a medication (often a new pharmaceutical) for an unproven use. Phase I trials are used to determine proper dosages and toxicity. A Phase II study is done on a limited number of patients to establish effectiveness. Phase III trials involve many patients and compare a new therapy against the current standard or best available therapy. Phase III trials precede the application for approval by the FDA to make the drug or treatment available to the general public.

COLLIMATOR: A device, often a tube-like structure, capable of organizing radiation to permit only parallel rays to emanate. See MLC or MULTILEAF COLLIMATOR.

COMBINATION THERAPY: See CHT or CHB; ADT with designation ADT_1 versus ADT_2 or ADT_3 is preferred since this communicates the number of drugs used in the androgen deprivation therapy. ADT also more clearly communicates the mechanism of this approach to treatment.

CONCORDANCE: The agreement in findings that support the accuracy of a particular investigation or treatment. Concordance is a critical concept in studies to diagnose, stage and treat PC. The principle of concordance is used in combining the results of endorectal MRI with magnetic resonance spectroscopy to enhance the accuracy of these investigations. Concordant drops in multiple biomarkers such as PSA and PAP or PSA and CGA are associated with a longer response time and survival.

CONFORMAL RADIOTHERAPY: The use of careful planning and delivery techniques designed to focus radiation on the areas of the prostate and surrounding tissue which need treatment and protect areas which do not need treatment. Three-dimensional conformal radiation therapy (3DCRT) is a sophisticated form of this method as is Intensity Modulated Radiation Therapy (IMRT).

COWPER'S GLANDS: Small sex accessory tissues that contribute to the fluid component of the ejaculate; a pair of pea-sized glands that lie below the prostate gland, named after the English surgeon William Cowper (1660-1709). Cowper's glands secrete an alkaline fluid that forms part of the semen and neutralizes the acidic environment of the urethra, thereby protecting the sperm.

CREATINE: A nitrogenous organic acid, $C_4H_9N_3O_2$, that is found in the muscle tissue of vertebrates mainly in the form of phosphocreatine and which supplies energy for muscle contraction.

CREATININE: The metabolic waste substance resulting from the breakdown of creatine in muscle. Creatinine is secreted in the urine and the measurement of serum creatinine in the blood correlates with kidney function (or possible urinary obstruction) since in the event of urinary obstruction this waste product is inadequately removed from the body .

CRYOABLATION: See CRYOSURGERY.

CRYOSURGERY: The use of liquid nitrogen or Argon gas circulated through hollow probes to freeze a particular organ to extremely low temperatures to kill the tissue, including any cancerous tissue. When used to treat prostate cancer, the cryoprobes are guided by transrectal ultrasound or MRI.

CRYOTHERAPY: See CRYOSURGERY.

CT SCAN: Computerized or computed tomography; see CAT SCAN.

CYSTOSCOPE: An instrument employing laser optics that is introduced via the urethra and allows the urologist to view the bladder interior and openings of the ureters into the bladder.

CYSTOSCOPY: A procedure in which the interior of the bladder can be visually inspected by means of an instrument, a cystoscope, which is inserted into the bladder via the urethra.

DEBULKING: Reduction of the volume of cancer by one of several techniques; most frequently used to imply surgical debulking.

DECILITER: One tenth of a liter or 100 ml. See ML.

DE-DIFFERENTIATED: See DIFFERENTIATION.

DENDRITIC CELLS (DC): Cells that process antigens (proteins) and present them to immune lymphocytes called T cells which play a major role in the initiation of the immune response against tumor and other types of abnormal cells. Antigen presenting cells; e.g. Provenge®, an investigational therapy employing DC.

DES: Diethylstilbestrol. A synthetic estrogen used in treating prostate cancer.

DHEA (DIHYDROEPIANDROSTERONE): An adrenal androgen precursor produced in the adrenal cortex and transformed into testosterone within prostate cells.

DHEA-S: The sulfated metabolite of DHEA. DHEA-S is a more reliable laboratory test than DHEA and is therefore preferred over DHEA when evaluating the adrenal androgen status. DHEA-S is metabolized to androstenedione and then to testosterone; see ANDROSTENEDIONE.

DHT: See DIHYDROTESTOSTERONE.

DIAGNOSIS: The evaluation of signs, symptoms and selected test results by a physician to determine the physical and biological causes of these signs and symptoms and whether a specific disease or disorder is involved.

DIFFERENTIATION: Degree of maturity; relates to the appearance or morphology of cells and their function. Mature cells are considered to be well-differentiated whereas more primitive and aggressive cells are of a lower degree of differentiation or are de-differentiated.

DIGITAL RECTAL EXAMINATION (DRE): The use by a physician of a lubricated and gloved finger inserted into the rectum to feel for abnormalities of the prostate and rectum.

DIHYDROTESTOSTERONE (DHT or 5 alpha-dihydrotestosterone): A male hormone 5 times more potent than testosterone that is converted from testosterone within the prostate by the enzyme 5-alpha reductase.

DIPLOID: Having one complete set of normally paired chromosomes, i.e., a normal amount of DNA. Diploid cancer cells tend to grow slowly and respond well to hormone therapy. A diploid number of chromosomes would equal 46, a haploid set would equal 23; also see HAPLOID.

DNA (DEOXYRIBONUCLEIC ACID): The basic biologically active chemical that defines the physical development and growth of nearly all living organisms; a complex protein that is the carrier of genetic information.

DOUBLING TIME: The time that it takes a particular focus of cancer to double in size.

DOWN-REGULATING (DOWN-REGULATION): Turning off a mechanism of action at the biochemical level in the body. A common example of down-regulation relates to turning off the pituitary hormone (LH) that normally stimulates the testicles to make testosterone. Also see UP-REGULATING.

DOWNSIZING: The use of hormonal or other forms of management to reduce the volume of prostate cancer in and/or around the prostate prior to attempted curative treatment.

DOWNSTAGING: The use of hormonal or other forms of management in the attempt to lower the clinical stage of prostate cancer prior to attempted curative treatment (e.g., from stage T3a to stage T2b).

DRE: See DIGITAL RECTAL EXAMINATION.

DT: Doubling time.

Dx: Standard abbreviation for diagnosis.

DYSURIA: Urination that is associated with pain or discomfort. Dysuria may occur with bladder infections or irritation of the bladder wall due to radiation injury.

EBRT (EXTERNAL BEAM RADIATION THERAPY): External beam radiation treatment that can include conventional photons, or use protons, neutrons, or electrons. This may be given conventionally or with 3D conformal techniques or via IMRT; see EXTERNAL BEAM RADIATION THERAPY; see IMRT.

ECE: An abbreviation for extra-capsular extension.

EJACULATION: The release of semen through the penis during orgasm. Ejaculation may be termed "dry" if there is scanty or no fluid component to the ejaculate resulting from destruction of the prostate gland by RT or surgery.

EJACULATORY DUCTS: The tubular passages through which semen reaches the prostatic urethra during orgasm, formed by the fusion of the ductus deferens carrying sperm from the testicles and the union with the seminal vesicle.

EMBOLISM: A blood clot that has traveled usually from a leg vein to the lung as in pulmonary embolism.

EMPOWERMENT: Taking responsibility for, and authority over one's own outcomes based on education and knowledge of the consequences and contingencies involved in one's own decisions. This focus provides the uplifting energy that can sustain in the face of crisis.

ENDOCRINE GLAND: Any of various glands producing hormonal secretions that pass directly into the bloodstream. Examples of endocrine glands include the thyroid, parathyroids, anterior and posterior pituitary, pancreas, adrenals, pineal, and gonads.

ENZYME: Any of a group of chemical substances which are produced by living cells and which cause particular chemical reactions to happen while not being changed themselves.

EOD (EXTENT OF DISEASE): An approach to standardize the reporting of the extent of cancer as seen on a bone scan; after work by Mark Soloway, M.D.

erMRI: See ENDORECTAL MRI.

ENDORECTAL MRI: Magnetic resonance imaging of the prostate done via a probe inserted into the rectum. May be combined with endorectal magnetic resonance spectroscopy (currently only being done at UC San Francisco and Memorial Sloan Kettering in New York City).

ENDOTHELIN-1: A prostate cancer cell product that stimulates osteoblasts and also acts as a vasoconstrictor that may be responsible for bone pain in metastatic PC.

EPITHELIAL CELL: A cell type within the prostate that lines the ducts and functionally secretes chemicals such as PSA into the blood stream or into the duct openings or lumens.

ESTRADIOL: The most potent of the natural estrogen compounds; compare with estriol and estrone which are other natural estrogenic hormones of lesser potency. Estradiol is metabolized from testosterone; estrone is metabolized from androstenedione, an adrenal androgen.

ESTROGEN: A female hormone or estrogen (e.g., diethylstilbestrol) used in the treatment of PC.

EULEXIN®: The brand or trade name of flutamide in the USA; an anti-androgen that blocks the androgen receptor and prevents testosterone and/or DHT from stimulating cell growth.

EXTERNAL BEAM RADIATION THERAPY (EBRT): A form of radiation therapy in which the radiation is delivered by a machine directed at the area to be radiated as opposed to radiation given within the target tissue such as brachytherapy.

FAMILIAL: Of first-degree relatives.

FDA: Food and Drug Administration.

FIBROBLAST: A cell type that is involved with producing fibrous or connective tissue; a connective-tissue cell that secretes proteins and molecular collagen from which the extracellular fibrillar matrix of connective tissue forms.

FINASTERIDE: An inhibitor of the enzyme (5-alpha reductase or 5-AR) that stimulates the conversion of testosterone to DHT. Used to treat BPH and PC; see PROSCAR®.

FISTULA: In the context of PC, an abnormal passage resulting from injury or disease that connects an abscess, cavity, or hollow organ to the body surface or to another hollow organ. For example, a fistula or connection between the rectum and bladder can occur in instances of significant damage to the rectal wall in proximity to the bladder.

FLARE REACTION: A temporary increase in tumor growth and symptoms (clinical flare) or in PSA only (biochemical flare) due to a testosterone surge caused by the initial use of an LHRH agonist. Can be mild to dangerous. May be prevented by taking an anti-androgen (Eulexin®, Casodex®, or Nilandron®) several days before starting a LHRH agonist (Lupron® or Zoladex®) or by the use of an LHRH antagonist such as abarelix (Plenaxis™) or by any maneuver that suppresses testosterone or blocks its action.

FLASHES: See FLUSHES.

FLUSHES: A transitory sensation of extreme heat (as in response to some drugs or in some physiological states). Flushes or flashes are due to dilation of blood vessels in the skin of the affected area.

FLUTAMIDE: Trade name is Eulexin®; an anti-androgen used in the palliative hormonal treatment of advanced prostate cancer and in the adjuvant and neoadjuvant hormonal treatment of earlier stages of prostate cancer. Normal dosage is two capsules (125 mg each) three times a day.

FREE PSA: PSA unbound to any major protein; free PSA relates to benign prostate growth. The percentage of free-PSA is the Free PSA divided by Total PSA x 100 and expressed as percent. Multiple studies have shown that men with free PSA % > 25%

had low risk of PC while those with < 10% free PSA % were likely to have PC.

FSH (FOLLICLE STIMULATING HORMONE): A hormone produced in the pituitary gland. In the male, stimulates the Sertoli cells of the testicle to make sperm. May be a factor in PC growth since FSH receptors have been identified on PC cells.

FUSION: Combining two or more inputs of data so that they can be overlaid one upon another to provide a sense of agreement or concordance; fusion-imaging studies such as ProstaScint-CT or ProstaScint-PET are examples.

GANTRY: Radiation therapy hardware from which the linear accelerator delivers its energy; the multileaf collimator (MLC) is attached to the gantry and modulates the radiation beam as it exits.

GENITOURINARY SYSTEM (GU SYSTEM): In the male, pertaining to the organs comprising the genital and urinary system. This includes the testicles, penis, seminal vesicles, urethra, bladder, ureters and kidneys.

D14 **GENITOURINARY TOXICITY:** RT damage to urinary and/or genital tissues or functions.

GLAND: A structure or organ that produces a substance which may be used in another part of the body. In the context of prostate cancer, also frequently used in reference to the prostate gland.

GLAND VOLUME (GV): The size in cubic centimeters or grams of the prostate gland.

GLEASON: After Donald Gleason, M.D.; the name of the physician who developed the Gleason grading system, one of the most important tools available to profile the aggressiveness of prostate cancer.

GLEASON SCORE: A widely used method for classifying the degree of loss of the normal glandular tissue architecture (size, shape and differentiation of glands). Two numbers, each from 1–5, are assigned successively to the two most predominant tissue patterns present in the examined tissue sample and are added together to produce the Gleason score. High numbers indicate poor differentiation and therefore more aggressive cancer.

GONADOTROPHINS: Trophic or growth promoting hormones from the anterior pituitary. The two major gonadotrophins are luteinizing hormone or LH which stimulates the Leydig cells in the testicles to make testosterone and follicle stimulating hormone or FSH which stimulates the Sertoli cells in the testicles to make sperm. LH and FSH receptors have been identified on PC cells.

GRADE: A means of describing the potential degree of severity of a cancer based on the appearance of the glandular architecture as seen using a microscope. The Gleason grade is classified as either the primary or secondary grade. The primary grade represents the tissue pattern that is present in 51% or more of the examined specimen. The secondary grade represents from 5% to 49% of the next most predominant pattern; see GLEASON SCORE.

Gy (Gray): A unit for radiation absorbed dose (rad) in any material. One Gy = 100 cGy = 100 rads. Use of the term Gy is not restricted to x- or gamma radiation, but can be used for all forms of ionizing radiation (see cGy).

GYNECOMASTIA: Enlargement or tenderness of the male breasts or nipples. A potential side-effect of any form of hormonal therapy which increases levels of estrogens as seen with DES, PC SPES™, Emcyt®, monotherapy with anti-androgens (Flutamide or Casodex®) or the combination of the latter with Proscar®. **D15**

HAPLOID: Having the same number of sets of chromosomes as a germ cell (sperm or egg) or half as many as a somatic cell (all remaining cells having to do with the body); having a single set of chromosomes; see DIPLOID.

HDK: High-dose ketoconazole; trade name is Nizoral®; an agent used in the treatment of PC that works against ADPC and AIPC. HDK lowers testicular and adrenal androgen levels and also has multiple effects on the tumor cell.

HDR BRACHYTHERAPY: High dose rate brachytherapy applied by a radioactive iridium wire inserted into the prostate gland after first using transrectal ultrasound guidance for placement of hollow plastic needles followed by CT evaluation for planning the dose. The iridium wire is inserted into the plastic needles.

HEMATURIA: Signifying that there is blood in the urine. This may be "gross hematuria" where the blood is obvious to the naked eye or "microscopic hematuria" where a microscopic evaluation reveals the presence of blood through the identification of red blood cells in the urine.

HEMORRHAGIC CYSTITIS: Bleeding into the urine due to injury to the bladder wall.

HEREDITARY: Inherited from one's parents and earlier generations.

HEREDITY: The historical distribution of biological characteristics through a group of related individuals via their DNA.

HORMONE: A substance, usually a peptide or steroid, produced by one tissue and conveyed by the bloodstream to another to effect physiological activity, such as growth or metabolism; testosterone and estrogen are examples.

HORMONE REFRACTORY PC: A loosely used term that really should apply to progressive PC in the setting of a testosterone level less than 20 ng/dl and when an ARM has been excluded; the preferred term is AIPC or androgen-independent PC; see ARM; see AIPC.

HOT FLASHES OR FLUSHES: See FLUSHES or FLASHES.

HYDRONEPHROSIS: The swelling of the kidney seen on x-ray examination and related to obstruction of urine flow beyond the kidney; usually the ureter is obstructed leading to both hydroureter and hydronephrosis.

HYPOTHALAMUS: A part of the regulatory system located in the brain above the area of the pituitary that serves as a master controller for most of the body's hormonal functions.

Hx: An abbreviation for "History". This is often used by physicians in their consultation reports.

IAD (INTERMITTENT ANDROGEN DEPRIVATION): The discontinuation of ADT that allows for recovery of natural testosterone production with the intent to allow the patient to recover from symptoms of androgen deprivation; same as IHT.

IATROGENIC: Caused by the action of the physician; relating usually to an adverse event that is doctor induced.

IMAGING: A radiology technique or method allowing a physician to see something that would not normally be visible.

IMPLANT: A device that is inserted into the body; e.g., a tiny container of radioactive material inserted in or near a tumor; also a device inserted in order to replace or substitute for an ability which has been lost; for example, a penile implant is a device which can be surgically inserted into the penis to provide rigidity for intercourse.

IMPOTENCE: The inability to have or to maintain an erection; also known as ED or erectile dysfunction.

IMRT (INTENSITY MODULATED RADIATION THERAPY): An approach to radiation delivery allowing the treatment team to specify the tumor target dose and the amount of radiation allowable to the nearby tissues; it uses sophisticated computer planning to arrive at acceptable equations. Sophisticated hardware is also incorporated into this planning that allows the radiation intensity to be modulated up or down as the delivery system rotates around the patient.

INTERMITTENT ANDROGEN DEPRIVATION (IAD): The discontinuation of ADT that allows for recovery of natural testosterone production with the intent to allow the patient to recover from symptoms of androgen deprivation; same as IHT.

IONIZING RADIATION: The release of energy caused by disruption of an electron from its orbit around the nucleus.

ISODOSE CONTOUR: A two or three-dimensional shape that contains the volume receiving a dose greater than or equal to a specified amount.

ISODOSE LINE: A two-dimensional line that circumscribes an area receiving a dose greater than or equal to a specified amount.

KEGEL EXERCISES: Pelvic floor exercises used to aid in regaining urinary continence after surgical removal of the prostate.

LAPAROSCOPIC LYMPHADENECTOMY: Laparoscopic surgical procedure in which some lymph nodes are removed and submitted for examination by a pathologist to exclude metastatic spread of PC to lymph node tissue. This is an invasive procedure usually undertaken only by patients at high risk of lymph node invasion.

LEVITRA®: Brand name for vardenafil, an oral phosphodiesterase type 5 (PDE5) inhibitor used in the treatment of impotence.

LH: Luteinizing hormone; a pituitary hormone that stimulates the Leydig cells of the testicles to make the male hormone testosterone. LH is blocked by LHRH agonists and antagonists as well as estrogens.

LHRH: Luteinizing hormone-releasing hormone (also known as GnRH or gonadotrophin releasing hormone); hormone from the hypothalamus that interacts with the LHRH receptor in the pituitary to release LH which in turn stimulates specific cells in the testicles (Leydig cells) to make testosterone.

LHRH AGONISTS (or ANALOGS): Synthetic compounds that are chemically similar to Luteinizing Hormone Releasing Hormone (LHRH), but are sufficiently different that they suppress testicular production of testosterone by binding to the LHRH receptor in the pituitary gland and either have no biological activity and therefore competitively inhibit the action of LHRH, or have LHRH activity that exhausts the production of LH by the pituitary. Used in the hormonal treatment of advanced prostate cancer and in the adjuvant and neoadjuvant hormonal treatment of earlier stages of prostate cancer. LHRH agonists mimic natural LHRH but then shut down LH production after continuous exposure; also abbreviated as LHRH-A.

LHRH ANTAGONIST: An agent that blocks the LHRH receptor by pure antagonism without the initial release of LH that is responsible for causing a testosterone surge seen with LHRH agonists; Abarelix (Plenaxis®) is an example of an LHRH Antagonist.

LIGAND: A protein or an enzyme that combines with its appropriate binding site or receptor. The interaction of a ligand with its receptor initiates a biochemical reaction leading to the synthesis of other substances, often proteins, hormones or enzymes. Almost all reactions in the human body involve ligands interacting with their appropriate receptors.

LINEAR ACCELERATOR (LINAC): A type of high energy x-ray machine that generates radiation fields for external beam radiation therapy. A linear accelerator is typically mounted with a collimator and/or a multileaf collimator in a gantry that revolves vertically around a treatment couch.

LITER: A unit of volume in the Metric system equivalent to 1000 milliliters (ml); a liter is roughly equivalent to one quart.

LOBE: A subdivision of a bodily organ or part bounded by fissures, connective tissue, or other structural boundaries (e.g., the prostate or the brain).

LOCALIZED: Restricted to a well-defined area.

LUPRON®: The USA trade or brand name of leuprolide acetate, a LHRH agonist.

LUTS: Lower Urinary Tract Symptoms such as difficulty in starting urination, slowness of the urinary stream, and incomplete emptying of the bladder; these symptoms are quantified in the AUA Symptom Score.

LYMPH NODES: The small glands which occur throughout the body and which filter the clear fluid known as lymph or lymphatic fluid; lymph nodes filter out bacteria and other toxins, as well as cancer cells.

MAB (mAb): Monoclonal antibody: an antibody directed against one specific protein (antigen).

MACROPHAGE: A mononuclear tissue cell that may be fixed or freely motile, is derived from a monocyte, and functions in the protection of the body against infection and noxious substances. Macrophages are phagocytic—they ingest foreign proteins, process them within their cell structure and are an important part of the body's immune response.

MAGNETIC RESONANCE: Absorption of specific frequencies of radio and microwave radiation by atoms placed in a strong magnetic field.

MAGNETIC RESONANCE IMAGING (MRI): The use of magnetic resonance with atoms in body tissues to produce distinct cross-sectional, and even three-dimensional images of internal organs. MRI is primarily of use in staging biopsy-proven prostate cancer.

D19

MALIGNANCY: A growth or tumor composed of cancerous cells.

MALIGNANT: Cancerous; tending to become progressively worse and to result in death; having the invasive and metastatic (spreading) properties of cancer.

MARGIN: Normally used to mean the "surgical margin", which is the outer edge of the tissue removed during surgery. If the surgical margin shows no sign of cancer ("negative margins"), then the prognosis is better than if the margin is positive or involved by cancer.

MCP: An abbreviation for modified citrus pectin, a synthetic derivative of pectin (a water soluble carbohydrate found in fruits) shown to lower PSA velocity in PC patients.

MEDICAL ONCOLOGIST: A physician certified in Internal Medicine who then undergoes additional specialty training to gain expertise in the diagnosis and treatment of various cancers or malignancies. Medical oncologists have skills in medical therapies to treat cancer as opposed to surgical treatments, which is the expertise of the surgical oncologist.

METASTASIS (plural is METASTASES): Secondary tumor formed as a result of a cancer cell or cells from the primary tumor site (e.g., the prostate) traveling through the body to a new site and then growing there.

METASTASIZE: Spread of a malignant tumor to other parts of the body.

METASTATIC: Having the characteristics of a secondary tumor.

METRA™ DPD: Laboratory test to detect excessive bone resorption; see Pyrilinks-D™ (Dpd).

MEV (MeV): Mega (million) electron-Volts.

MICROVESSEL DENSITY: An objectified measurement of angiogenesis.

ML: Milliliter, a unit of volume equivalent to one thousandth of a liter; abbreviated as ml; see LITER.

MLC: See MULTILEAF COLLIMATOR.

MOAB: See MAB.

MOTILITY: Relating to the ability to move around, to travel, to be motile; cell motility relates to the tendency for the cell to move through other cells and tissues.

MRI: See MAGNETIC RESONANCE IMAGING.

MULTILEAF COLLIMATOR (MLC): A type of collimator that can define irregularly shaped radiation fields. An MLC has two rows of narrow metal blocks (leaves) that can be independently driven in or out of the radiation beam from opposite sides under computer control.

NADIR: See PSA Nadir.

NECROSIS: Death of cells or tissues through injury or disease, especially in a localized area of the body.

NEOADJUVANT: The use of a different kind of therapy before the use of what is considered a definitive therapy, e.g. the use of neoadjuvant androgen deprivation therapy (ADT) prior to radiation therapy of PC or the use of neoadjuvant chemotherapy before surgery for breast cancer. Neoadjuvant is contrasted to adjuvant, which relates to the use of another therapy after the so-called more definitive therapy, e.g. ADT after RT.

NEOADJUVANT HORMONE BLOCKADE (NHB): Use of ADT

prior to other therapies such as radiation therapy, surgery or possibly chemotherapy to reduce tumor volume and/or prostate gland volume with the goal to allow these other therapies to work better; also called NHT (Neoadjuvant Hormone Therapy).

NERVE-GRAFTING: In the context of a radical prostatectomy, using a small section of the sural nerve taken from near the patient's ankle and using it to create a bridge to replace the section of one or both of the cavernous nerves removed during RP when nerve-sparing is not possible.

NERVE-SPARING: Used to describe a procedure during the course of a radical prostatectomy in which the surgeon saves the nerves that affect sexual and related functions. Nerve-sparing may be done on one side of the prostate (unilateral) or both sides (bilateral).

NEUROVASCULAR BUNDLE: See NVB.

NEUTRON BEAM RT: A type of radiation therapy using the neutron as the particle to deliver energy to destroy DNA. Neutron beam RT acts directly upon DNA and is defined as high linear energy transfer (high LET) radiation as opposed to photon, electron and proton RT that act upon DNA (low LET) indirectly via activated hydroxyl radicals.

D21

NG: Nanogram, a unit of measurement that is one billionth of a gram or 10-9 grams. Nanograms are indicated in lower case as "ng". Testosterone is usually measured in ng/dl or nanograms per deciliter; see DECILITER.

NOCTURIA: Getting up at night to urinate. Nocturia is expressed, for example, as "Nocturia times 3" or "Nocturia x 3" to indicate that the patient routinely gets up three times at night to urinate.

NOMOGRAM: A graphic representation, often used in analyzing data, consisting of several lines marked off to scale. A straight-edge is used to connect known values on two lines so that an unknown value can be read at the point of intersection with another line.

NON-INVASIVE: Not requiring any incision or the insertion of an instrument or substance into the body.

NSE: Neuron-specific enolase; a neuroendocrine marker ; an enzyme produced by neuroendocrine cells found in more aggressive types of PC.

NTCP: Normal Tissue Complication Probability. A term used in reference to the probability of injuring normal tissues surrounding the prostate that are exposed to radiation during the course of radiation to the prostate gland itself. As the radiation dose increases, the NTCP increases unless the radiation beam conforms to the prostate gland targeted by RT. Also see TCP (TUMOR CONTROL PROBABILITY).

NVB: Neurovascular Bundle; the capsular veins and arteries of the prostate and the cavernous nerves derived from branches of the pelvic plexus.

ONCOGENES: Genes relating to tumor growth.

ONCOLOGY: The branch of medical science dealing with tumors. An oncologist is a specialist in the study of cancer and the treatment of the patient with cancer.

ORCHIECTOMY (ORCHIDECTOMY): The surgical removal of the testicles; surgical castration.

ORGAN: A group of tissues that work in concert to carry out a specific set of functions (e.g., the heart or the lungs or the prostate).

ORGAN-CONFINED DISEASE (OCD): PC that is apparently confined to the prostate clinically or pathologically; not going beyond the confines of the prostatic capsule.

OSTEOPENIA: A reduction in the bone density that is more than one standard deviation from the normal bone density. Using the T-score, it is within the range of -1.0 to -2.4 SD. Once the T-score is -2.5 or more, the patient is defined as having osteoporosis.

OSTEOPOROSIS: A reduction in bone density resulting in a T-score of -2.5 or more. A loss of bone due to increased osteoclastic activity leading to bone resorption.

OVERSTAGING: The assignment of an overly high clinical stage at initial diagnosis because of the difficulty of assessing the available information with accuracy (e.g., stage T3b as opposed to stage T2b).

PALPABLE: Capable of being felt during a physical examination by an experienced physician; in the case of prostate cancer, this normally refers to some form of abnormality of the prostate which can be felt during a digital rectal examination (DRE).

PALPATE: To feel with the finger or fingers as part of a physical assessment, usually in reference to part of the human body; from the Latin "to touch gently".

PAP (PROSTATIC ACID PHOSPHATASE): An enzyme or bio-marker secreted by prostate cells associated with a higher probability of disease outside the prostate when pretreatment levels are 3.0 or higher. PAP elevations of this degree connote that the disease is not OCD (organ-confined disease).

PARASYMPATHOLYTIC: Tending to oppose the physiological results of parasympathetic nervous activity or of parasympathomimetic drugs.

PARENTERAL: A route of administration of a drug or medicine that is not via the mouth. Parenteral administration could be intravenous, intramuscular, subcutaneous, via the rectum, etc.

PARTIN TABLES: Tables constructed based on results of the PSA, clinical stage and Gleason score and associating those values with the findings at radical prostatectomy. Data involving thousands of men with PC used to predict the probability that the prostate cancer has penetrated the capsule, spread to the seminal vesicles or lymph nodes, or remains confined to the prostate. Developed by a group of scientists at the Brady Institute for Urology at Johns Hopkins Medical Center.

PBRT: Proton beam radiation therapy; a form of external radiation using the proton particle as the source of energy.

PC: Prostate cancer. Not to be confused with Personal Computer.

PC SPES™: A herbal therapy for PC with estrogenic activity comprised of eight herbs with evidence of efficacy against androgen-dependent and androgen-independent PC.

Pd: Pyridinoline; a bone resorption marker; a bone collagen breakdown product.

PELVIS: A basin-shaped structure of the vertebrate skeleton, composed of the innominate bones on the sides, the pubis in front, and the sacrum and coccyx behind, that rests on the lower limbs, supporting the spinal column.

PENILE: Of the penis.

PENIS: The male organ used in urination and intercourse.

PEPTIDASE: An enzyme capable of breaking down a peptide into amino acids.

PERIPROSTATIC: Pertaining to the soft tissues immediately adjacent to the prostate.

PET SCAN: Positron emission tomography using a radioactive isotope that is taken up by tumor tissue showing that the tumor is functionally active.

PG: Picogram or one trillionth (10-12) of a gram. The abbreviation is in lower case as "pg".

PHOTON: The quantum of electromagnetic energy, regarded as a discrete particle having zero mass, and no electric charge. X-rays are examples of relatively high-energy photons used for their penetrating power in radiography, radiology, radiotherapy, and scientific research.

PIN: Prostatic intraepithelial neoplasia; a pathologically identifiable condition believed to be a possible precursor of prostate cancer; broken down into high-grade PIN or PIN 2 and PIN 3 or low-grade PIN or PIN 1. High grade PIN is associated with having PC.

PLANNING TARGET VOLUME (PTV): Equivalent to the clinical target volume plus a margin to account for uncertainty in immobilization and localization of the patient anatomy during treatment.

PLOIDY: A term used to describe the number of sets of chromosomes in a cell; see DIPLOID and ANEUPLOID.

PROCTITIS: Inflammation of the rectum; in PC therapy proctitis may be an adverse effect of radiation therapy.

PROGNOSIS: The prospect of survival and recovery from a disease as anticipated from the usual course of that disease or indicated by special features of the case.

PROLACTIN (PRL): A trophic hormone produced by the pituitary that increases androgen receptors, increases sensitivity to androgens and regulates production and secretion of citrate; prolactin is increased by estrogens.

PROSCAR®: Brand name of finasteride; a 5AR inhibitor that blocks the conversion of testosterone to DHT; see DHT.

PROSTAGLANDIN: Hormone-like substances that stimulate target cells into action. They differ from hormones in that they act locally, near their site of synthesis, and they are metabolized very rapidly. Any of various oxygenated unsaturated cyclic fatty acids of animals that have a variety of hormone-like actions (as in controlling blood pressure or smooth muscle contraction).

PROSTASCINT: A monoclonal antibody (mAb) tagged with a radioactive isotope that is used to detect prostate cancer particularly within lymph nodes. The ProstaScint mAb is directed against the prostate specific membrane antigen (PSMA). PSMA is associated with androgen-independent PC. A few centers are using the ProstaScint scan to identify PC within the prostate gland.

PROSTATE: The gland surrounding the urethra and immediately below the bladder in males.

PROSTATECTOMY: Surgical removal of part or all of the prostate gland.

PROSTATE-SPECIFIC ANTIGEN (PSA): A protein secreted by the epithelial cells of the prostate gland including cancer cells. An elevated level in the blood indicates an abnormal condition of the prostate gland, either benign or malignant. It is used to detect potential problems in the prostate gland and to follow the progress of PC therapy; see SCREENING.

PROSTATIC ACID PHOSPHATASE (PAP): An enzyme or biomarker secreted by prostate cells associated with a higher probability of disease outside the prostate when pretreatment levels are 3.0 or higher. PAP elevations connote that the disease is not OCD (organ confined disease).

PROSTATITIS: Infection or inflammation of the prostate gland treatable by medication and/or prostate massage.

PROTOCOL: A precise set of methods by which a research study is to be carried out.

PROTON BEAM RADIATION THERAPY: A form of RT that uses the proton, a positively charged nuclear particle with a mass 1836 times that of an electron, to deliver ionizing radiation. The proton can be programmed to stop at a particular volume of depth within tissue resulting in the delivery of its radiation payload.

PSA (PROSTATE-SPECIFIC ANTIGEN): A protein secreted by the epithelial cells of the prostate gland including cancer cells. An elevated level in the blood indicates an abnormal condition of the prostate gland, either benign or malignant. It is used to detect potential problems in the prostate gland and to follow the progress of PC therapy; see SCREENING.

PSA BUMP (also called PSA bounce): A rise in PSA after first having a decline in PSA after RT.

PSAD: PSA density. The amount of PSA per unit volume of the prostate gland. PSAD is derived by dividing the serum PSA reading by the volume of the prostate in cubic centimeters (cc). For accuracy, the gland volume should be determined by transrectal ultrasound or by endorectal MRI.

PSA NADIR (PSAN): The lowest value the PSA reaches during or after a particular treatment. A progressive rise after a PSA nadir has been reached usually indicates biologic activity of PC.

PSA RELAPSE-FREE SURVIVAL: Survival of the PC patient that relates to no evidence of biochemical relapse based on a rising PSA as seen in three consecutive determinations; also called biochemical relapse-free survival (bRFS).

PSAR: PSA recurrence; a rise in PSA after a treatment intended to eradicate or control PC.

PSAV: PSA velocity; rate of increase in PSA expressed in nanograms per milliliter per year.

PSM: Prostate specific membrane antigen. An antigen that is found in benign disease (PSM´) and prostate cancer (PSM).

PSMA: Prostate specific membrane antigen; see PSM.

PYRILINKS-D™ (Dpd): A urine test that quantitates bone resorption. Dpd or deoxypyridinoline is a metabolic breakdown product of the bone matrix. It is important to distinguish Dpd from pyridinoline (Pd). The former is a more accurate assessment of bone resorption than the latter since it is subject to less biological variation. To test for Dpd, the second-voided urine specimen of the day is ideal to use. Other markers of bone resorption are ICTP and N-telopeptide. Elevated Dpd levels prior to treatment of PC are associated with an increased risk of metastatic disease.

qCT or QCT: Quantitative CT bone densitometry. A superior way to evaluate bone density versus the DEXA scan. QCT is not falsely elevated due to calcium deposits in blood vessels or due to degenerative joint disease (arthritis) and therefore gives a truer picture of the mineralization of the bone.

RADIATION ONCOLOGIST: A physician trained in the use of radiation therapy to treat cancer. This is not to be confused with a "Radiologist" who is trained to use radiologic imaging such as X-rays, CT, MRI, nuclear scans, ultrasound and other tests in the evaluation and diagnosis of illness.

RADIATION PROCTITIS: Inflammation of the rectal mucosa lining due to the ionizing effects of radiation therapy.

RADIATION THERAPY (RT): The use of x-rays and other forms of radiation to destroy malignant cells and tissue.

RADIATION URETHRITIS: Inflammation of the urethra caused by the ionizing effects of radiation therapy.

RADICAL: In the context of surgery, directed at the cause of a disease; thus, radical prostatectomy is the surgical removal of the prostate with the intent to cure the problem believed to be caused by or within the prostate.

RADICAL PROSTATECTOMY (RP): An operation to remove the entire prostate gland and seminal vesicles.

RBE: Relative biological effectiveness; a scale to compare the intensity of radiation of various nuclear particles. Neutrons for example have a higher RBE compared to photons or protons due to their ability to cause lethal double-stranded breaks in DNA, whereas photons and protons predominantly cause a single-stranded break.

RCOG: Radiotherapy Clinics of Georgia. One of the centers of excellence for radiation treatment of PC.

RECEPTOR: A docking site which interacts with a ligand. Receptors may be on the cell membrane or within the cell cytoplasm or nucleus. Estrogen receptors and androgen receptors are examples. All cells have multiple receptors.

RECTAL EXAM: See DIGITAL RECTAL EXAM.

RECTUM: The final part of the intestines that ends at the anus.

RECURRENCE: The reappearance of disease. This can be manifested clinically as findings on the physical examination (e.g. DRE) or as a laboratory recurrence (e.g. rise in PSA).

REFRACTORY: Resistant to therapy; e.g., hormone refractory prostate cancer (AIPC) is resistant to forms of treatment involving hormone manipulation.

REMISSION: The real or apparent disappearance of some or all or the signs and symptoms of cancer. The period (temporary or permanent) during which a disease remains under control, without progressing. Even complete remission does not necessarily indicate cure.

RESORPTION: Loss of bone through increased breakdown via osteoclasts or other mechanisms causing a reduction in bone mass.

RISK: The chance or probability that a particular event will or will not happen.

RP: See RADICAL PROSTATECTOMY.

RT: See RADIATION THERAPY.

RTOG: Radiation Therapy Oncology Group. An organization which is responsible for conducting many clinical trials and comparison studies in the field of radiation.

Rx: Standard abbreviation for treatment.

SAB: See SEQUENTIAL ANDROGEN BLOCKADE.

SCREENING: Evaluating populations of people who have no symptoms of the disease for which they are being evaluated, in an effort to diagnose disease early.

SEMINAL: Related to the semen; for example, the seminal vesicles are structures at the base of the bladder and connected to the prostate that provide nutrients for the semen.

SEMINAL VESICLES (SV): Glandular structures located above and behind the prostate that secrete and store seminal fluid. The seminal vesicles connect with the ejaculatory ducts. The seminal fluid contains nutrients for the sperm that improves their viability and mobility.

D28 **SENSITIVITY:** The probability that a diagnostic test can correctly identify the presence of a particular disease assuming the proper conduct of the test; specifically, the number of true positive results divided by the sum of the true positive results and the false negative results; see SPECIFICITY.

SEQUENTIAL ANDROGEN BLOCKADE (SAB): A combination of medications that provides androgen deprivation by blocking the androgen receptors and also the conversion of testosterone to DHT. A combination of Flutamide or Casodex with Proscar is an example of SAB. Used by many patients because it maintains high serum testosterone levels and is said to allow for sexual potency in about 50% of men.

SERIES: A number of things or events of the same class coming one after another in spatial or temporal succession; a series of patients relates to a collection of patients undergoing a specific treatment within a certain time frame or a collection of patients having a common basis for study.

SEXTANT: Having six parts; thus, a sextant biopsy is a biopsy that takes sample from six regions of the prostate gland: right and left base, right and left midgland and right and left apex.

SI: Seed Implantation; insertion of radioactive seeds, usually Iodine-125 or Palladium-103, into the prostate tissue to destroy prostate cancer.

SIDE-EFFECT: A reaction to a medication or treatment (most commonly used to mean an unnecessary or undesirable effect).

SPECIFICITY: The probability that a diagnostic test can correctly identify the absence of a particular disease assuming the proper conduct of the test; specifically, the number of true negative results divided by the sum of the true negative results and the false positive results.

STAGE: A term used to define the size and physical extent of a cancer.

STAGING: The process of determining extent of disease in a specific patient in light of all available information. It is used to help determine appropriate therapy. There are two staging methods: the Whitmore-Jewett staging classification (1956) and the more detailed TNM (tumor, nodes, metastases) classification (1992) of the American Joint Committee on Cancer and the International Union Against Cancer. Staging should be subcategorized as clinical staging and pathologic staging. Pathologic stage usually relates to what is found at the time of **D29** surgery after a microscopic review of the tissues by a pathologist. The TNM system is now most commonly used.

Whitmore-Jewett   Stage A becomes TNM T1
                          Stage B becomes T2
                          Stage C becomes T3

Whitmore-Jewett Stages:

Stage A is clinically undetectable tumor confined to the gland and is an incidental finding at prostate surgery which was undertaken to resolve BPH or a similar, presumably non-malignant, condition.

A1:   Well-differentiated with focal involvement.

A2:   Moderately or poorly differentiated or involves multiple foci in the gland.

Stage B is tumor confined to the prostate gland.

B0:   Nonpalpable, PSA-detected.

B1:   Single nodule in one lobe of the prostate.

B2:   more extensive involvement of one lobe or involvement of both lobes

Stage C is a tumor clinically localized to the periprostatic area but extending through the prostatic capsule; seminal vesicles may be involved.

C1: Clinical extracapsular extension.

C2: Extracapsular tumor producing bladder outlet or ureteral obstruction.

Stage D is metastatic disease.

D0: Clinically localized disease (prostate only) but persistently elevated enzymatic serum acid phosphatase.

Dl: Regional lymph nodes only.

D2: Distant lymph nodes, metastases to bone or visceral organs.

D3: D2 prostate cancer patients who relapse after adequate endocrine therapy.

TNM Stages:

D30 Primary Tumor (T)

T_X: Primary tumor cannot be assessed.

T_0: No evidence of primary tumor.

T1: Clinically inapparent tumor not palpable or visible by imaging.

Tla: Tumor incidental histologic finding in ≤ 5% of tissue resected via TURP.

Tlb: Tumor incidental histologic finding > 5% of tissue resected via TURP.

T1c: Tumor identified by needle biopsy (e.g., because of elevated PSA).

T2: Tumor palpable but confined within the prostate.

T2a: Tumor involves half of a lobe or less.

T2b: Tumor involves more than half a lobe, but not both lobes.

T2c: Tumor involves both lobes.

T3: Tumor extends through the prostatic capsule.

T3a: Unilateral extracapsular extension.

T3b: Bilateral extracapsular extension.

T3c: Tumor invades the seminal vesicle(s).

T4: Tumor is fixed or invades adjacent structures other than the seminal vesicles.

T4a: Tumor invades any of bladder neck, external sphincter or rectum.

T4b: Tumor invades levator muscles and/or is fixed to the pelvic wall.

STENT: A rod or catheter inserted into a tubular structure, such as a blood vessel (coronary artery) or ureter, to provide support during or after anastomosis or to maintain an open and unobstructed state, i.e. patency.

SYSTEMIC: Throughout the whole body; affecting the entire body.

Sx: An abbreviation for symptom.

T1a, T1b, T1c, T2a, T2b, T2c, T3a, T3b, T3c, T4: See TNM STAGES.

T-CELL: An immune-system cell that orchestrates an immune response to infected or malignant cells, sometimes by direct contact with the abnormal cells. T-cells are lymphocytes that develop in the thymus and circulate in the blood and lymphatic system; see DENDRITIC CELL.

TCP: Tumor Control Probability; a term used in radiation therapy; the goal of the radiation oncologist is to achieve the highest TCP while minimizing the normal tissue complication probability; see NTCP. The ratio of TCP to NTCP relates to the therapeutic index whereby the effectiveness of the treatment is related to the side-effects of treatment. In the setting of RT, this can be expressed as Therapeutic Index = TCP÷NTCP.

TENESMUS: The sense that the rectum or bladder needs to be urgently emptied but attempts are unsuccessful.

TELANGIECTASIA: Tiny blood vessels reflecting the formation of new blood vessels and seen commonly on the skin as a result of radiation.

TESTIS (plural is TESTES): One of two male reproductive glands located inside the scrotum that are the primary sources of the male hormone testosterone.

TESTICLE: See TESTIS.

TESTOSTERONE (T): The male hormone or androgen which

comprises most of the androgens in a man's body. Chiefly produced by the testicles. May be produced in tissues from precursors such as androstenedione. T is essential to virtually every male function from the brain to toe nails.

TGF-b (Transforming Growth Factor Beta): A bone-derived growth factor that stimulates the PC cell and osteoblast. Plasma elevations of TGFb-1 have been associated with occult metastatic PC.

THERAPEUTIC INDEX (TI): Treatment benefit divided by treatment side-effects.

THROMBOTIC: Related to blood clotting; having a tendency to cause blood clotting.

TID (tid): A Latin abbreviation for "Ter In Die", meaning three times a day. In prescriptions for medication or treatment, it is written as "tid".

TNM (tumor, nodes, metastases): See STAGING.

TOMOTHERAPY: Rotational radiotherapy delivery using an intensity-modulated fan beam. Intensity-modulated delivery is achieved by moving multiple collimator vanes into and out of the fan beam. The length of time that a leaf spends out of the beam is proportional to the intensity of radiation allowed through that particular portion of the beam.

TRANSRECTAL: Through the rectum as in Transrectal Ultrasound of the Prostate (TRUSP).

TRANSURETHRAL: Through the urethra.

TRUSP or TRUS (TRANSRECTAL ULTRASOUND): A method that uses echoes of ultrasound waves (far beyond the hearing range) to image the prostate by inserting an ultrasound probe into the rectum. Commonly used to visualize and guide prostate biopsy procedures.

T-SCORE: A designation used in evaluation bone mineral density that relates the patient's bone density to that found in a healthy person 25 years of age. The T-score is in contrast to the "Z-Score", which relates the patient's bone density to a pooled population of an age similar to the patient. The T-score is the desired test result. See Z-SCORE.

TUMOR: An excessive growth of cells caused by uncontrolled and disorderly cell replacement. An abnormal tissue growth that can be either benign or malignant; see BENIGN, MALIGNANT.

TURP (TRANSURETHRAL RESECTION OF THE PROSTATE): A surgical procedure to remove tissue obstructing the urethra. The technique involves the insertion of an instrument called a resectoscope into the penile urethra, and is intended to relieve obstruction of urine flow due to enlargement of the prostate.

TUR/P: See TURP.

ULTRASOUND (US): Sound waves at a particular frequency (far beyond the hearing range) whose echoes bouncing off tissue can be used to image internal organs or events (e.g., a baby in the womb).

UNDETECTABLE PSA (UD-PSA): Defined in our research as a PSA of < 0.05 ng/ml using a hypersensitive assay such as DPC Immulite 3rd generation PSA or Tosoh assay.

UNDERSTAGING: The assignment of an overly low clinical stage at initial diagnosis because of the difficulty of assessing the available information with accuracy (e.g., stage T2b as opposed to stage T3b).

UP-REGULATING (UP-REGULATION): Turning on or increasing a mechanism of action at the biochemical level in the body. Also see DOWN-REGULATING.

UREMIA: A severe toxic condition that usually occurs in severe kidney disease characterized by accumulation in the blood of constituents normally eliminated in the urine. Uremia causes severe elevations in BUN and Creatinine.

URETERAL: Pertaining to the ureter, the hollow tube that allows passage of urine from the kidneys to the bladder.

URETHRA: The tube that drains urine from the bladder through the prostate and out through the penis.

UROLOGIST: A surgically trained doctor who specializes in disorders of the genitourinary system.

USPIO PARTICLE SCANNING (ultra-small paramagnetic iron oxide scan): A staging method that involves the intravenous injection of iron nanoparticles followed by magnetic resonance imaging (MRI). The iron particles are taken up within the lymph nodes. In the presence of metastases they are displaced, leaving a white filling defect; also called MR lymphography. In the USA, the trade name is Combidex and in Europe it is Sinerem. This staging technique will replace CT of the abdomen and pelvis, the ProstaScint scan and laparoscopic lymphadenectomy.

VASECTOMY: Operation to make a man sterile by cutting the vas deferens, thus preventing passage of sperm from the testes to the prostate.

VASOACTIVE: Causing constriction or dilation of blood vessels. Vasoactive substances are used to increase erectile ability in men with impotence by means of causing dilation of blood vessels (vasodilation) within the body of the penis (corpus cavernosum).

VASODILATION: Dilation of a blood vessel, as by the action of a nerve or drug.

VEGF: Vascular Endothelial Growth Factor; A substance known to stimulate blood vessel growth or angiogenesis and hence stimulate PC growth.

VESICLE: A small sac containing a biologically important fluid as in seminal vesicle.

VIADUR® (leuprolide acetate): An LHRH agonist (LHRH-A) that is implanted under the skin and releases the LHRH-A over the course of one year. See LHRH ANALOGS.

D34

VIAGRA®: Brand name for sildenafil, an oral phosphodiesterase type 5 (PDE5) inhibitor used in the treatment of impotence.

WATCHFUL WAITING (WW): Active observation and regular monitoring of a patient without actual treatment. (Watchful waiting in many publications, however, involves use of ADT. This is not WW.)

XINLAY™: Tentative brand name for atrasentan, a drug manufactured by Abbott Laboratories, which is in clinical trials with FDA approval pending. Approval expected in late 2005 for use in patients with advanced prostate cancer.

X-RAY: A type of high-energy radiation that can be used at low levels to make images of the internal structures of the body and at high levels for radiation therapy.

ZOLADEX®: Trade or brand name for goserelin acetate, an LHRH agonist or LHRH-A.

Z-SCORE: A designation of bone mineral density that relates the patient's bone density to that of a pooled population of similar age. See T-SCORE.

ZONE: Part or area of an organ usually defined as a region or territory.

Appendix

References

1. Giovannucci E, Rimm EB, Colditz GA, et al: A prospective study of dietary fat and risk of prostate cancer. J Natl Cancer Inst 85:1571-9, 1993.

2. Gann PH, Hennekens CH, Sacks FM, et al: Prospective study of plasma fatty acids and risk of prostate cancer. J Natl Cancer Inst 86:281-6, 1994.

3. Sellers TA, Potters L, Rich SS, et al: Familial clustering of cancers of the breast and prostate in a population-based sample of postmenopausal women. Proc Annu Meet Am Assoc Cancer Res 35:A1724, 1994.

4. Keetch DW, Rice JP, Suarez BK, et al: Familial aspects of prostate cancer: a case control study. J Urol 154:2100-2, 1995.

5. Harris CH, Dalkin BL, Martin E, et al: Prospective longitudinal evaluation of men with initial prostate specific antigen levels of 4.0 ng/ml or less. J Urol 157:1740-3, 1997.

6. Crawford ED, Chia D, Andriole G, et al: PSA changes as related to the initial PSA: data from the prostate, lung, colorectal and ovarian cancer (PLCO) screening trial. Proc Am Soc Clin Oncol 20:177a, 2001.

7. Catalona WJ, Partin AW, Finlay JA, et al: Use of percentage of free prostate-specific antigen to identify men at high risk of prostate cancer when PSA levels are 2.51 to 4 ng/ml and digital rectal examination is not suspicious for prostate cancer: an alternative model. Urology 54:220-4, 1999.

8. Komatsu K, Wehner N, Prestigiacomo AF, et al: Physiologic (intraindividual) variation of serum prostate-specific antigen in 814 men from a screening population. Urology 47:343-6, 1996.

9. Oremek GM, Seiffert UB: Physical activity releases prostate-specific antigen (PSA) from the prostate gland into blood and increases serum PSA concentrations. Clin Chem 42:691-5, 1996.

10. Tchetgen MB, Song JT, Strawderman M, et al: Ejaculation increases the serum prostate-specific antigen concentration. Urology 47:511-6, 1996.

11. Herschman JD, Smith DS, Catalona WJ: Effect of ejaculation on serum total and free prostate-specific antigen concentrations. Urology 50:239-43, 1997.

12. Brackin PS, Diamond SM, Hartanto VH, et al: Avoid unnecessary prostate biopsy: the role of antibiotics in improving PSA specificity. J Urol 165:315A, 2001.

13. Southwick PC, Catalona WJ, Partin AW, et al: Prediction of post-radical prostatectomy pathological outcome for stage T1c prostate cancer with percent free prostate specific antigen: a prospective multicenter clinical trial. J Urol 162:1346-51, 1999.

14. Arcangeli CG, Humphrey PA, Smith DS, et al: Percentage of free serum prostate-specific antigen as a predictor of pathologic features of prostate cancer in a screening population. Urology 51:558-64; discussion 564-5, 1998.

15. Carter HB, Partin AW, Luderer AA, et al: Percentage of free prostate-specific antigen in sera predicts aggressiveness of prostate cancer a decade before diagnosis. Urology 49:379-84, 1997.

16. Pannek J, Rittenhouse HG, Chan DW, et al: The use of percent free prostate specific antigen for staging clinically localized prostate cancer. J Urol 159:1238-42, 1998.

17. Horninger W, Rogatsch H, Reissigl A, et al: Correlation between preoperative predictors and pathologic features in radical prostatectomy specimens in PSA-based screening. Prostate 40:56-61, 1999.

18. Jhaveri FM, Klein EA, Kupelian PA, et al: Declining rates of extracapsular extension after radical prostatectomy: evidence for continued stage migration. J Clin Oncol 17:3167-72, 1999.

19. Jani AB, Vaida F, Hanks G, et al: Changing face and different countenances of prostate cancer: racial and geographic differences in prostate-specific antigen (PSA), stage, and grade trends in the PSA era. Int J Cancer 96:363-71, 2001.

20. Eskew LA, Bare RL, McCullough DL: Systematic 5 region prostate biopsy is superior to sextant method for diagnosing carcinoma of the prostate. J Urol 157:199-202; discussion 202-3, 1997.

21. Daniel O, Van Zyl JJW: Rise of serum acid phosphatase level following palpation of the prostate. Lancet i:998, 1952.

22. Moul JW, Connelly RR, Perahia B, et al: The contemporary value of pretreatment prostatic acid phosphatase to predict pathological stage and recurrence in radical prostatectomy cases. J Urol 159:935-40, 1998.

23. Dattoli M, Wallner K, True L, et al: Prognostic role of serum prostatic acid phosphatase for 103Pd-based radiation for prostatic carcinoma. Int J Radiat Oncol Biol Phys 45:853-6, 1999.

24. Kahn D, Williams RD, Haseman MK, et al: Radioimmunoscintigraphy with In-111-labeled capromab pendetide predicts prostate cancer response to salvage radiotherapy after failed radical prostatectomy. J Clin Oncol 16:284-9, 1998.

25. Ellis RJ, Kim EY, Conant R, et al: Radioimmunoguided imaging of prostate cancer foci with histopathological correlation. Int J Radiat Oncol Biol Phys 49:1281-6, 2001.

26. Scheidler J, Hricak H, Vigneron DB, et al: Prostate cancer: localization with three-dimensional proton MR spectroscopic imaging–clinicopathologic study. Radiology 213:473-80, 1999.

27. D'Amico AV, Schnall M, Whittington R, et al: Endorectal coil magnetic resonance imaging identifies locally advanced prostate cancer in select patients with clinically localized disease. Urology 51:449-54, 1998.

28. Kaji Y, Kurhanewicz J, Hricak H, et al: Localizing prostate cancer in the presence of postbiopsy changes on MR images: role of proton MR spectroscopic imaging. Radiology 206:785-90, 1998.

29. Veltri RW, Partin AW, Epstein JE, et al: Quantitative nuclear morphometry, Markovian texture descriptors, and DNA content captured on a CAS-200 Image analysis system, combined with PCNA and HER-2/*neu* immunohistochemistry for prediction of prostate cancer progression. J Cell Biochem Suppl 19:249-58, 1994.

30. Chybowski FM, Keller JJ, Bergstralh EJ, et al: Predicting radionuclide bone scan findings in patients with newly diagnosed, untreated prostate cancer: prostate specific antigen is superior to all other clinical parameters. J Urol 145:313-8, 1991.

31. Oesterling JE: Using prostate-specific antigen to eliminate unnecessary diagnostic tests: significant worldwide economic implications. Urology 46:26-33, 1995.

32. Aihara M, Lebovitz RM, Wheeler TM, et al: Prostate specific antigen and gleason grade: an immunohistochemical study of prostate cancer. J Urol 151:1558-64, 1994.

33. Huncharek M, Muscat J: Serum prostate-specific antigen as a predictor of radiographic staging studies in newly diagnosed prostate cancer. Cancer Invest 13:31-5, 1995.

34. Flanigan RC, McKay TC, Olson M, et al: Limited efficacy of preoperative computed tomographic scanning for the evaluation of lymph node metastasis in patients before radical prostatectomy. Urology 48:428-32, 1996.

35. Albertsen PC, Hanley JA, Harlan LC, et al: The positive yield of imaging studies in the evaluation of men with newly diagnosed prostate cancer: a population based analysis. J Urol 163:1138-43, 2000.

36. Lee N, Newhouse JH, Olsson CA, et al: Which patients with newly diagnosed prostate cancer need a computed tomography scan of the abdomen and pelvis? An analysis based on 588 patients. Urology 54:490-4, 1999.

37. Tarle M, Kovacic K: Bone scans, PSA, PAP and CEA values in a multivariable analysis of prostate cancer heterogeneity and aggressiveness, Second International Conference of Anticancer Research. Saronis, Greece, October 1988, pp 11-15.

38. Kadmon D, Thompson TC, Lynch GR, et al: Elevated plasma chromogranin-A concentrations in prostatic carcinoma. J Urol 146:358-61, 1991.

39. Kim IY, Ahn HJ, Lang S, et al: Loss of expression of transforming growth factor-beta receptors is associated with poor prognosis in prostate cancer patients. Clin Cancer Res 4:1625-30, 1998.

40. Kim IY, Ahn HJ, Zelner DJ, et al: Loss of expression of transforming growth factor beta type I and type II receptors correlates with tumor grade in human prostate cancer tissues. Clin Cancer Res 2:1255-61, 1996.

E3

41. Morton DM, Barrack ER: Modulation of transforming growth factor beta 1 effects on prostate cancer cell proliferation by growth factors and extracellular matrix. Cancer Res 55:2596-602, 1995.

42. Thompson TC, Truong LD, Timme TL, et al: Transforming growth factor beta 1 as a biomarker for prostate cancer. J Cell Biochem Suppl 16H:54-61, 1992.

43. Lee C, Sintich SM, Mathews EP, et al: Transforming growth factor-beta in benign and malignant prostate. Prostate 39:285-90, 1999.

44. Shariat SF, Shalev M, Menesses-Diaz A, et al: Preoperative plasma levels of transforming growth factor beta(1) (TGF-beta(1)) strongly predict progression in patients undergoing radical prostatectomy. J Clin Oncol 19:2856-64, 2001.

45. Seay TM, Blute MC, Zincke H: Radical prostatectomy and early adjuvant hormonal therapy for pTxN+ adenocarcinoma of the prostate. Urology 50:833-7, 1997.

46. Frazier HA, Robertson JE, Paulson DF: Does radical prostatectomy in the presence of positive pelvic lymph nodes enhance survival? World J Urol 12:308-12, 1994.

47. Bauer JJ, Sesterhenn IA, Mostofi FK, et al: Elevated levels of apoptosis regulator proteins p53 and bcl-2 are independent prognostic biomarkers in surgically treated clinically localized prostate cancer. J Urol 156:1511-6, 1996.

48. Matsushima H, Kitamura T, Goto T, et al: Combined analysis with bcl-2 and P53 immunostaining predicts poorer prognosis in prostatic carcinoma. J Urol 158:2278-83, 1997.

49. Walsh PC, Donker PJ: Impotence following radical prostatectomy: insight into etiology and prevention. J Urol 128:492-7, 1982.

50. Walsh PC, Epstein JI, Lowe FC: Potency following radical prostatectomy with wide unilateral excision of the neurovascular bundle. J Urol 138:823-7, 1987.

51. Kim ED, Nath R, Kadmon D, et al: Bilateral nerve graft during radical retropubic prostatectomy: 1-year followup. J Urol 165:1950-6, 2001.

52. Zippe CD, Jhaveri FM, Klein EA, et al: Role of Viagra after radical prostatectomy. Urology 55:241-5, 2000.

53. Zagaja GP, Mhoon DA, Aikens JE, et al: Sildenafil in the treatment of erectile dysfunction after radical prostatectomy. Urology 56:631-4, 2000.

54. Hong EK, Lepor H, McCullough AR: Time dependent patient satisfaction with sildenafil for erectile dysfunction (ED) after nerve-sparing radical retropubic prostatectomy (RRP). Int J Impot Res 11 Suppl 1:S15-22, 1999.

55. Munding MD, Wessells HB, Dalkin BL: Pilot study of changes in stretched penile length 3 months after radical retropubic prostatectomy. Urology 58:567-9, 2001.

56. Montorsi F, Guazzoni G, Strambi LF, et al: Recovery of spontaneous erectile function after nerve-sparing radical retropubic prostatectomy with and without early intracavernous injections of alprostadil: results of a prospective, randomized trial. J Urol 158:1408-10, 1997.

57. Scholz M, Strum S: Re: Recovery of spontaneous erectile function after nerve-sparing radical retropubic prostatectomy with and without early intracavernous injections of alprostadil: results of a prospective, randomized trial. J Urol 161:1914-5, 1999.

58. Montague DK, Angermeier KW, Paolone DR: Long-term continence and patient satisfaction after artificial sphincter implantation for urinary incontinence after prostatectomy. J Urol 166:547-9, 2001.

59. Venn SN, Greenwell TJ, Mundy AR: The long-term outcome of artificial urinary sphincters. J Urol 164:702-6; discussion 706-7, 2000.

60. Haab F, Trockman BA, Zimmern PE, et al: Quality of life and continence assessment of the artificial urinary sphincter in men with minimum 3.5 years of followup. J Urol 158:435-9, 1997.

61. Gousse AE, Madjar S, Lambert MM, et al: Artificial urinary sphincter for post-radical prostatectomy urinary incontinence: long-term subjective results. J Urol 166:1755-8, 2001.

62. Litwiller SE, Kim KB, Fone PD, et al: Post-prostatectomy incontinence and the artificial urinary sphincter: a long-term study of patient satisfaction and criteria for success. J Urol 156:1975-80, 1996.

63. Clemens JQ, Bushman W, Schaeffer AJ: Urodynamic analysis of the bulbourethral sling procedure. J Urol 162:1977-81; discussion 1981-2, 1999.

64. Clemens JQ, Bushman W, Schaeffer AJ: Questionnaire based results of the bulbourethral sling procedure. J Urol 162:1972-6, 1999.

65. Schaeffer AJ, Clemens JQ, Ferrari M, et al: The male bulbourethral sling procedure for post-radical prostatectomy incontinence. J Urol 159:1510-5, 1998.

66. Kao TC, Cruess DF, Garner D, et al: Multicenter patient self-reporting questionnaire on impotence, incontinence and stricture after radical prostatectomy. J Urol 163:858-64, 2000.

67. Park R, Martin S, Goldberg JD, et al: Anastomotic strictures following radical prostatectomy: insights into incidence, effectiveness of intervention, effect on continence, and factors predisposing to occurrence. Urology 57:742-6, 2001.

68. Elliott DS, Boone TB: Combined stent and artificial urinary sphincter for management of severe recurrent bladder neck contracture and stress incontinence after prostatectomy: a long-term evaluation. J Urol 165:413-5, 2001.

69. Long JP, Bahn D, Lee F, et al: Five-year retrospective, multi-institutional pooled analysis of cancer-related outcomes after cryosurgical ablation of the prostate. Urology 57:518-23, 2001.

70. Zelefsky MJ, Leibel SA, Gaudin PB, et al: Dose escalation with three-dimensional conformal radiation therapy affects the outcome in prostate cancer. Int J Radiat Oncol Biol Phys 41:491-500, 1998.

71. Ragde H, Elgamal AA, Snow PB, et al: Ten-year disease free survival after transperineal sonography-guided iodine-125 brachytherapy with or without 45-gray external beam irradiation in the treatment of patients with clinically localized, low to high Gleason grade prostate carcinoma. Cancer 83:989-1001, 1998.

E5

72. D'Amico AV, Whittington R, Malkowicz SB, et al: Biochemical outcome after radical prostatectomy, external beam radiation therapy, or interstitial radiation therapy for clinically localized prostate cancer. JAMA 280:969-74, 1998.

73. Noldus J, Graefen M, Haese A, et al: Stage migration in clinically localized prostate cancer. Eur Urol 38:74-8, 2000.

74. Narayan P, Gajendran V, Taylor SP, et al: The role of transrectal ultrasound-guided biopsy-based staging, preoperative serum prostate-specific antigen, and biopsy Gleason score in prediction of final pathologic diagnosis in prostate cancer. Urology 46:205-12, 1995.

75. Merrick GS, Butler WM, Lief JH, et al: Efficacy of sildenafil citrate in prostate brachytherapy patients with erectile dysfunction. Urology 53:1112-6, 1999.

76. Weber DC, Bieri S, Kurtz JM, et al: Prospective pilot study of sildenafil for treatment of postradiotherapy erectile dysfunction in patients with prostate cancer. J Clin Oncol 17:3444-9, 1999.

77. Zelefsky MJ, McKee AB, Lee H, et al: Efficacy of oral sildenafil in patients with erectile dysfunction after radiotherapy for carcinoma of the prostate. Urology 53:775-8, 1999.

78. Kedia S, Zippe CD, Agarwal A, et al: Treatment of erectile dysfunction with sildenafil citrate (Viagra) after radiation therapy for prostate cancer. Urology 54:308-12, 1999.

79. Critz FA, Williams WH, Levinson AK, et al: Simultaneous irradiation for prostate cancer: intermediate results with modern techniques. J Urol 164:738-41; discussion 741-3, 2000.

80. Blasko JC, Grimm PD, Sylvester JE, et al: Palladium-103 brachytherapy for prostate carcinoma. Int J Radiat Oncol Biol Phys 46:839-50, 2000.

81. Critz FA, Williams WH, Benton JB, et al: Prostate specific antigen bounce after radioactive seed implantation followed by external beam radiation for prostate cancer. J Urol 163:1085-9, 2000.

82. Cavanagh W, Blasko JC, Grimm PD, et al: Transient elevation of serum prostate-specific antigen following 125I/103Pd brachytherapy for localized prostate cancer. Semin Urol Oncol 18:160-5, 2000.

83. Hanlon AL, Pinover WH, Horwitz EM, et al: Patterns and fate of PSA bouncing following 3D-CRT. Int J Radiat Oncol Biol Phys 50:845-9, 2001.

84. Ghafar MA, Johnson CW, De La Taille A, et al: Salvage cryotherapy using an argon based system for locally recurrent prostate cancer after radiation therapy: the Columbia experience. J Urol 166:1333-7; discussion 1337-8, 2001.

85. Rogers E, Ohori M, Kassabian VS, et al: Salvage radical prostatectomy: outcome measured by serum prostate specific antigen levels. J Urol 153:104-110, 1995.

86. Gheiler EL, Tefilli MV, Tiguert R, et al: Predictors for maximal outcome in patients undergoing salvage surgery for radio-recurrent prostate cancer. Urology 51:789-795, 1998.

87. Cheng L, Sebo TJ, Slezak J, et al: Predictors of survival for prostate carcinoma patients treated with salvage radical prostatectomy after radiation therapy. Cancer 83:2164-71, 1998.

88. Mate TP, Gottesman JE, Hatton H, et al: High dose rate afterloading 192Iridium prostate brachytherapy: feasability report. Int J Radiat Oncology Biol Phys 41:525-533, 1998.

89. Kovács G, Galalae R, Loch T, et al: [High dosage brachytherapy and external irradiation of localized prostate carcinoma–results at the Kiel University Clinic] [Article in German]. Schweiz Rundsch Med Prax 90:1617-22, 2001.

90. Kovács G, Galalae R, Loch T, et al: Prostate preservation by combined external beam and HDR brachytherapy in nodal negative prostate cancer. Strahlenther Onkol 175 Suppl 2:87-8, 1999.

91. Keyser D, Kupelian PA, Zippe CD, et al: Stage T1-2 prostate cancer with pretreatment prostate-specific antigen level < or = 10 ng/ml: radiation therapy or surgery? Int J Radiat Oncol Biol Phys 38:723-9, 1997.

92. Hanks GE, Hanlon AL, Schultheiss TE, et al: Conformal external beam treatment of prostate cancer. Urology 50:87-92, 1997.

93. Zelefsky MJ, Fuks Z, Hunt M, et al: High dose radiation delivered by intensity modulated conformal radiotherapy improves the outcome of localized prostate cancer. J Urol 166:876-81, 2001.

94. Consensus statement: guidelines for PSA following radiation therapy. American Society for Therapeutic Radiology and Oncology Consensus Panel. Int J Radiat Oncol Biol Phys 37:1035-41, 1997.

95. Zelefsky MJ, Fuks Z, Happersett L, et al: Clinical experience with intensity modulated radiation therapy (IMRT) in prostate cancer. Radiother Oncol 55:241-9, 2000.

96. Teh BS, Woo SY, Butler EB: Intensity modulated radiation therapy (IMRT): a new promising technology in radiation oncology. Oncologist 4:433-42, 1999.

97. Lattanzi J, McNeeley S, Pinover W, et al: A comparison of daily CT localization to a daily ultrasound-based system in prostate cancer. Int J Radiat Oncol Biol Phys 43:719-25, 1999.

98. Lattanzi J, McNeeley S, Donnelly S, et al: Ultrasound-based stereotactic guidance in prostate cancer–quantification of organ motion and set-up errors in external beam radiation therapy. Comput Aided Surg 5:289-95, 2000.

99. Slater JD, Yonemoto LT, Rossi CJ, Jr., et al: Conformal proton therapy for prostate carcinoma. Int J Radiat Oncol Biol Phys 42:299-304, 1998.

100. Laramore GE, Krall JM, Thomas FJ, et al: Fast neutron radiotherapy for locally advanced prostate cancer. Final report of Radiation Therapy Oncology Group randomized clinical trial. Am J Clin Oncol 16:164-7, 1993.

101. Russell KJ, Caplan RJ, Laramore GE, et al: Photon versus fast neutron external beam radiotherapy in the treatment of locally advanced prostate cancer: results of a randomized prospective trial. Int J Radiat Oncol Biol Phys 28:47-54, 1994.

102. Häggström S, Lissbrant IF, Bergh A, et al: Testosterone induces vascular endothelial growth factor synthesis in the ventral prostate in castrated rats. J Urol 161:1620-5, 1999.

103. Mukherjee P, Sotnikov AV, Mangian HJ, et al: Energy intake and prostate tumor growth, angiogenesis, and vascular endothelial growth factor expression. J Natl Cancer Inst 91:512-23, 1999.

104. Mazzucchelli R, Montironi R, Santinelli A, et al: Vascular endothelial growth factor expression and capillary architecture in high-grade PIN and prostate cancer in untreated and androgen-ablated patients. Prostate 45:72-9, 2000.

105. Huggins C, Hodges CV: Studies on prostatic cancer. I. The effect of castration, of estrogen and androgen injection on serum phosphatases in metastatic carcinoma of the prostate. Cancer Res 1:293-7, 1966.

106. McLeod D, Zinner N, Tomera K, et al: A phase 3, multicenter, open-label, randomized study of abarelix versus leuprolide acetate in men with prostate cancer. Urology 58:756-61, 2001.

107. Garnick MB, Campion M: Abarelix Depot, a GnRH antagonist, v LHRH superagonists in prostate cancer: differential effects on follicle-stimulating hormone. Abarelix Depot study group. Mol Urol 4:275-7, 2000.

108. Ben-Josef E, Yang SY, Ji TH, et al: Hormone-refractory prostate cancer cells express functional follicle-stimulating hormone receptor (FSHR). J Urol 161:970-6, 1999.

109. Coleman RE, Purohit OP, Vinholes JJ, et al: High dose pamidronate: clinical and biochemical effects in metastatic bone disease. Cancer 80:1686-90, 1997.

110. Coleman RE, Vinholes J, Purohit OP, et al: Effect of pamidronate on tumour marker levels in breast and prostate cancer-correlation with clinical and biochemical response. Proc Am Soc Clin Oncol 16:330a, 1997.

111. Shipman CM, Rogers MJ, Apperley JF, et al: Bisphosphonates induce apoptosis in human myeloma cell lines: a novel anti-tumour activity. Br J Haematol 98:665-72, 1997.

112. van der Pluijm G, Vloedgraven H, van Beek E, et al: Bisphosphonates inhibit the adhesion of breast cancer cells to bone matrices in vitro. J Clin Invest 98:698-705, 1996.

113. Hughes DE, Wright KR, Uy HL, et al: Bisphosphonates promote apoptosis in murine osteoclasts in vitro and in vivo. J Bone Miner Res 10:1478-87, 1995.

114. Sahni M, Guenther HL, Fleisch H, et al: Bisphosphonates act on rat bone resorption through the mediation of osteoblasts. J Clin Invest 91:2004-11, 1993.

115. Adami S, Bhalla AK, Dorizzi R, et al: The acute-phase response after bisphosphonate administration. Calcif Tissue Int 41:326-31, 1987.

116. Strum SB, Scholz MC, McDermed JE: Intermittent androgen deprivation in prostate cancer patients: factors predictive of prolonged time off therapy. Oncologist 5:45-52, 2000.

117. Andriole GL, Guess HA, Epstein JI, et al: Treatment with finasteride preserves usefulness of prostate-specific antigen in the detection of prostate cancer: results of a randomized, double-blind, placebo-controlled clinical trial. PLESS Study Group. Proscar Long-term Efficacy and Safety Study. Urology 52:195-201; discussion 201-2, 1998.

118. Strum SB, McDermed JE, Madsen L, et al: Intermittent androgen deprivation (IAD) with finasteride (F) given during the induction and maintenance periods results in prolonged time off IAD in patients with localized prostate cancer (LPC). Proc Amer Soc Clin Oncol 18:353A, 1999.

119. Staiman VR, Lowe FC: Tamoxifen for flutamide/finasteride-induced gynecomastia. Urology 50:929-33, 1997.

120. Strum SB, Scholz MC, McDermed JE: The Androgen Deprivation Syndrome: the incidence and severity in prostate cancer patients receiving hormone blockade. Proc Amer Soc Clin Oncol 17:316A, 1998.

121. Strum SB, McDermed JE, Scholz MC, et al: Anaemia associated with androgen deprivation in patients with prostate cancer receiving combined hormone blockade. Br J Urol 79:933-41, 1997.

122. Hall MC, Fritzsch RJ, Sagalowsky AI, et al: Prospective determination of the hormonal response after cessation of luteinizing hormone-releasing hormone agonist treatment in patients with prostate cancer. Urology 53:898-902; discussion 902-3, 1999.

123. Nejat RJ, Rashid HH, Bagiella E, et al: A prospective analysis of time to normalization of serum testosterone after withdrawal of androgen deprivation therapy. J Urol 164:1891-4, 2000.

124. Herr HW, O'Sullivan M: Quality of life of asymptomatic men with non-metastatic prostate cancer on androgen deprivation therapy. J Urol 163:1743-6, 2000.

125. Hsieh T, Chen SS, Wang X, et al: Regulation of androgen receptor (AR) and prostate specific antigen (PSA) expression in the androgen-responsive human prostate LNCaP cells by ethanolic extracts of the Chinese herbal preparation, PC-SPES. Biochem Mol Biol Int 42:535-44, 1997.

126. Halicka HD, Ardelt B, Juan G, et al: Apoptosis and cell cycle effects induced by extracts of the Chinese herbal preparation PC SPES. Int J Oncol 11:437-448, 1997.

127. Kameda H, Small EJ, Reese DM: A phase II study of PC SPES, an herbal compound, for the treatment. of advanced prostate cancer (PCa). Proc Amer Soc Clin Oncol 18:320a, 1999.

128. Oh WK, George DJ, Hackmann K, et al: Activity of the herbal combination, PC-SPES, in the treatment of patients with androgen-independent prostate cancer. Urology 57:122-6, 2001.

129. Varnehorst E, Wallentin L, Risberg B: The effects of orchiectomy, oestrogens and cyproterone-acetate on the antithrombin-III concentration in carcinoma of the prostate. Urol Res 9:25-8, 1981.

130. Emtage LA, George J, Boughton BJ, et al: Haemostatic changes during hormone manipulation in advanced prostate cancer: a comparison of DES 3 mg/day and goserelin 3.6 mg/month. Eur J Cancer 26:315-9, 1990.

131. Ross RW, Kussmaul S, Small EJ: The effect of the herbal supplement PC-SPES on bone mineral density in men with prostate cancer. Proc Am Soc Clin Oncol 20 (part2):151b (abstract), 2001.

132. Albertsen PC, Fryback DG, Storer BE, et al: Long-term survival among men with conservatively treated localized prostate cancer. JAMA 274:626-31, 1995.

133. D'Amico AV, Propert KJ: Prostate cancer volume adds significantly to prostate-specific antigen in the prediction of early biochemical failure after external beam radiation therapy. Int J Radiat Oncol Biol Phys 35:273-9, 1996.

134. D'Amico AV, Chang H, Holupka E, et al: Calculated prostate cancer volume: the optimal predictor of actual cancer volume and pathologic stage. Urology 49:385-91, 1997.

135. Goluboff ET, Prager D, Rukstalis D, et al: Safety and efficacy of exisulind for treatment of recurrent prostate cancer after radical prostatectomy. J Urol 166:882-6, 2001.

136. Small EJ, Fratesi P, Reese DM, et al: Immunotherapy of hormone-refractory prostate cancer with antigen-loaded dendritic cells. J Clin Oncol 18:3894-903, 2000.

137. Ferrer FA, Miller LJ, Lindquist R, et al: Expression of vascular endothelial growth factor receptors in human prostate cancer. Urology 54:567-72, 1999.

138. Freeman MR, Schneck FX, Gagnon ML, et al: Peripheral blood T lymphocytes and lymphocytes infiltrating human cancers express vascular endothelial growth factor: a potential role for T cells in angiogenesis. Cancer Res 55:4140-5, 1995.

139. Kitahara S, Yoshida K, Ishizaka K, et al: Stronger suppression of serum testosterone and FSH levels by a synthetic estrogen than by castration or an LH-RH agonist. Endocr J 44:527-32, 1997.

140. Nelson JB, Hedican SP, George DJ, et al: Identification of endothelin-1 in the pathophysiology of metastatic adenocarcinoma of the prostate. Nat Med 1:944-9, 1995.

141. Bagnato A: Endothelins as autocrine regulators of tumor cell growth. TEM 9:378-383, 1998.

142. Nelson JB, Carducci MA, Zonnenberg B, et al: The endothelin-A receptor antagonist atrasentan improves time to clinical progression in hormone refractory prostate cancer patients: a randomized, double-blind, multi-national study. J Urol 165:168A, 2001.

143. Nelson JB, Carducci MA, Padley RJ, et al: The endothelin-a receptor antagonist atrasentan (ABT-627) reduces skeletal remodeling activity in men with advanced, hormone refractory prostate cancer. Proc Am Soc Clin Oncol 20:4a, 2001.

144. Koga H, Naito S, Koto S, et al: Use of bone turnover marker, pyridinoline cross-linked carboxyterminal telopeptide of type I collagen (ICTP), in the assessment and monitoring of bone metastasis in prostate cancer. Prostate 39:1-7, 1999.

145. Takeuchi S, Arai K, Saitoh H, et al: Urinary pyridinoline and deoxypyridinoline as potential markers of bone metastasis in patients with prostate cancer. J Urol 156:1691-5, 1996.

146. Berruti A, Dogliotti L, Bitossi R, et al: Incidence of skeletal complications in patients with bone metastatic prostate cancer and hormone refractory disease: predictive role of bone resorption and formation markers evaluated at baseline. J Urol 164:1248-53, 2000.

147. Rodriguez R, Schuur ER, Lim HY, et al: Prostate attenuated replication competent adenovirus (ARCA) CN706: a selective cytotoxic for prostate-specific antigen-positive prostate cancer cells. Cancer Res 57:2559-63, 1997.

148. Elliott WL, Roberts BJ, Howard CT, et al: Chemotherapy with [SP-4-3-(R)]-[1,1-cyclobutanedicarboxylato(2-)](2- methyl-1,4-butanediamine-N,N')platinum (CI-973, NK121) in combination with standard agents against murine tumors in vivo. Cancer Res 54:4412-8, 1994.

149. DeWeese TL, van der Poel H, Li S, et al: A phase I trial of CV706, a replication-competent, PSA selective oncolytic adenovirus, for the treatment of locally recurrent prostate cancer following radiation therapy. Cancer Res 61:7464-72, 2001.

150. Yu DC, Chen Y, Dilley J, et al: Antitumor synergy of CV787, a prostate cancer-specific adenovirus, and paclitaxel and docetaxel. Cancer Res 61:517-25, 2001.

151. Tamm I, Dorken B, Hartmann G: Antisense therapy in oncology: new hope for an old idea? Lancet 358:489-97, 2001.

152. Crooke ST: Molecular mechanisms of antisense drugs: RNase H. Antisense Nucleic Acid Drug Dev 8:133-4, 1998.

153. Jansen B, Schlagbauer-Wadl H, Brown BD, et al: bcl-2 antisense therapy chemosensitizes human melanoma in SCID mice. Nat Med 4:232-4, 1998.

154. Miyake H, Tolcher A, Gleave ME: Antisense bcl-2 oligodeoxynucleotides inhibit progression to androgen-independence after castration in the Shionogi tumor model. Cancer Res 59:4030-4, 1999.

155. Miyake H, Tolcher A, Gleave ME: Chemosensitization and delayed androgen-independent recurrence of prostate cancer with the use of antisense bcl-2 oligodeoxynucleotides. J Natl Cancer Inst 92:34-41, 2000.

156. Gleave M, Tolcher A, Miyake H, et al: Progression to androgen independence is delayed by adjuvant treatment with antisense bcl-2 oligodeoxynucleotides after castration in the LNCaP prostate tumor model. Clin Cancer Res 5:2891-8, 1999.

157. Chi KN, Gleave ME, Klasa R, et al: A phase I dose-finding study of combined treatment with an antisense bcl-2 oligonucleotide (Genasense) and mitoxantrone in patients with metastatic hormone-refractory prostate cancer. Clin Cancer Res 7:3920-7, 2001.

E11

E12

Appendix

Useful Forms

The Importance of Objectified Reporting

Introduction

Communication and Balance are the essence of a healthy and happy life. This is true at all levels from that of the cell to the universe at large. Within your world of prostate cancer, communication of your medical story is a key to unlocking pathways leading to optimal care. Information must be conveyed properly, reported objectively, assimilated, and re-presented clearly. In the words of Jack Webb: "The facts ma'am, just the facts."

F1

We are in a computer age that allows wonderful graphical presentation of data. The reporting formats we should now be using must be reviewed and updated to convey our current ability to present *factual information, trends or changes over time, comparison of present studies to past,* and *clear presentation of final impressions.*

Currently, most reporting remains in the "narrative" format. The use of narrative (story-telling) reporting in the medical arena is subject to serious problems due to the subjectivity of this style of reporting.

Objectified reporting should be a foundational principle and reality of quality medicine. **The improvement in outcomes that can be achieved with such an approach are monumental.** The physician has much to gain as well, since the knowledge attained via such information management reestablishes the true spirit of medicine—realizing new insights into disease diagnosis, evaluation, and treatment—in the context of helping our humankind. Please review the forms presented here and incorporate them into your strategy for success.

What Forms are Shown in This Appendix?

Consider the forms as integral parts of your medical chart — keystones to reporting your medical log. These can be broken down into the major headings of Diagnosis, Evaluation, Staging, Treatment, and Surveillance.

Diagnosis
- The TransRectal UltraSound of the Prostate (TRUSP) Form
- The Diagnostic Biopsy Form

Evaluation
- The Biomarkers, Hormones, Bone Integrity and Other Labs Form
- The AUA Symptom Score Form

F2   Staging
- The Bone Scan Form
- The PC Laboratory Form
- The ProstaScint-CT Fusion Form
- The Endorectal MRI with Spectroscopy Form

Treatment (integration of the above into a medical strategy)
- The Helpline Medical Form (HMF) Form
- The Flow Sheets Form(s)

Surveillance
- The Summary and Surveillance Form

A database structured in this manner provides you and the physicians you consult with an incredible wealth of information from which you can understand PC in much more detail. If you add the enhancement tools manifested as "HMF" and "Flow Sheets", you now have a means to refine your care at the very highest level. This is what we want to bring to you—a way for you to do the very best and have a wonderful outcome.

Our Goals for You
Your medical findings lend themselves to a logical analysis.

This is a key to good care. Your understanding of the information conveyed in these forms is part of the empowerment that will have you feeling more confident about a successful outcome. You will enter into a new relationship with your care givers because you are now a key participant on the healthcare team. Organization of these forms into a Medical Chart should be your logical next step. This Chart or Log should accompany you on all your physician visits. Your life depends upon it.

The Transrectal Ultrasound of the Prostate (TRUSP) Report
The TRUSP involves imaging the prostate by means of an ultrasound probe inserted into the rectum. This allows visualization of the prostate using sound waves. This approach, called TRUSP or TRUS, is the method used by most urologists and/or radiologists to guide the biopsy needle in order to obtain samples of prostatic tissue for the purpose of diagnosing PC.

Most urologists use the TRUSP solely for PC diagnosis. However, the TRUSP can provide additional valuable information that includes, but is not limited to:

- Calculation of the **Gland Volume**

- **Assessment of hypoechoic areas** (regions of abnormal ultrasound pattern within the prostate that produce less of an echo pattern, i.e. having less echogenicity, which are associated with a higher probability of PC involvement.

- Evaluation of the prostate capsule for **evidence of capsular penetration.**

- **Assessment of the seminal vesicles** for PC involvement.

- **Determination of PSA density** (PSA divided by gland volume).

Such information should be conveyed formally in a TRUSP report—an official document. Unfortunately, this is rarely found in the medical record. Instead, a hand-written note amounting to one or two lines in the office chart indicating that a TRUSP was done is what is most commonly found. We should optimize the information conveyed from studies that relate to our lives and expect such information to be more formally pre-

F3

sented. The TRUSP report presented here (Form F-1) is a first-generation attempt to do this.

The gland volume is an important piece of information. Most radiation oncologists use such information to decide whether to use ADT (androgen deprivation therapy) to reduce the gland volume for the purpose of minimizing radiation scatter to the bladder and/or rectum. Gland volumes greater than 40 cc or grams are considered too high. Within three to six months after starting ADT, the gland volume can be reduced dramatically with volumes of 100 cc brought down to 30 to 40 cc and starting volumes of 50 cc not uncommonly reduced to 12 cc.

Secondly, the gland volume directly relates to the expression of benign-related PSA. **The formula used is GV x 0.066 = the amount of PSA related to the contribution of benign prostate cells.** If we subtract this amount from the total PSA we are left with the "excess" PSA, that most likely relates to the malignant prostate cell population—the PC. If, in addition, we have obtained a Gleason score that has been validated by a PC pathology expert (see form at http://www.pcri.org/tools/forms/pathology_biopsy_form.html), we can determine the PSA leak—the amount of PSA that is leaked into the bloodstream in relation to the Gleason score. If we divide the "excess PSA" by the "PSA leak", we have a *calculated PC tumor volume*. This is an approximation of the amount of PC present. All of this is shown in detail in the software for PC tumor calculation on the PCRI Web site at www.pcri.org. Go to the Software section of the main menu on the home page and download this Excel program which is based on peer-reviewed medical publications.

Currently, the "sextant" biopsy approach is the most commonly used strategy to target the prostate for the purpose of diagnosis of PC. This divides the prostate into six sectors. These include (from top to bottom) the base (right and left sides), the midgland (right and left sides) and the apex (right and left sides). The TRUSP form depicts this graphically. The sextant approach is being replaced with the 5-region biopsy or the 11 multi-site biopsy or other approaches that now incorporate significantly more sampling of prostate tissue, especially the later-

F4

al portions of the peripheral zone of the prostate. These approaches significantly increase the ability to diagnose prostate cancer earlier and avoid repetitive biopsy procedures that are stressful, uncomfortable and costly to the patient and the healthcare industry. The 5-region biopsy approach was discussed and illustrated in Chapter 3 of *The Primer*.

Form F-1: The Transrectal Ultrasound of the Prostate (TRUSP) Form.	
Patient Name (last, first)	Smith, Joseph
Date	7/4/01
PSA (ng/ml)	10.0
TRUSP Gland Volume (GV) in cc	40.0
PSA Density (PSA ÷ GV)	0.25
Number of biopsy cores taken *	12
Seminal vesicles normal (Yes vs. No)	No
Capsular penetration (Yes vs. No)	Yes – left midgland
PSA attributed to benign prostate cells (GV x 0.066)	2.64
Excess PSA (total PSA minus PSA attributed to benign prostate cells)	7.36

*⊠ Please check box if biopsy specimens each are placed in separate vials containing fixative.

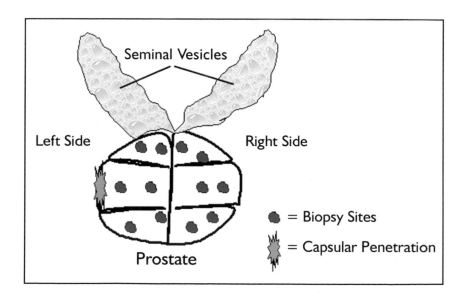

Seminal Vesicles

Left Side   Right Side

● = Biopsy Sites

⚡ = Capsular Penetration

Prostate

The Diagnostic Biopsy Report

The biopsy report (Form F-2) conveys substantial information about the biologic expression of the tumor. When tissue
is removed from your body and is sent to a pathologist, an
official document, a biopsy report, must be created. **You
should request all such reports, share them with all the doctors who are involved with your care and keep copies of
these reports along with other pertinent reports in your
medical chart.**

F6

The pathologic diagnosis of prostate cancer may represent
significant challenges for some pathologists. If the microscopic diagnosis of PC is an issue and questions are raised
concerning the diagnosis of PC, you should obtain a second
opinion from a recognized expert in PC pathology.

In established cases of PC, expert pathology review is also
essential. Since the Gleason score (GS) is a critical item and
a key variable in virtually every prognostic and treatment algorithm, an accurate GS mandates that you obtain an official
second opinion from a PC pathology expert. The ones that
we are most familiar are listed on page 50 of *The Primer.*

The full addresses for these pathologists or specialty laboratories are listed under PCAB (Prostate Cancer Address Book)
on the PCRI homepage in the "Resources" section
(http://www.pcri.org/resource/state.html).

A second opinion on the pathology is usually covered by insurance but if not, runs about $300-500. A copy of the orig-

inal pathology *report* with the actual *slides* and often the tissue *block* is sent to the outside reviewer. A copy of the insurance information is usually sent along with this. Your primary care doctor or specialist can initiate such a second opinion. Additionally, other prognostic tests such as p53, p27, bcl-2, Ki 67 and ploidy (DNA analysis) can also be done by some of the above pathologists using the tissue blocks. The tissue blocks represent the sampled tissue that has been placed into paraffin wax and stored in this manner. Such material is the source for microscopic glass slides that the pathologist uses to view the cancer material under the microscope. These tissue blocks, if stored under proper conditions, last indefinitely.

There are new treatments for prostate cancer that also require examination of the paraffin-embedded tissue. For example, the monoclonal antibody treatment involving the HER-2/*neu* oncogene requires that HER-2/*neu* antigen be present in the PC tissue. The Dendreon trial using dendritic **F7** cells requires the confirmation of PAP (prostatic acid phosphatase) staining in the tissue block containing prostate cancer that has been obtained from the diagnostic biopsy, the radical prostatectomy (assuming an RP has been done), or other tissue that demonstrated PC. Some hospitals are discarding the paraffin blocks after eight years. You should therefore call the facility that was involved with your pathology specimen and make sure you know what their policy is regarding retention of this valuable resource. Many facilities will turn over the tissue blocks to the patient after obtaining a signed release. Call their pathology department and find out. Your ability to enter a clinical trial may be at stake.

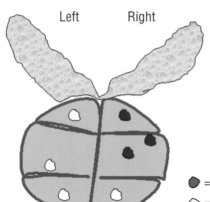

Left   Right

Patient Name (Last, first): Smith, John	
Date of biopsies	July 10, 2001
Number of cores obtained *	7

*☒ Check here if each core placed in separate vial.

● = Prostate Cancer
○ = No Prostate Cancer

Form F-2: The Diagnostic Biopsy Form.

This is a hypothetical example of a patient having 7 cores of tissue obtained at the time of diagnostic biopsy. The report shows clearly the length of each core, the presence or absence of PC, the amount and percentage involvement of each core involved by PC and calculations of percentage involvement of the entire specimen as well as the cumulative percent of each core involved with PC. Of course, the Gleason score is indicated as well.

Site	Length (mm)	PC (Yes/ No)	PC (mm) (%)	Gleason score
1 left base	10	N	-	-
2 left mid	7	N	-	-
3 left apex	5	N	-	-
4 right base	5	Y	5 (100)	3,3
5 right mid	8	Y	4 (50)	3,4
6 right mid	7	Y	7 (100)	3,3
7 right apex	12	N	-	-
Totals	57 mm	3/7	16mm (250%) 28% (of specimen)	-

DESCRIPTION:

In the specimen showing a Gleason score of (3,4), the amount of Gleason grade 4 was estimated at 20%. Extensive perineural invasion was seen in this specimen.

Jack Frost, M.D.

The Biomarkers, Hormones, Bone Integrity and Other Labs Form

This form is a magnified portion of the *flow sheet* (see page F37). This form (F-3) concentrates on the biologic markers (biomarkers) and hormone levels associated with PC. It also emphasizes bone integrity biomarkers and other pertinent labs. Durable responses as a result of treatment are more likely if all biologic expressions of cancer growth are minimized.[1] PC cells make innumerable products of which we only measure a few. It makes a great deal of sense to identify the biomarkers of disease activity and determine if our treatments suppress all of these products if the goal of our therapy is to induce complete remissions of disease in the patient with PC.

Typical "garden-variety" PC produces mostly PSA. However, as the tumor undergoes mutation and as more primitive cell populations are expressed within the cancer cell population, other markers such as PAP, CGA, NSE and CEA are produced. Form F-3 directs our attention to such markers and calls for their baseline measurement. In essence, we are assessing the tumor cell population for products that indicate more aggressive variants of PC. If we find elevations of any of these biomarkers, it would be appropriate to obtain levels of these markers over the course of therapy and to identify sites of disease activity associated with such biomarker expression.

PAP, not uncommonly, is elevated in PC that has spread to the bone. This may be related to the fact that PAP is an enzyme (a phosphatase) that digests (hydrolyzes) phosphates within the bone marrow. This enzyme is most active in an acid pH environment and therefore it is called prostatic "acid" phosphatase or PAP. The growth and spread of PC may be facilitated by PAP production by the PC cell population. **In other words, the substances that are being tested to monitor disease activity and response to treatment are also functional enzymes or proteins that support the growth of the tumor.**

CGA and NSE elevations, especially in concert, are associated with a small cell variant of PC. In such patients, looking for disease activity in the liver and/or lungs is reasonable. Patients with small cell PC (SCPC) often have bone metastases that are not readily seen on bone scan but they are seen as "lytic" or destructive lesions on plain x-rays or on CT scans. SCPC is often characterized by relatively little PSA production, and the "expression" of PSA in the blood is often surprisingly low with values under 2.0 ng/ml not at all uncommon.

The middle section of Form F-3 relates to the endocrine aspects of PC. PC is an endocrine disease for the most part. When we use androgen deprivation therapy (ADT), we deprive the tumor of needed androgens. We cannot intelligently treat this type of a disease unless we monitor endocrine function as it relates to PC cell growth and response to treatment. It is imperative during ADT that men have their testosterone (T) levels checked to see if therapy has reduced T to castrate levels (< 20 ng/dl or less than 0.69 nM/L). Once this has been confirmed, there is usually little need to repetitively test the testosterone level during ADT.

If T is not suppressed to this level, PC tumor regression via ADT may not be complete. LH suppression by the LHRH agonists like Lupron® or Zoladex® should drop LH levels to < 1.0. If this is found, then pituitary suppression by the LHRH agonist or antagonist is adequate and not the cause of the inability to lower testosterone to less than 20 ng/dl. The adrenal glands may be the source of the testosterone that has not been suppressed by the LHRH agonist. Measuring DHEA-S and androstenedione blood levels may indicate high production of either or both of these adrenal androgen precursors. Such hormones are metabolized within the PC cell to T and from there to DHT. Both T and DHT contribute to PC cell growth. Measuring these agents gives us clues as to ways we can manipulate the tumor cell population. This is also true if we find the prolactin level to be elevated. This form, therefore, focuses on the biology and endocrinology of PC. Other measurements are indicated as well for evaluating cholesterol, thyroid status, homocysteine, and iron stores.

Form F-3: The Biomarkers, Hormones, Bone Integrity and Other Labs Form.

Biomarkers or Hormones	Normal Range	Enter Data Below						
Date Obtained	m/d/yr							
PSA 3rd Gen DPC								
PAP	0-3.5							
NSE	< 12.5							
CEA	< 4.0							
CGA (units/Liter)	< 14.3							
TGF-β_1								
IL-6sR								
Testosterone ng/dl	200-1600							
SHBG	13-71							
FAI (T ÷ SHBG)*								
DHT	30-100							
DHEA-S	80-560							
Androstenedione	50-250							
LH	1.4-7.7							
Prolactin (fasting AM)	2.5-17							
DPD (Pyrilinks-D)**	< 5.4							
BMD T-score								
(note QCT								
or DEXA scan)								
HDL	> 34							
Homocysteine	< 7.0							
UltraSensitive-TSH	0.4-4.0							
Ferritin	18-370							
Soluble Transferrin Receptor (sTfR)	< 28							

*FAI = free androgen index, T = testosterone, SHBG = sex hormone binding globulin.
**DPD = deoxypyridinoline (trade names Pyrilinks-D™ or Metra™ DPD.)

F11

The American Urological Association (AUA) Symptom Score Form

The development of lower urinary tract symptoms (LUTS) certainly impairs quality of life. LUTS may include problems of frequency, urgency, and hesitancy in urination as well as getting up at night to urinate, a lessening in the force of the urinary stream, a sense of incomplete emptying, straining to empty the bladder and urinary flow that may stop and start again. LUTS may result from diseases such as BPH, prostatitis, PC, and also from illnesses that affect the blood vessel and/or nerve supply to the prostate and bladder. These urinary symptoms are enumerated in the AUA Symptom Score Form (F-4). Those completing this form are asked to objectify these symptoms by assigning a number relating to the severity of the urinary symptom under evaluation. The results for each symptom are totaled to give the AUA symptom score.

F12 This objectification of medical information is a desired goal throughout all aspects of medicine. Thus, the AUA Symptom Score Form, widely accepted by all specialists involved in prostate health, serves as an important prototype of the concept of "Objectified Medical Reporting."

LUTS and its representation via the AUA symptom score is important to the man with PC who is involved in the decision-making process of selecting a primary treatment for his disease. Should he choose radical prostatectomy, some form of radiation therapy, cryosurgery, androgen deprivation, or watchful waiting? If the AUA symptom score is greater than 10, there is an increasing risk of urinary complications resulting from radiation therapy or cryosurgery. The higher the AUA symptom score, the more likely such complications will seriously impact the quality of life of the man undergoing these treatments. This is because the early toxicities associated with all forms of RT and cryosurgery often involve irritation of the urethra with obstructive symptoms and may also involve tissue swelling or edema of prostatic tissue surrounding the urethra that further inhibits urine flow due to compression of the urethra. In such instances, the insult of further toxicity inherent in such therapies as RT or cryosurgery is added to the injury that has already affected the prostate due to diseases such as BPH, PC, prostatitis, vascular disease from diabetes, hypothyroidism, arteriosclerosis and other causes.

Trying to reduce such symptoms prior to initiating RT or cryosurgery is helpful, and the use of androgen deprivation therapy (ADT) to reduce PC volume, gland volume, and lessen symptoms of BPH may result in a striking reduction in the AUA symptom score. To reduce obstructive symptomatology, the use of other agents such as alpha-1 blockers (e.g. Hytrin®, Cardura®, Flomax® and others) or approaches to reduce signs and symptoms of prostatitis and/or cystitis (e.g. antibiotics, Elmiron®, Prelief®, and dietary changes) are worthy considerations. However, if LUTS are severe, the man with PC may consider a different choice of local PC therapy. The selection of a radical prostatectomy, performed by a urologist highly skilled in this procedure, will usually eradicate organ-confined PC and at the same time eliminate lower urinary tract symptoms that are caused by BPH, prostatitis, and/or PC. Therefore, the AUA symptom score is an important factor in the decision-making crossroads encountered by the man with PC.

F13

✏️

_____

_____

_____

_____

_____

_____

_____

_____

_____

_____

_____

Form F-4: The AUA Symptom Score Form.*

Last Name	First Name	Date

Circle the response correct for you and indicate your result in the far right box for all SEVEN questions.

1. **Incomplete emptying:** Over the past month, how often have you had a sensation of not emptying your bladder completely after you finished urinating?

Not at all	Less than 1 time in 5	Less than half the time	About half the time	More than half the time	Almost always	Your Result
0	1	2	3	4	5	

2. **Frequency:** Over the past month, how often have you had to urinate again less than 2 hours after you finished urinating?

Not at all	Less than 1 time in 5	Less than half the time	About half the time	More than half the time	Almost always	Your Result
0	1	2	3	4	5	

3. **Intermittency:** Over the past month, how often have you found that you stopped and started again several times when you urinated?

Not at all	Less than 1 time in 5	Less than half the time	About half the time	More than half the time	Almost always	Your Result
0	1	2	3	4	5	

4. **Urgency:** Over the past month, how often have you found it difficult to postpone urination?

Not at all	Less than 1 time in 5	Less than half the time	About half the time	More than half the time	Almost always	Your Result
0	1	2	3	4	5	

5. **Weak-stream:** Over the past month, how often have you had a weak stream?

Not at all	Less than 1 time in 5	Less than half the time	About half the time	More than half the time	Almost always	Your Result
0	1	2	3	4	5	

6. **Straining:** Over the past month, how often have you had to push or strain to begin urination?

Not at all	Less than 1 time in 5	Less than half the time	About half the time	More than half the time	Almost always	Your Result
0	1	2	3	4	5	

7. **Nocturia:** Over the past month or so, how many times did you get up to urinate from the time you went to bed until the time you got up in the morning?

F15

None	1 time	2 times	3 times	4 times	5 or more times	Your Result
0	1	2	3	4	5	

Add up your results for AUA Score = _____

Quality of Life Due to Urinary Symptoms:
If you were to spend the rest of your life with your urinary condition just the way it is now, how would you feel about that? (Circle or Underline.)

Delighted	Pleased	Mostly Satisfied	Mixed	Mostly Dissatisfied	Unhappy	Terrible

* Adapted from: Barry MJ, Fowler FJ, Jr., O'Leary MP, et al: The American Urological Association symptom index for benign prostatic hyperplasia. The Measurement Committee of the American Urological Association. J Urol 148:1549-57, 1992.

The Bone Scan Report(s)

The bone scan is a tool used in staging PC and in monitoring the patient's course of illness, including the response to any of a variety of treatments. There are limitations to this radiologic imaging examination. Uptake of the radioactive isotope (Technetium 99) is not specific to PC and may be due to traumatic causes (e.g. past or recent fracture or bone injury) and degenerative causes (e.g. arthritis, bone curvature). In addition, there are significant variations in the quality of the bone scan from hospital to hospital as well as variations between bone scans taken at different times within the same hospital or imaging center. The changes in the bone scan that result from a response to therapy or that reflect PC disease progression require a significant amount of time. The actual status within the bone tissue precedes the picture presented by the bone scan. In other words, the bone scan is "yesterday's news". Most importantly, despite these recognized limitations, there has been no standardization in the way that information within the bone scan study is presented to the clinician. **Moreover, there is not a standard format for the comparison of serial bone scans.** In today's world of impressive technological advances, we too often do not optimize the tools we have at hand. In the context of a human life, such a shortcoming should be corrected. This can easily be done with savings in life and in healthcare dollars.

Others have recognized the above limitations of the bone scan and tried to improve the objectivity of this important tool. As long as 30 years ago, there were reports on how to *quantify* the bone scan by reading isotope activity in counts per second. This approach was termed *quantified bone scanning* (QBS) and was first reported in 1972 by Galasko et al[2] and then two years later by Citrin et al.[3] A report on computerization of bone scanning was published by Drelichman et al from Wayne State University in 1984.[3]

Objectified bone scanning (OBS) is a simpler concept and basically involves a methodical approach in reporting the findings of the bone scan. OBS facilitates and enhances the clinician's evaluation of the bone scan(s) by making the bone scan report a discipline. This is accomplished through:

1) Using a table format.
2) Comparing, over time, the sites of increased isotope uptake on serial bone scans.
3) Graphically portraying isotope uptake activity.
4) Using an index of suspicion (ios) for PC to categorize areas of isotope uptake.
5) Using plain x-rays, CT or MRI studies to confirm or refute bone scan sites that are suspicious for malignancy.
6) Employing the traditional narrative description.

The narrative description in the OBS report is used to emphasize and/or clarify issues about the scan findings. Too often, areas of isotope activity on the scan are simply "written off" as traumatic in origin, as arthritis or some other form of degenerative disease. Meanwhile, an objective format that provides a comparison over time has not been done. This is true for other studies that may involve radiology, laboratory and/or pathology reporting. **The take-home message here is "We are not using our powers of observation to note changes over time to enhance our understanding of the patient's medical reality."** The truth is out there; let us discover it.

F17

Forms F-5 and F-6 are examples of an approach involving OBS in a hypothetical patient with known prostate cancer (PC) who has undergone two bone scans. The scans and their dates are shown, as are the interpretations by the radiologist(s) of these scans as they relate to:

1) Traumatic causes.
2) Degenerative bone and joint disease.
3) Moderate suspicion for PC.
4) PC.

In the context of a patient with known PC, the radiologist is able to further objectify the extent of disease (EOD) using the classification of Soloway et al.[5] This is obviously important in the analysis of the patient's clinical course, not only as it relates to standard therapy of PC, but most certainly in the evaluation of new agents used in clinical trials.

Form F-5: The Objectified Bone Scan (OBS) Form–Report #1.

Patient Name: JOHN DOE
Scan Date: 2/10/98
Dx: Prostate Cancer

F18

Abnormal uptake	IOS*	Confirmation	Conclusion
1) Skull–right parietal	4	plain films–no lesion seen	4
2) Skull–right mandible	3	plain films–no lesion seen	4
3) Cervical spine–C4-5	3	plain films–degenerative changes	1
4) Rib–left 5th anterior	1	plain film–old fracture	1
5) Lumbar spine–L3	4	plain film–sclerotic	4
6) Wrist–left	1	plain films–old fracture	1
7) Femur–right proximal	4	plain film–sclerotic change	4
8) Foot–right calcaneal area	1	plain films–spur	1

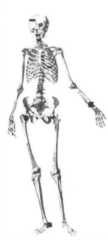

Scan Date 2/10/98
** EOD = 1

Description: Multiple areas of increased isotope uptake are designated by #1 through 8 in the table. Uptake of isotope at sites #1 and 2 (right parietal area of the skull and right mandible) are not explained on the plain x-rays and are therefore regarded as metastatic prostate cancer until proven otherwise. Uptake at sites #3, 4, 6 and 8 are all consistent with traumatic change or degenerative joint disease (arthritic changes). Follow-up bone scans will clarify these issues. The extent of disease (EOD) as it relates to prostate cancer is "1" since a total of five lesions are seen that are consistent with PC. The lumbar vertebra at L-3 is counted as two lesions because the entire vertebra is involved (see Soloway Index below).
Jack Frost, M.D.

* IOS = Index of Suspicion after Strum

1 = Traumatic changes.
2 = Degenerative changes.
3 = Moderate suspicion for PC.
4 = Very high probability of PC.

** EOD after Soloway et al [5]

0 = No bone mets
1 = 1 to 5 lesions (involvement of one half of a vertebra is counted as one lesion).
2 = 6 to 20 lesions.
3 = More than 20 lesions but less than a "super scan."
4 = "Super scan"- defined as more than 75% of the ribs, vertebrae and pelvic bones.

Form F-6: The Objectified Bone Scan (OBS) Form–Report #2.

Patient Name: JOHN DOE
Scan Date: 3/12/99
Dx: Prostate Cancer

Abnormal uptake	IOS*	Confirmation	Conclusion
1) Skull– right parietal	4	not done	4
2) Skull– right mandible	3	not done	4
3) Cervical spine– C4-5	2	not done	2
4) Rib–left 5th anterior	1	not done	1
5) Lumbar spine– L3	4	not done	4
6) Wrist–left	1	not done	1
7) Femur– right proximal	see below		lesion resolved
8) Foot–right calcaneal area	1	not done	1

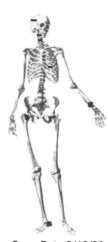

F19

Scan Date 3/12/99
** EOD = 1

Description: On 3/12/99, a second bone scan was performed on John Doe and compared to the study done on 2/10/98. The right parietal skull lesion (# 1) has decreased in the intensity of isotope uptake by about 50%. This is consistent with a bone metastasis responding to therapy. The right mandibular area of uptake (# 2) is unchanged. Evaluation of that area has provided no explanation for this uptake and malignancy is still a consideration. Mild uptake in the cervical spine at C4-5 (# 3) remains unchanged and is consistent with degenerative changes. Uptake in the left 5th rib (#4) also remains unchanged. This was the site of a previous rib fracture. Uptake at L-3 (#5) is unchanged. Sites (#6) and (#8) are unchanged and are likely traumatic in nature. There has been complete disappearance of uptake in the right proximal femur (# 7) consistent with response to treatment. EOD = 1 since there are a total of four lesions consistent with PC. The lumbar vertebra at L-3 is counted as two lesions because the entire vertebra is involved (see Soloway Index below).
Jack Frost, M.D.

* IOS = Index of Suspicion after Strum	** EOD after Soloway et al [5]
1 = Traumatic changes. 2 = Degenerative changes. 3 = Moderate suspicion for PC. 4 = Very high probability of PC.	0 = No bone mets 1 = 1 to 5 lesions (involvement of one half of a vertebra is counted as one lesion). 2 = 6 to 20 lesions. 3 = More than 20 lesions but less than a "super scan." 4 = "Super scan"- defined as more than 75% of the ribs, vertebrae and pelvic bones.

The Laboratory Reports

Laboratory results, including blood, urine and other testing, are expressions of the biology of the various health systems within your body. Reports of such testing should be sorted by date. As physicians' offices convert to electronic charting, such reports will be automatically faxed to you from your doctor's office(s). Until then, you should request copies of all lab reports and keep them in a three-ring binder. Your laboratory results should also be entered onto a flow sheet form (see Form F-11). We hope, assuming that progress will be made in this realm of medical reporting, that lab results will soon automatically be imported into a flow sheet format. The concept of flow sheets will be discussed later.

You should share your laboratory results with *all* doctors involved in your care. This will decrease unnecessary laboratory testing and the expenses involved and save you the pain of venapuncture, the loss of blood, and the misuse of a lab technician's time in the event that your doctors have ordered duplicate studies. This commonly occurs. Healthcare cannot afford this waste.

Please be aware that not all laboratories are equal in their testing of specimens. This is especially important in the realm of prostate cancer. The PSA assays differ in their sensitivity. The more sensitive assays such as the Tosoh and DPC assays give you longer lead times to document a change in your status, especially after radical prostatectomy or during ADT.[6] This lead-time, up to two years using an ultrasensitive PSA after RP, not only alerts you to a possible problem, but also enables you to initiate changes in your lifestyle or medical therapy or to join a clinical trial. Tosoh's PSA has a threshold of undetectability at 0.05 ng/ml. DPC's 3rd generation Immulite assay has a threshold of 0.003 ng/ml. Dianon and UroCor, two national laboratories of excellence for pathology review and prostate cancer laboratory reporting, use the Tosoh assay.

Form F-7: The PC Laboratory Form.

DATE ORDERED: _____ PATIENT NAME: _____

SSN: _____ DATE COLLECTED: _____

ORDERING PHYSICIAN: _____

Check or Circle Tests to be Drawn

PC BIOMARKERS	BONE MARROW	SERUM LEVELS
PSA	CBC and Platelet Count	Nizoral
PAP		Selenium
NSE	**COAGULATION**	Vitamin D
CGA	PT	
CEA	PTT	

HORMONE LEVELS	HEALTH PANELS	NEW TUMOR MARKERS
LH	Chemistry panel	TGF-β_1
Prolactin (fasting AM)	Lipid panel	IGF-1
Testosterone	Liver panel	IGF-BP 2
SHBG		IGF-BP 3
DHT	**ANEMIA ANALYSIS**	IL-6
ACTH	Ferritin	IL-6sR
Cortisol (fasting AM)	Soluble Transferrin Receptor	
DHEA-S	B-12	
Androstenedione	Folate	
	US-TSH	
	Stool OB	

BONE INTEGRITY	URINE ANALYSIS	Add Ons
Dpd (2nd voided urine)	Urine Analysis (Micro)	
Ionized Calcium	Urine Analysis (DIP)	
Spot Urine Calcium		

The ProstaScint-CT Fusion Report and the Endorectal MRI with Spectroscopy Report

The desired goal of a report is one of conveying information to the physician so that he or she can more fully comprehend the patient's situation. The patient clearly is the beneficiary in such circumstances. We have suggested that this be accomplished by:

- **Objectifying the results of reporting** by the use of a table format that requires a specific response or responses.
- **Portraying results using computer graphics** to reinforce their findings to the patient-physician team.
- **Fusing the imaging outputs of complimentary radiologic studies** such as ProstaScint, CT, MRI, PET and/or bone scans based on technological advances in the field of image analysis.
- Invoking the concept of **concordance of findings** as an important means to increase the accuracy of any kind of analysis.

ProstaScint-CT Fusion Report

The ProstaScint fusion scan and its reporting format shown in Form F-8 embody these concepts. Fusing the radiologic computer image outputs of the ProstaScint and the CT scan into one image provides an enhanced anatomic orientation and yields more accurate results.[7] The routine adoption of such technology will provide a clearer understanding of the patient's stage. The studies to confirm this are in progress. The table within Form F-8 shows the various anatomic sites (lymph node areas and prostate gland) that the radiologist reading the study must, by the very nature of the table, comment on. In addition, the reporting format provides a graphic of the patient's actual ProstaScint-CT fusion study (or graphic of any study being performed on the patient). The graphic is marked to clearly indicate areas of abnormal uptake of ProstaScint isotope and to orient the viewer. A normal schematic of the lymphatics of the abdomen and pelvis are shown below that to educate those viewing the report. The narrative description provides further details that may not be covered in the table-reporting format and allows the radiologist to expound on fine details.

Patient's ProstaScint-CT Fusion Image

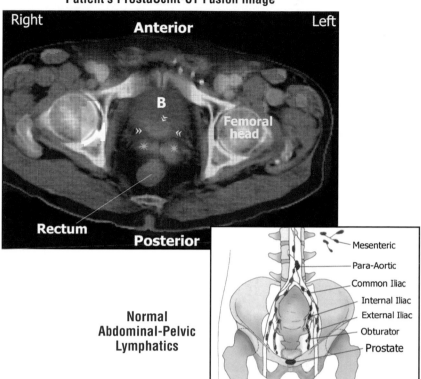

Right **Anterior** Left

B

Femoral head

Rectum **Posterior**

Normal
Abdominal-Pelvic
Lymphatics

Mesenteric
Para-Aortic
Common Iliac
Internal Iliac
External Iliac
Obturator
Prostate

F23

Form F-8: The ProstaScint-CT Fusion Form.				
Highlight or Circle Area(s) of Abnormal Uptake in Red				
Anatomic Site	**Right Side**		**Left Side**	
Mesenteric node(s)	+	–	+	–
Para-aortic node(s) at L1 to 3	+	–	+	–
Para-aortic node(s) at L4 to 5	+	–	+	–
Common Iliac node(s)	+	–	+	–
External iliac node(s)	+	–	+	–
Internal Iliac node(s)	+	–	+	–
Obturator node(s)	+	–	+	–
Prostate or Fossa	+	–	+	–
Seminal vesicle(s)	+	–	+	–

Description: Patient MK was injected with Indium-111-tagged ProstaScint™ monoclonal antibody on 3/29/02. Four days later, ProstaScint scanning with a dual-headed camera was performed along with non-contrast CT of the pelvis. Co-registration of the ProstaScint SPECT images and CT images was performed by software and the fusion images were created. The graphical sample (top figure on page F23) shows areas of abnormal ProstaScint uptake in the left and right seminal vesicles (✳). The left seminal vesicle is larger, likely indicating more involvement than the right. The rectum is seen posterior to the seminal vesicles. Avid uptake of ProstaScint in the rectum, which normally occurs, is clearly demonstrated. Anterior to the seminal vesicles, the bladder (B) is visualized. The base of the prostate gland pushing into the posterior aspect of the bladder demonstrates uptake of ProstaScint. This area is marked by three yellow double arrows **«**. No lymph node uptake was discerned on ProstaScint scanning nor was there any evidence of pathologic nodal enlargement (> 1.0 cm) on the CT scan.

Read by Samuel Kipper, M.D. _____
Date of Study: 4/1/02
Date of Report: 4/2/02.

Endorectal MRI with Spectroscopy

The concept of *concordance* is a scientific way of saying "If it looks like a zebra, runs like a zebra, and has stripes, it probably is a zebra." The endorectal MRI with spectroscopy is an example of the use of concordance to improve the accuracy of results. Upon reviewing Form F-9, one can see the findings of concordance presented in words and in picture. In this sample form, the findings of the MRI are presented in column one, those of the spectroscopic study in column two, and the presence or absence of concordance is shown in the third column.

The anatomic regions of the prostate are represented as if a sextant biopsy were being done with the "base", "midgland" and "apex" on both the left (L) and right (R) sides shown. The graphic portrayal of the table results shown at the right of the table allow the radiologist to paint a picture of what he is seeing for the physician. An actual computer screenshot of the study could be done and pasted into the report with the needed call-outs to tag the areas of pathology. For now, the simple graphic analysis using a sextant model of the prostate is provided.

F25

Beneath the table are additional inputs of information relating to:

- ECE (extra-capsular extension) and specific locations if present
- Seminal vesicle involvement and
- Lymph node involvement in the pelvic area within the scope of the endorectal MRI's range of detection.

Finally, the stages of disease based on (1) endorectal MRI (erMRI) findings, (2) spectroscopy findings, and (3) the stage based on abnormalities that are concordant, are shown.

Sites of dominant lesions that might be pertinent insofar as potential treatment with a radiation therapy boost using brachytherapy (seed implantation or HDR) or IMRT can be seen graphically and commented on in the narrative (comments) section. Referring to Form F-9 while reading along with the above discussion will enable one to more clearly understand the goals of such objectified and visualized reporting.

Form F-9: The Endorectal MRI and Spectroscopy Form.

Patient's Name (last, first)	Exam Date	PSA	Volume	PSA Density
Doe, John	**6/9/99**	**4.6**	**33 cc**	**0.139**

Indicate in each anatomic area the presence of cancer (yes) or the absence (no) by circling or highlighting the appropriate response.

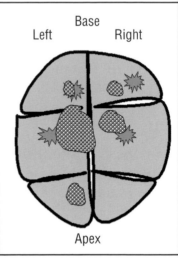

Base
Left   Right

Apex

MRI Findings	Spectroscopy Findings	Concordance
Right Base Yes vs. No	Right Base Yes vs. No	Yes vs. No
Right Mid Yes vs. No	Right Mid Yes vs. No	Yes vs. No
Right Apex Yes vs. No	Right Apex Yes vs. No	Yes vs. No
Left Base Yes vs. No	Left Base Yes vs. No	Yes vs. No
Left Midgland Yes vs. No	Left Midgland Yes vs. No	Yes vs. No
Left Apex Yes vs. No	Left Apex Yes vs. No	Yes vs. No

Extra-Capsular Extension Yes No   Indicate Site(s) of ECE:

Seminal Vesicle Involvement   **Right** Yes vs. No   **Left** Yes vs. No

Lymph Node Involvement

R obturator Yes vs. No	**R int iliac** Yes vs. No	**R ext iliac** Yes vs. No
L obturator Yes vs. No	**L int iliac** Yes vs. No	**L ext iliac** Yes vs. No

Stage per erMRI	**Stage** per Spectroscopy	**Stage** per Concordance
T2a, T2b, T2c, T3a, T3b, T3c	T2a, T2b, T2c, T3a, T3b, T3c	T2a, T2b, T2c, T3a, T3b, T3c

Comments:
Dominant disease per MRI is in left midgland with extension across midline to right. Concordant abnormalities are found in the right and left base and midgland. No extra-capsular extension (ECE) is seen.

James Roberts, M.D.

The Helpline Medical Form (HMF)

This document, the HMF, embodies 30 years of front-line work with patients on the battlefield of medical oncology. The HMF is not copyrighted; it can be used by any patient or by any physician and optimally by the two working together as a team. Many physicians have incorporated the HMF into their prostate cancer practice.

The HMF (Form F-10a-g) is a 7-part document. The seven parts include:

- Baseline Enrollment and Disclaimer
- Call Log
- Basic Medical Information
- Prediagnostic History
- Diagnosis and Staging
- Algorithms
- Detailed Clinical Chronological Review (DCCR)   **F27**

For the HMF to provide optimal value, *patient involvement is needed* in completing this form to the best of the patient's ability. If patients are passive onlookers in their treatment, they will learn far less about how to combat this disease. Their outcome will likely be less than optimal. This communication tool can and should be used by the patient and his team, and it is intended to be shared with your physicians to highlight outstanding aspects of your medical history and smooth the way for clear communication. The form can be e-mailed to anyone involved in your care, it can be printed out in hard-copy for in-depth review, and it can be faxed or mailed as well.

The **baseline enrollment and sample disclaimer** is self-explanatory. The essentials of your personal contact information are needed to communicate with you. The disclaimer portion of the HMF is both for your protection and to protect those who are providing guidance. Read the disclaimer carefully; it will tell you what you can and cannot expect from a helpline.

Form F-10a: The HMF–Baseline Enrollment and Disclaimer.

Doe	John	9/17/1942	Katie	516-743-2110	516-743-2113	
Last Name	First Name	Birth Date	Spouse's Name	Telephone	Fax	
DoeJohn@aol.com	365 Adams Avenue			West Hempstead	NY	11010
E-mail Address	Street Address	Suite/Apt	City or Province		State	Zip Code

(For non-physician Staff)

Disclaimer:

Dear _____, This information is being provided by the XYZ Helpline. The information is provided solely as a gratuitous public service. The information that will be presented to you during this communication is based on peer-reviewed medical literature, the experiences of other patients with prostate cancer or the experience of the XYZ medical advisors. What is communicated to you is not intended as a medical consultation or as a substitute for an established doctor-patient relationship. We do not have your full medical records and we are essentially here to provide you with information to discuss with your physicians. We can present hypothetical information to you and hope that this improves your understanding and leads to a better outcome for you. This is accomplished by asking more informed questions of your doctors. Do you understand our function here at the XYZ Helpline and your responsibility to share and discuss what is presented to you with your M.D. advisors? (If the caller answered in the affirmative without hesitation, check here: ☐

F28

The **Call Log** is used by the helpline staff. It briefly indicates that the HMF has been accessed. It shares with you the effort that is being expended to improve your outcome with details as to what has been done. Any communication with your physicians is also indicated.

Form F-10b: The HMF–Call Log. (Entries by Helpline Staff Only)					
Call	**Date**	**Staff**	**Time**		**Action(s):** Booklet, Conference, Refer, Review, Revise, Tape, Telephone, Update, Webcast, Website, other.
			Start	End	
1	6/8/01	VG	11:00 AM	12:00 PM	Call from John and HMF e-mailed to him.
					He will complete to the best of his ability
					and e-mail back to the Help Desk.
2	6/10/01	VG	9:00 AM	9:45 AM	Reviewed HMF with data provided by John.
					Discussed with John preliminary findings.
					HMF sent to Medical Advisor for his review.
3	6/12/01	SS	2:30 PM	3:00 PM	Reviewed HMF; suggestions made. To
					arrange conference call with John. John to
					print out HMF and give to his physician.

F29

The third part of the HMF relates to **basic medical information.** How old is he? Does he have any allergies? What are this patient's primary diagnoses? Who are his doctors? How do we contact them?

Form F-10c: The HMF–Basic Medical Informaion.		
Age: 59	**Allergies:** Penicillin	**Dx 1:** Prostate cancer
MD name-spec & Tel: Glenn Tisman–Med Onc: 555-444-3232		**Dx 2:** Hypertension
MD name-spec & Tel: Ralph Jones–Uro: 555-888-4567		**Dx 3:** Hyperlipidemia
MD name-spec & Tel:		**Dx 4:**

Prediagnostic History establishes a sense of how long the PC process may have been going on and the nature of the PC. Past PSA levels and determinations of PSA velocity (PSAV) and PSA doubling time (PSADT) are very important clues as to the occurrence and the subsequent behavior of the PC. A PSAV of 0.75 ng/ml/yr or greater is highly indicative of PC, as is a PSADT of less than 12 years. These values require multiple inputs over time. They can be calculated using the PC Tools software on the PCRI Web site (www.pcri.org). A PSADT of 6 months or less at diagnosis or after primary treatment by RP or RT or Cryosurgery most often relates to systemic (metastatic) disease. Miscellaneous information relating to past urinary illnesses or symptoms can also be entered in this section. Additional rows can be inserted pending the amount of information that is available from times before the diagnosis of PC was established.

Form F-10d: The HMF–Prediagnostic History.				
Date	PSA	PSADT	PSAV	Additional Information
4/1/92	2.5			

Diagnosis and Staging relates key baseline information of prognostic significance. This includes the baseline PSA and PAP, the Gleason score, gland volume, core involvement and clinical stage. The Gleason score must be validated by an expert in PC pathology. This section of the HMF contains the critical biologic expressions that are used in the algorithm section; additional information that is pertinent to risk assessment is also part of this section.

Form F–10e: The HMF–Diagnosis and Staging.							
9/00	197	"normal"	6/6	(4,3)	(4,3)	Diagnostic Labs	Bostwick
PC diagnosis date	bPSA	bPAP	Cores with PC/ cores biopsied	Gleason score (GS)-original	Gleason score expert review	Original GS Reviewer ID	Expert GS Reviewer ID
T3a	30 cc	Not done	100%	66.9 cc	Negative	Negative	?
Clinical stage (CS)	Gland volume (GV)	Ploidy	% greatest core involved	Tumor volume calculation	Bone scan + vs. -	ProstaScint scan + vs. -	CT scan + vs. -
B2	6.6	4	320%	Endorectal MRI-Spectroscopy Findings:			
Narayan stage	PSA density	AUA symptom score	Sum % all cores involved				
Specifics of staging if study(ies) abnormal (e.g. date of study, findings):							

F31

The abbreviations used in this discussion include the following:

bPSA = what the PSA was immediately prior to the biopsies that established the diagnosis.

bPAP = what the PAP was immediately prior to the biopsies that established the diagnosis, or a PAP taken 5 to 6 weeks after a diagnostic biopsy before any treatment has been initiated.

Ploidy = DNA analysis from the diagnostic biopsy and/or radical prostatectomy specimen.

CT = computerized tomography of the pelvis and/or abdomen; positive (+) indicates abnormal; negative (-) indicates normal.

Narayan stage = B1 if tumor is microscopically found in one lobe of the prostate versus B2 if both sides are involved.

PSA density = bPSA divided by gland volume; this expresses tumor density within the gland.

AUA score = objective measurement of lower urinary tract symptoms that has bearing on treatment modalities such as RT, seeds, cryosurgery and indirectly RP.

erMRI + spec = endorectal MRI with spectroscopy.

Form F-10f: **The HMF–Algorithms.** (See below for abbreviations)

Predictions of Outcome After RP Using Pre-RP Inputs

D'Amico: OCD based on tumor volume calculation per diagnosis and staging section: 34%

Stamey: Cure with RP assuming calculated tumor volume accurate: 6%

Partin Tables 2001: OCD, CP, SV, LN, at RP using GS, bPSA, CS:
No data for clinical stage T3a

Narayan: OCD, ECE, SV, LN, at RP using GS, bPSA, biopsy findings: 20, 60, 45, 50

D'Amico: OCD using GS and bPSA: No data for this presentation

D'Amico: OCD using GS, bPSA and core %: No data for this presentation

Bluestein: LN at RP using GG, bPSA, CS (<3% = negligible): Not Negligible

Gao: ECE/SM, by Average CA in sum of cores: No data by Max CA in any core:
No data by core %: No data

Gilliland- ECE using age, PSA, GS: 73% with range of 60-82% (using PSA of 25)

D'Amico: 4 Yr PSA relapse-free survival after RP using core %, GS, bPSA: No data for T3a

Predictions of Outcome After RP Using Findings at RP and/or Post RP

Partin II : Local vs. Systemic Relapse using bPSA, GS at RP, RP findings, post RP
PSAV: NA

Kattan: 7 YFFR using preRP PSA, findings at RP: NA

Pound: FF-Mets at 3,5,7 yrs after RP when PSA recurrence occurs: Not applicable (NA)

Lerner: 5 YFFR if apparent OCD at RP using PSA, GS, Ploidy:
If Diploid: 58%   If Aneuploid: 39%

Stamey: FF PSA relapse after RP: No data

D'Amico: FF PSA relapse after RP at 2 yrs: No data

Predictions of Outcome After RT Using Pre-RT Inputs

Kattan: 5 YFFR after 3D Conformal RT using 72 Gy + ADT x 3 mos: **24.3%**

Pisansky: 5 YFFR after 74 Gy 3D Conformal RT: 26%

Kattan: 5 YFFR after seed implants with and without EBRT: program being prepared

Predictions of Outcome After RP or RT Using Pre-RT and Pre-RP Inputs

D'Amico: 5 YFFR using GS, bPSA, CS, Risk Category: No data for T3a clinical stage
RP: RT: SI+ADT: SI only:

F32

OCD (organ confined disease); CP (capsular penetration);
SV (seminal vesicle involvement); LN (lymph node involvement);
ECE (extra-capsular extension); SM (surgical margins); CA (cancer);
Gy (Gray-units of radiation); CS (clinical stage);
5 YFFR (5 year freedom from any kind of relapse including PSA);
ADT (androgen deprivation therapy); FF (freedom from);
RP (radical prostatectomy); RT (radiation therapy); SI (seed implant).

These algorithms are data derived from peer-reviewed medical publications that relate human experience to outcome. Most of them are expressions of statistical analytic approaches. The value of these calculations is that they provide a *risk assessment* of the patient on a more individualized basis since they incorporate the hard data of the "Diagnosis and Staging" section. In the forms shown, areas of concern for this patient are shown in red. All of these findings are factors that determine *what further testing may be indicated and what treatments should be given greater or lesser consideration.*

F33

The **Detailed Clinical Chronological Review (DCCR)** section of the HMF contains the important events of the patient's medical history as it relates to PC or issues highly pertinent to PC. Treatments are designated as "Rx" and are bolded for emphasis. The suggestions from the helpline are identified as such. The patient adds information to the HMF, encouraging its use as an important navigational tool for all involved in the patient's care. Using the DCCR as a means of group communication focuses energy on areas of concern given a particular patient's database. This approach, grounded in hard factual information, avoids generic suggestions "to operate", "radiate" or "do nothing", and it promotes an evidence-based methodology to support diagnostic studies and treatment modes. Such an approach, if extensively adopted, would help to improve the outcome of the patient and ease his path to that outcome. This is the essence of good treatment strategy.

F34

_____

_____

_____

_____

_____

_____

_____

_____

_____

_____

_____

_____

Form F-10g: Detailed Clinical Chronological Review (DCCR).

Date	Occurrence	Details of Clinical History
9/00	Dx PC	bPSA(max) 197, GS (4,3)–reviewed by Bostwick; CST3a; GV 30 cc.
9/6/00	Bone scan #1 ProstaScint #1	"Negative" "Negative"
9/25/00	PAP 2.5	Normal less than 3.0
10/00	Rx1: ADT_3	Zoladex, Casodex (50), Proscar 5 bid: bPSA 197
11/5/00	erMRI with spec	UCSF: after one month on ADT_3: probably ECE (extra-capsular extension) at left apex
1/01	Bone scan #2	"Negative"
5/01	PSA 0.11	Need info on any prior PSA levels drawn before 5/01
6/12/01	Helpline Medical Advisor	1. Suggest evaluate bone integrity with 2 tests: QCT bone density and Pyrilinks-D (Dpd) urine test. Info on QCT is at **www.qct.com** or **www.image-analysis.com**. Info on Dpd at **www.pcri.org** in Jan 1999 issue of PCRI *Insights*.
		2. Check testosterone level to ensure less than 20 ng/dl
		3. If PSA does not reach < 0.05, consider probable androgen independent PC (AIPC)
		4. If PSA does not reach < 0.05, consider ProstaScint-CT Fusion study.
		5. If AIPC, treatment options include stopping Casodex and using HDK + HC, or DES (with coumadin on board).
		6. If ProstaScint fusion study shows no lymph node uptake, consider repeat erMRI with spectroscopy to see if any residual PC in prostate and correlate with ProstaScint-CT fusion study. Consider targeted biopsies to confirm this (assuming PSA does not reach <0.05) and if so, consider RT to prostate and observe PSA. RT given could be in the form of IMRT or 3D Conformal RT.
		7. Our Medical Advisor will be glad to call your physician at his convenience. Please print out HMF and share with your physician(s).

The Flow Sheet

Flow sheets are critical to the management of any patient, no matter what the illness. The concepts involved with flow sheets are simple, but often totally missed by many doctors. **The flow sheet looks at the patient's medical story over time. It relates specific treatment(s) and allows visual correlation of a treatment with parameters (indicators) of response.**

Simply put, the flow sheet gives a timetable of the patient's medications or procedures and correlates them with laboratory studies (response parameters) to point out any changes reflecting either the presence or lack of the desired biologic effect. At the same time, bodily functions are monitored using laboratory tests. This monitoring warns the doctor-patient team of any developing drug toxicity or tissue damage, which may be due to the treatment and/or the disease. An example of this would be John Doe treated with Flutamide and Lupron for metastatic PC.

F36
An example of his flow sheet is included in Form F-11. Note how the flow sheet not only acts as a treatment record, but the columns also show the time-related effects of therapy on the CBC (hematocrit dropping) due to androgen deprivation therapy as well as a desired therapeutic effect on the PSA. The worsening liver function test (SGPT–a liver enzyme) is forecasting problems secondary to liver toxicity, which may be due to Flutamide. The flow sheet is declaring this in advance because the physician or the patient can see the test result going from low normal to high normal before entering the flagged abnormal range. Similarly, the alkaline phosphatase (due to bone metastases) is showing a response to ADT and is falling from the initial 456 toward the normal range < 125). Even within the normal range, it continues to drop lower and lower.

The concepts here relate to baseline, trends, the issue of changes within the "normal" range and that of treatment versus response parameter.

We suggest that physicians designate the patient as the primary recipient of any consultation report. Hard copies of any laboratory data generated in the physician's office, as well as copies of flow sheets and biomarker forms should be sent to the patient. **The empowered patient asks for such documentation from his physician. A true physician welcomes such a request.**

Form F-11: The Flow Sheet Form.
(Front)

Last name: Doe   **First:** John   **Ht:** 68 in   **Wt:** 160   **BSA:** 1.88   Page # 1

Month/day	2/1	2/28	3/28	4/25	5/23	Dietary Adjuncts
Flutamide	250 mg TID	√	√	Hold	√	ß Carotene 25,000 units day
Lupron	7.5 mg	7.5 mg	7.5 mg	7.5 mg	7.5 mg	C 1000 mg TID
Proscar	5 mg BID	√	√	√	√	Ca++ (Bone Assure®)
Fosamax			70 mg/wk	√	√	Cernilton®
Procrit	10 K q WK	√	Hold	√	√	CoQ$_{10}$ 200 mg QD
Vasotec	5 mg QD	√	√	√	√	E 400 QD (d-alpha)
Prilosec	20 mg QD	√	√	√	√	E 210 mg QD (gamma)
Silymarin				200/D		Genistein
						Green Tea
						L-Carnitine
						Lycopene 10 mg TID
						Selenium 400mcg QD
Coumadin Dose						
PT I INR	I	I	I	I	I	
WBC	5.5	5.9	5.7	6.3	6.0	
PMNs I LYMPHS	I	I	I	I	I	
HCT %	37	36	39	37	35	
PLATELETS	180	212	188	234	177	
Na+ I K+	I	I	I	I	I	
BUN I CREAT	I	I	I	I	I	
GLUCOSE/ LDH						
CA++ I PHOS--	I	I	I	I	I	
Albumin I Globulin	I	I	I	I	I	
Bilirubin I Alk Phos	I 456	I 245	I 188	I 143	I 92	(alk phos normal < 125)
SGOT I SGPT	18 I 18	20 I 24	26 I 33	55 I 78	35 I 40	
PSA I PAP	122 I 29	60 I 12	14 I 2.5	0.5 I 2.2	<0.05 I 2.0	
TESTO I SHBG	345 I	<20 I	<20 I	I	I	
Pyrilinks-D *	4.3		6.5	4.0		
DHEA-S I Androstenedione	89 I 125	I	I	I	I	
Prolactin I DHT	8.9 I 55	I	I <30	I	I	
CEA CGA NSE	2.0 4.8 7.8	I I	I I	I I	I I	
Weight	160	162	163	168	170	

F37

*Pyrilinks-D = Dpd or deoxypyridinoline or Metra™ DPD.

Form F-11: **The Flow Sheet Form.**
(Back)

Chest X-rays (Include Dates for **all** report results)

1/23/01 normal
9/17/01 normal

KUB + Plain Films

ENDORECTAL MRI with or without spectroscopy; plain MRI, CT (specify)

HEAD:
CHEST:
CT Abdomen/Pelvis: 9/17/01 no lymph node enlargement in pelvis or abdomen; liver normal
ENDORECTAL MRI + SPECTROSCOPY: 1/15/01– gland volume 24 cc, no ECE, concordant MRI and MRS abnormalities in right and left base, right midgland and right apex. No regional nodes seen.

F38

ULTRASOUND (Including TRUSP)

12/22/99 – gland volume 30 cc; hypoechoic lesions in right and left base; capsule intact, no SV involvement

NUCLEAR MEDICINE
(BS= bone scan; PS = ProstaScint scan; PET = positron emission tomography)

BS #1: 1/22/01- no abnormal uptake: normal scan

BONE MARROW BIOPSY and ASPIRATE (include pathology number)

BIOPSY:
ASPIRATE:

PATHOLOGY REPORTS (include pathology number)

The Summary and Surveillance Form

Introduction

This form (F-12) focuses attention on what additional studies have been done that are important to the patient as part of either evaluation of disease activity and extent, response to treatment or to surveillance as it relates to preventive health measures. The concept is for him to be aware of evaluations that can change the course of his life. A colonoscopy, for example, can detect pre-malignant polyps. At the time of colonoscopy, your gastroenterologist can remove polyps and prevent the development of colon cancer. We would like to see a focus on such periodic testing where it is applicable to the patient. **This form is a reminder to enhance the complete care of the patient.**

What "Procedures" are Included

The list of "Procedures" are what we suggest be used in the management of patients with prostate cancer.

F39

Physical exam: especially important if active disease or treatment toxicity is a concern.

DRE: done at least annually to exclude local pathology.

Past/Fam/Soc Hx: additional new information about your past history, family or social history.

Chest X-ray: especially important with a history of tobacco abuse or respiratory disease.

EKG: an annual EKG in the chart is very helpful in case of findings on the electro- cardiogram (EKG) that need comparison to see if the changes are new.

Urine analysis: a test to exclude infection, or systemic manifestations of disease.

OB X 3: occult blood in the stool done on three occasions; a way to detect occult bleeding that may be occurring anywhere along the gastrointestinal tract from the mouth to the anus.

Colonoscopy: visualization of the entire colon to rule out precancerous changes and other lesions.

Dpd (Pyrilinks-D™ or Metra™ DPD): a laboratory test to detect excessive bone resorption using the second-voided urine of the day.

Bone Density (BMD): used to evaluate treatment of osteopenia or osteoporosis or rechecked if the baseline BMD is borderline. It can be repeated annually or semi-annually pending circumstances.

ProstaScint: a monoclonal antibody scan used to detect PC within soft tissue, e.g. prostate, lymph nodes; it may be used as part of staging or in follow-up to determine a change in status of the patient as a result of treatment or disease progression.

Bone scan: an isotope scan to follow patients with an abnormal bone scan or as a baseline study to rule out overtly metastatic disease.

Stress EKG: used for annual monitoring of your heart's functional status.

Eye exam: an annual exam to exclude glaucoma, the most common cause of blindness.

Skin exam: a check by your internist or dermatologist to exclude curable skin cancer.

US-TSH: an ultra-sensitive thyroid stimulating hormone level to rule out low thyroid function or to evaluate appropriate dosing for those taking thyroid medication.

Homocysteine: a blood test that indicates excessive levels of a substance implicated in heart disease, diabetes, vascular disease and Alzheimer's disease.

Ferritin: a measurement of tissue iron; too little indicates iron lack and too much, overload.

Flu vaccine: given annually in September to October to prevent influenza epidemics.

Pneumovax: a vaccine against pneumococcal pneumonia given every ten years.

This form can be modified to suit your individual needs.

Share all these forms with your doctor(s).

Form F-12: The Summary and Surveillance Form.

Procedure	Date	Date	Date	Date	Date	Date	Date	Date
Physical Exam								
DRE								
Past/Fam/Soc Hx								
Chest X-ray								
EKG								
Urine analysis								
OB X 3								
Colonoscopy								
Pyrilinks-D								
Bone Density (BMD)								
ProstaScint								
Bone Scan								
Stress EKG								
Eye Exam								
Skin Exam								
US-TSH								
Homocysteine								
Ferritin								
Flu Vaccine								
Pneumovax								

F41

References

1. Steineck G, Kelly WK, Mazumdar M, et al: Acid phosphatase: defining a role in androgen-independent prostate cancer. Urology 47:719-26, 1996.

2. Galasko CS, Doyle FH: The response to therapy of skeletal metastases from mammary cancer. Assessment by scintigraphy. Br J Surg 59:85-8, 1972.

3. Citrin DL, Bessent RG, Tuohy JB, et al: Quantitative bone scanning: a method for assessing response of bone metastases to treatment. Lancet 1:1132-3, 1974.

4. Drelichman A, Decker DA, Al-Sarraf M, et al: Computerized bone scan. A potentially useful technique to measure response in prostatic carcinoma. Cancer 53:1061-5, 1984.

5. Soloway MS, Hardeman SW, Hickey D, et al: Stratification of patients with metastatic prostate cancer based on extent of disease on initial bone scan. Cancer 61:195-202, 1988.

6. Arai Y, Okubo K, Aoki Y, et al: Ultrasensitive assay of prostate-specific antigen for early detection of residual cancer after radical prostatectomy. Int J Urol 5:550-5, 1998.

7. Scheidler J, Hricak H, Vigneron DB, et al: Prostate cancer: localization with three-dimensional proton MR spectroscopic imaging--clinicopathologic study. Radiology 213:473-80, 1999.

Appendix

Clinical Stages of PC Illustrated

Staging is the process of determining extent of disease in a specific patient in light of all available information. It is used to help determine appropriate therapy. There are two staging methods: the Whitmore-Jewett staging classification (1956) and the more detailed TNM (tumor, nodes, metastases) classification (1992) of the American Joint Committee on Cancer and the International Union Against Cancer. Staging should be subcategorized as clinical staging and pathologic staging. Pathologic stage usually relates to what is found at the time of surgery. **The TNM system is now most commonly used.** In the Whitmore-Jewett classification, the:

Whitmore-Jewett stage A becomes TNM stage T1.
Whitmore-Jewett stage B becomes TNM stage T2.
Whitmore-Jewett stage C becomes TNM stage T3.

The Whitmore-Jewett classification, still being used by some physicians, is described below, and the TNM classification follows.

Whitmore-Jewett Stages

Stage A is clinically undetectable tumor confined to the gland and is an incidental finding at prostate surgery, e.g. TURP.

A1: Well-differentiated with focal involvement.
A2: Moderately or poorly differentiated or involves multiple foci in the gland.

Stage B is tumor confined to the prostate gland.

B0: Nonpalpable, PSA-detected.

B1: Single nodule in one lobe of the prostate.

B2: More extensive involvement of one lobe or involvement of both lobes.

Stage C is a tumor clinically localized to the periprostatic area but extending through the prostate capsule; the seminal vesicle(s) may be involved.

C1: Clinical extracapsular extension.

C2: Extracapsular tumor producing bladder outlet or ureteral obstruction.

Stage D is metastatic disease.

D0: Clinically localized disease (prostate only) but persistently elevated enzymatic serum acid phosphatase.

D1: Regional lymph nodes only.

D2: Distant lymph nodes, metastases to bone or visceral organs.

D3: D2 prostate cancer patients who relapse after adequate endocrine therapy.

TNM Stages

Primary Tumor (T)

TX: Primary tumor cannot be assessed.

T0: No evidence of primary tumor.

T1: Clinically inapparent tumor <u>not palpable</u> or visible by imaging.

T1a: Tumor incidental histologic finding in ≤ 5% of tissue resected via TURP.

T1b: Tumor incidental histologic finding in > 5% of tissue resected via TURP

T1c: Tumor identified by needle biopsy (e.g., because of elevated PSA).

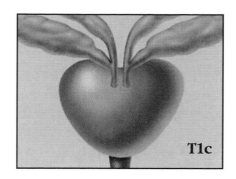

T2: Tumor palpable but confined within the prostate.

T2a: Tumor involves half of a lobe or less.

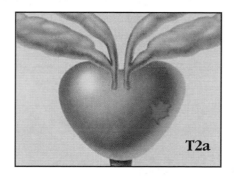

G3

T2b: Tumor involves more than half a lobe, but not both lobes.

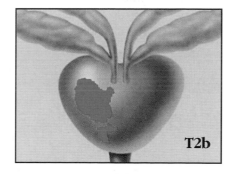

T2c: Tumor involves both lobes.

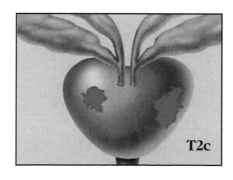

T3: Tumor extends through the prostatic capsule.

T3a: Unilateral extracapsular extension.

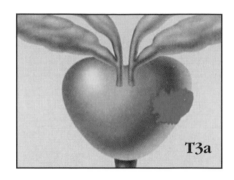

T3b: Bilateral extracapsular extension.

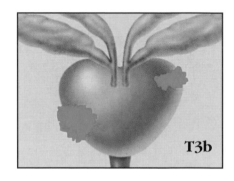

T3c: Tumor invades the seminal vesicle(s).

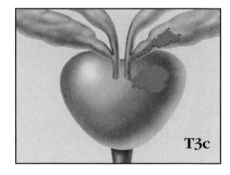

T4: Tumor is fixed or invades adjacent structures other than the seminal vesicles.

T4a: Tumor invades bladder neck, external sphincter, or rectum.

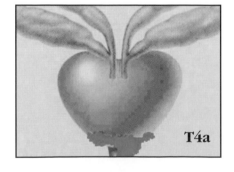

T4b: Tumor invades
levator muscles
and/or is fixed
to the pelvic
wall.

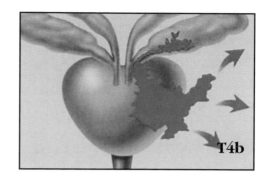

Regional Lymph Nodes (N)

NX: Regional lymph nodes cannot be assessed.

N0: No regional lymph node metastasis.

N1: Metastasis in a single lymph node, 2 cm or less in greatest dimension.

N2: Metastasis in a single lymph node, more than 2 cm but not more than 5 cm in greatest dimension; or multiple lymph node metastases, none more than 5 cm in greatest dimension.

N3: Metastasis in a lymph node more than 5 cm in greatest dimension.

Distant Metastases (M)

MX: Presence of distant metastasis cannot be assessed.

M0: No distant metastasis.

M1: Distant metastasis.

M1a: Nonregional lymph node(s).

M1b: Bone(s).

M1c: Other site(s).

G5

G6

Appendix

Figures, Tables, Physician's Notes and Forms Listed

Within the *Primer*, there are 133 different graphic presentations. The following lists of Figures, Tables, Physician's Notes and Forms should facilitate your finding a particular item.

List of Figures

H2

H3

List of Tables

H5

List of Physician's Notes

List of Forms

H8

Index

A

I1

anti-thrombin III deficiency, 154
  aspirin, lack of efficacy, 154–155
  Coumadin®, efficacy of, 154
aorta, 43
aortic bifurcation node, 55
apex, 27, 42, 45, 52
apoptosis, 66, 171, B8
  inhibitors of, Bcl-xL and mcl-1, B9
  promoters of, Bax, Bad, Bcl-xS, B9
APR (acute phase response), 143
Aptosyn® (exisulind), 160
Aredia® (pamidronate), 143, 179, B25
Argon gas, 83, 86
Arimidex® (anastrozole), prevention
  of gynecomastia, 150
Arnot, Dr. Bob, A10
Aromasin® (exemestane), 150
aromatase, 150–151
arteriosclerosis, F13
arthritis, 60
artificial urinary sphincter, 81–82
ASO (antisense oligonucleotides)
  AIPC, used against, 170
  bcl-2 ASO, 172
  bcl-2 ASO trials, Vancouver,
    San Antonio, 174
  bcl-2 ASO, decrease in bcl-2
    mRNA, 173
  bcl-2 ASO, inhibition of time to
    AIPC, 173
  bcl-2 ASO, synergy with Taxol®,
    173
  bcl-2 ASO, synergy with
    Taxotere®, 174
  directed against EGF, VEGF,
    Her-2/neu receptors, 174
  EGFR (epidermal growth factor
    receptor) antisense, 174
  Genasense®, 173
    clinical trials in Vancouver, 173
    Novantrone®, used with, 173
    reduction in lymphocyte bcl-2,
      173
    reduction in PSA, 173
  nucleotide base pairing, 172
  mRNA targeting, 172

atomic mass, 125
  definition of, B19
atomic number, 125, B19
Atrasentan®, 163–165
  AIPC clinical trials, 164–165
  biomarkers (PAP, LDH, alkaline
    phosphatase), effect on, 164
  clinical progression of PC, delay
    of, 164
  dose response, 164
  prevention of bone resorption, 165
  Web site, 165
  Xinlay™, 165
atrophy, 79
AUA symptom score, 75, F12, F31
  effects on choice of local therapy,
    F12
  form, F12, F14
AUS, see artificial urinary sphincter
autosomal dominant gene, B1
Avodart® (dutasteride), 136, 144, 149,
  B22

B

Bagnato, Dr. Anna, 164
Bahn, Dr. Duke, 87
Barken, Dr. Israel, 41
basal cells, 63
base, of prostate gland, 42, 45
baseline:
  baseline PAP, F31
  baseline PSA, F31
  baseline PSA, importance in seed
    implantation (SI) studies, B14
  baseline testing, 33, 36, 52–53, 64,
    95
basement membrane, 37
basic information, F31
Bastacky, Dr. Sheldon I., B2
BAT™ (B-mode acquisition and
  targeting, 18
  PowerPoint presentation about, 115
  prostate gland location using, 115
  reduction of RT side-effects, 115
Bauer, Dr. John, 73
Baylor College of Medicine, 114, C1
bcl-2, 35, 73–74, 171, B8, F7
  antisense oligonucleotides (ASO),
    see ASO, bcl-2

I3

bone scan, *(cont.)*
degenerative arthritis in, F17
extent of disease, F17–F18
index of suspicion, F17
objectified report and example, F16–F19
quantified bone scanning, F16
Soloway index, F18
trauma and, F17
bones, 29–30, 44
Bonkhoff, Professor Dr. Helmut, 50
Bostwick Labs, 74, B9
Bostwick, Dr. David, 50, 52, 118, A4
bowel problems, 12–13,
BPH, 37-38, A4, F13
brachytherapy, *see* radiation therapy, brachytherapy
brachytherapy, high dose rate, *see* radiation therapy, brachytherapy, high dose rate (HDR)
brachytherapy, seed implantation, *see* radiation therapy, brachytherapy seed implantation (SI)
Bragg peak, 121
breast cancer, 25, 31, 36,
bromocriptine, *see* Parlodel®
Brufsky, Dr. Adam, B22
bulbourethral glands (Cowper's glands), 26, 27, 80

C

Calydon virus, 167
Cancer Treatment Centers of America, Web site, A9
Cancerfacts™, A3
capillary, 37
capillary permeability, 162
capsular penetration, 52, 62, 96, F3
soft tissue extension, and degree of, B11
capsule, 29, 57
carcinogenesis, 28, 31
cardiovascular disease and Viagra®, 78
Cardura® (doxazosin), 78, F13
Casodex® (bicalutamide), 65, 105, 118, 135, 140, B22, B24

castration:
chemical, *see* ADT (androgen deprivation therapy)
surgical, *see* orchiectomy
CAT, *see* CT (computerized tomography)
catheters for seeding, 94
Caverject® (alprostadil), 79
cavernous nerve, 76, B11
CEA, 35, 53, 64–65, 68, 126, B6, F9, F11
cell cycle and neutron beam RT, 126
Cell Genesys™, 166–167
cell growth and regulation, B8
cell motility, 67
Cell Pathways, Inc.™, 160
cell signaling and communication, 66, 171
Center of Radiotherapy and Oncology (Barcelona), B13
cervical spine, 61
Cetrotide® (cetrorelix), 135
CG7060, *see* oncolytic viruses
CG7870, *see* oncolytic viruses
CGA, 35, 53, 63–66, 68, 126, B5, B6, F9, F11
kidney function affecting, B5
chemistry panel, 35
chemotherapy, 59, 136, 159, 170
PC review, 159
supportive care, importance of, 184
Chinn, Dr. Douglas, 84, 87
choice of an artist, 16–18, 50, 71–72, 77, 81, 83, 87, 91, 99, 106, 177, 182, F6
brachytherapists (HDR), 108
pathologists, B15
choline, 57–58
choosing a doctor, 15
chromogranin A (*see* CGA), B4
chromosome, 58
Cialis® (tadalafil), 78-79, 87
drug interactions and, 78
Cipro® (ciprofloxacin), 38
citrate, 57–58
Citrin, Dr. D.L., F16
Civantos, Dr. Francisco, 50

I8

brachytherapy–high dose rate (HDR) healthcare costs, 46, 61–62, 74, 99, B20, B22, F16, F20, F33
Helpap, Professor, 50
Helpline Medical Form (HMF), F27
HER-2/*neu*, 73, B8, F7
   antisense to, 174
hereditary PC (HPC), 28, B1–B2
hesitancy, *see* LUTS (lower urinary tract symptoms)
Hexadrol® (dexamethasone), 137
high dose rate brachytherapy, *see* radiation therapy, brachytherapy–high dose rate (HDR)
homeostasis, 67
homocysteine, F10–F11, F40
Hong, Dr. Eugene, 78
Honvan® (fosfestrol), *see* estrogens
Hormone Refractory Prostate Cancer, Web site, A13
hot flashes or flushes, *see* ADS (androgen deprivation syndrome)

I10

HPC, *see* hereditary PC
Huang, Dr. Andrew, B9–B10
Huggins, Dr. Charles Brenton, 132–133
human sexuality, 80
humanity, 12, 14, 22–23
humerus, 61
hybridization, 172
hydrocortisone, 137
Hypertext Guide to PC, A3
hypophysectomy, reduction of LH, 133
hypothalamic-pituitary axis, B19
hypothyroidism, F13
Hytrin® (terazosin), 78, F13

I

IAD (intermittent androgen deprivation), 144–145
   biologic end-point defined, 147
   PSAR, outstanding results treating, 148
   two drug regimens (IAD$_2$), 146
      Strum study of, 146
   three drug regimens (IAD$_3$), 147
      Leibowitz study, 148–149

Proscar® maintenance, 149
   IAD$_3$ versus IAD$_2$, 147
   Strum study, 147
   undetectable PSA duration, importance of, 146–147
iceball, *see* cryosurgery
IGF-1, in bone loss, B21
IGF-BP3 (insulin-like growth factor-binding protein 3), F21
IGF-BP5 (insulin-like growth factor-binding protein 5), 174
IL-6 (interleukin 6), F21
IL6sR (interleukin 6 soluble receptor), F11
ilia, 61
immobilization of patient, 109–110
immune function, 67
immunologic balance, 74
immunostaining, 74, B8
immunosuppression, 67
implanted seeds, *see* radiation therapy, brachytherapy (SI)
impotence, 75, 151
IMRT, *see* radiation therapy, intensity modulated RT (IMRT)
incidence of PC, 10
incontinence, 80–81
   after dilation, 82
   during intercourse, 81
   National Association for Continence Web site, A10
   pads worn in, 82
Indium-111, 54
insurance help, A13
intensity modulated RT, *see* radiation therapy, intensity modulated RT (IMRT)
intercourse, 80
intermittent androgen deprivation, *see* IAD (Intermittent Androgen Deprivation)
internal iliac node, 30, 43–44
intracrinology of PC (*see* also endocrinology of PC), 133–134
invasive cancer, 28

Narayan, Dr. Perry, 97
National Association for Continence, 81
nerve grafting, 76, B10
nerve-sparing RP, see radical prostatectomy
neural net (artificial neural net, ANN), B2
neuroendocrine, 63
  differentiation, B4
neurovascular bundles (NVB), 75–76, 86–87, B11
  capsular penetration and, B11
  location of, B11
  organ-confined disease, in, B11
  preservation of, B12
  surgical margin positive cases and, B12
neutron beam RT, see radiation therapy, neutron beam
neutrons, B19
NFκB, 174
Nilandron® (nilutamide), see anti-androgens
nipple sensitivity, 150
nitrate compounds, 78
nitroglycerine, 78
nitroglycerine and Viagra®, 78
Nizoral® (ketoconazole), 78, 136
  serum level determinations of, F21
nocturia, see LUTS (lower urinary tract symptoms)
nodes, see lymph nodes
Nolvadex® (tamoxifen), 150
  gynecomastia, prevention of, 150
noninvasive cancer, 28
normal tissue complication probability, see NTCP
Novantrone® (mitoxantrone), 170
novel therapies, 184
NSE, 35, 53, 64–65, 68, B6, F9, F11
NTCP (normal tissue complication probability), 91
N-telopeptides, 165
nucleotides, 170

Nucleotron™, A9
nucleus of cell, 48–49, 54
  structure of, 125
NuLytely® (polyethylene glycol), 56
nutritional intervention, B2
NVB, see neurovascular bundle

O

objectified observation, see watchful waiting, 157
objectified reporting, F1
obturator nodes (see also lymph nodes), 43
occult blood (OB), F39
OCD, see organ-confined disease (OCD)
Olsson, Dr. Carl, 87
oncogene, 73–74
oncolytic viruses, 165, 167
  E1A, E1B, E3, 167
  CG7060, 167
    clinical trial, results of, 168
    PSA decline with, 168
    PSA doubling time prolonged with, 168
    PSA tissue staining decreased with, 168
  CG7870, 167
    amplification of p53 (wild type) due to, 169
    clinical trial for metastatic PC described, 168
    clinical trial, early results of, 168
    Taxotere®, Taxol®, synergy with, 169
    toxicity, associated with, 169
  CN706, see CG7060
  CN787, see CG7870
  CV702, 167
  ONYX-15, 166, 169
  Web sites, 169
Onik, Dr. Gary, 87
ONYX-15, see oncolytic viruses
Oppenheimer, Dr. Jonathan, 50
opportunity in crisis, 12
options, 12
oral sex, 80

I15

I18

see VEGF
VCD, *see* vacuum constriction device
VED, *see* vacuum erection device
VEGF (Vascular Endothelial Growth
  Factor), 35, 162, B25
  ADPC (androgen-dependent PC),
    relation to, 162
  androgens, stimulation by, 162
  antisense to, 174
  ET-1 (endothelin-1), relation to,
    164
  metastatic disease, correlation
    with, B25
  production sites in PC, 162
VePesid® (etoposide), 170
Viadur® (leuprolide acetate), 135, 138,
  140, 141
Viagra® (sildenafil), 77–79, 87, 99, B10
  blood pressure and Viagra®, 78
  cardiovascular disease and, 78
  nitroglycerine and, 78
vinorelbine, *see* Navelbine®, 170
viral construct, 167
viral replication promoter, 167
Virgil's Prostate On-line, A4, A8
Vitamin D, B25
Vitamin E, B2
  suppositories, 118
VSV (vesiculo-stomatitis-virus), 166,
  169

W

Walsh, Dr. Patrick, 76, A8–A9, B12,
  C1–C2
  nerve grafting versus nerve
    sparing, B11
watchful waiting, 14, 156–157
  email discussion list, A12
  PSA velocity and PSA doubling
    time, value in, 157
  software (PC Tools I), 157–158
Wayne State University, 128, F16
Wernert, Professor, 50
Wheeler, Dr. Ronald, B24
Whitmore-Jewett staging, *see* staging,

Whitmore-Jewett
wholistic medicine, 22
Worthington, Janet, A8–A9

XYZ

Xinlay™, *see* Atrasentan
x-rays, 60
YB-1, 174
Young, Robert, A3
Zagaja, Dr. Gregory, 78
Zelefsky, Dr. Michael, 112, 116–117
Zippe, Dr. Craig, 77
Zoladex® (goserelin), 131, F10
Zometa® (zoledronic acid), 143, 152,
  179

124